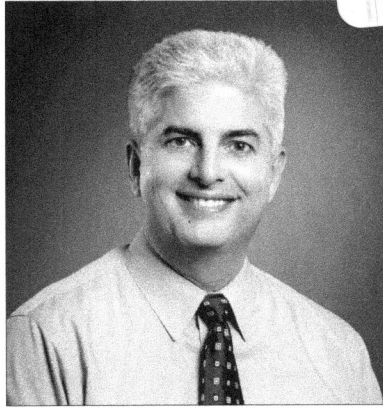

Dr. Julio Gonzalez

CORONALESSONS

Dr. Julio Gonzalez is an orthopedic surgeon, former State Representative in the Florida House of Representatives, and attorney.

Born in Miami, Florida, to parents who fled Castros' communist regime, Dr. Gonzalez obtained his medical degree from the University of Miami School of Medicine and his law degree from Stetson University College of Law. He served as a flight surgeon in the United States Navy, deploying twice aboard the U.S.S. America to the Mediterranean Sea, the Persian Gulf, Yugoslavia, and Somalia. His prior publications include *The Case For Free Market Healthcare*, *Dictionary of Orthopaedic Terminology*, *Health Care Reform: The Truth*, and *The Federalist Pages: A Constitutional Path to Restoring America's Greatness*.

Dr. Gonzalez is married to Dr. Gina Arabitg, a gynecologist,

Dr. Gonzalez is available for speaking engagements and may be contacted at *gonzopod@gmail.com*.
Learn more at *www.thefederalistpages.com*.

Aragon Publishers, LLC.

CORONALESSONS

ISBN 978-1-938842-50-4

Copyright ©2020 by Julio Gonzalez, M.D., J.D.

Published by Aragon Publishers, LLC

Cover design by Zelika Kojic

To My Country

May It Always Serve
as a Beacon for Freedom
and a Promoter of Good

Other books

*THE CASE FOR FREE MARKET
HEALTHCARE*

THE FEDERALIST PAGES
*A Constitutional Path
to Restoring America's Greatness*

HEALTH CARE REFORM: THE TRUTH

*DICTIONARY OF
ORTHOPAEDIC TERMINOLOGY*

CORONALESSONS

Hidden Insights On Where We Have Failed & Where We Have Succeeded From This Global Pandemic

(A Real-Time Analysis of the COVID-19 Pandemic)

Julio Gonzalez, M.D., J.D.

Contents

List of Abbreviations

ACE 2 receptor	angiotensin-converting enzyme 2 receptor
AIDS	Acquired Immunodeficiency Syndrome
BCG vaccine	bacille Calmette-Guerin vaccine
CARES Act	Coronavirus Aid, Relief and Economic Security Act
CDC	Centers for Disease Control and Prevention
CGTN	Chinese Global Television Network
CMS	Center for Medicare and Medicaid Services
COVID-19	Coronavirus Disease 2019
CWHTF	Coronavirus White House Task Force
DJIA	Dow Jones Industrial Average
DOJ	Department of Justice
EU	European Union
EUA	Emergency Use Authorization
FDA	Food and Drug Administration
FEMA	Federal Emergency Management Agency
GDP	gross domestic product
HIV	Human Immunodeficiency Virus
IHME	University of Washington's Institute for Health Metrics and Evaluation
MERS	Middle Eastern Respiratory Syndrome
NIH	National Institutes of Health
PCR	polymerase chain reaction
PRC	People's Republic of China
PPE	Personal Protective Equipment
PPP	Paycheck Protection Program
RT-PCR	reverse transcriptase polymerase chain reaction
SARS	Severe Acute Respiratory Syndrome
SARS-CoV-1	Severe Acute Respiratory Syndrome Coronavirus 1
SARS-CoV-2	Severe Acute Respiratory Syndrome Coronavirus 2
SCTF	Supply Chain Task Force
SNS	Strategic National Stockpile
WHO	World Health Organization

COVID-19 Timeline[i]

Dec. 16, 2019:	First patient with symptoms in Wuhan.
Dec. 21, 2019:	Wuhan doctors identify a cluster of cases.
Dec. 25, 2019:	Strong evidence accumulates of human-to-human contact in China.
ca. Dec. 25, 2019:	Increasing number of cases untraceable to the Wuhan Seafood Wholesale Market identified.
Dec. 30, 2019:	Dr. Li sends out message warning of a possible outbreak of a SARS type illness.
Dec. 31, 2019:	Wuhan Municipal Health Commission denies any obvious human-to-human transmission.
	China contacts the WHO.
Jan. 1, 2020:	Dr. Li is accused of spreading false rumors by Chinese authorities.
	Seven are arrested in China for spreading false rumors.
	An official from the Hubei Provincial Health Commission orders a genomics company to stop testing and destroy samples.
Jan. 2, 2020:	Study published showing 27/41 infected patients had contact with Wuhan Market.
	Wuhan Institute of Virology maps the genome of SARS-CoV-2, but does not share the information.
Jan. 3, 2020:	Chinese National Health Commission institutes order not to publish information regarding the COVID-19.
	CDC Director first gets reports of new disease.
	Wuhan Municipal Health Commission states no clear evidence of human-to-human transmission.

---

[i] Acknowledgment: In reconstructing these events, the author relied on information summarized *National Review*. Jim Geraghty, "The Comprehensive Timeline of China's COVID-19 Lies," *National Review* (blog), Mar. 23, 2020, accessed Apr. 20, 2020, https://www.nationalreview.com/the-morning-jolt/chinas-devastating-lies/.

Jan. 5, 2020:	Wuhan Municipal Health Commission again states no clear evidence of human-to-human transmission.
Jan. 6, 2020:	CDC issues travel watch regarding China; offers to send team to China to assist in investigation.
Jan. 8, 2020:	China reports having identified the virus; claims there is no evidence of human-to-human transmission.
	The WHO touts notable achievement on the part of China in identifying SARS-CoV-2, but does not make recommendations for travelers.
Jan. 10, 2020:	Dr. Li Wenling develops upper respiratory symptoms.
	NYT publishes article repeating the claim that there is no evidence the virus can spread among humans."
Jan. 11, 2020:	Wuhan City Health Commission claims that all 739 cases were reviewed and no new cases have en detected in Wuhan since Jan. 3. No medical staff infections have been found. No clear evidence of human-to-human transmission.[1]
Jan. 12, 2020:	Dr. Li is hospitalized.
Jan. 13, 2020:	Thailand detects virus in a Chinese woman who had visited Wuhan, but not the Wuhan market.
Jan. 14, 2020:	Wuhan health authorities: No medical cases have been found amongst close contacts.
	WHO: preliminary investigations by Chinese authorities show no clear evidence of human-to-human transmission.
Jan. 15, 2020:	First case reported in Japan. No contact with the Wuhan Market.
	Wuhan Municipal Health Commission admits, for the first time, that the there is a possibility of "limited" human-to-human transmission.
Jan. 17, 2020:	CDC announces travelers from Wuhan will undergo screeing at three US airports.
	Wuhan Municipal Health Commission still reporting no related cases found among close contacts.

Jan. 18, 2020:	Wuhan Lunar New Year celebration is held without restrictions. Over 40,000 people attend.
	SecHHS Azar has first discussions regarding COVID-19 with Pres. Trump.
Jan 20, 2020:	Wuhan Municipal Health Commission's last statement that no related cases had been found amongst close contacts is made.
	Head of Chinese National Health Commission reports two cases in Guangdong province was caused by human-to-human transmission.
Jan. 21, 2020:	CDC announces first case in the US occurring in Snohomish County, Wash., in a resident who visited China six days earlier.
Jan. 22, 2020:	WHO Dir. Gen. praises China on its handling of COVID-19.
	WHO Emergency Committee meeting concluded Wuhan events did not constitute a Public Health Emergency of International Concern.
	Pres. Trump: We have it under control.
Jan. 23, 2020:	Chinese announce quarantine of Wuhan; all international flights to and from the city cease.
Jan. 24, 2020:	Vietnam reports human-to-human transmission.
	Second case in Chicago.
Jan. 30, 2020:	WHO declares the outbreak in Italy a public health emergency of international concern.
Jan. 31, 2020:	Two confirmed cases appear in Rome.
	Italy suspends flights to China; declares national emergency.
	Sec. Azar declares a public health emergency in the United States.
	First confirmed case in Spain.

Feb. 1, 2020:	Dr. Li tests positive.
	Woman with flu-like symptoms disembarks the Diamond Princess in Hong Kong. She eventually tests positive for COVID-19.
	The Westerdam departs Hong Kong with 1,455 passengers.
Feb. 3, 2020:	CDC submits an EUA request before the FDA for coronavirus testing.
Feb. 4, 2020:	FDA issues EUA for testing.
	Mayor of Florence encourages Italians to hug Chinese people to encourage them in the fight against the SARS-CoV-2.
	The Westerdam arrives in Kaohsiung, Taiwan.
Feb. 5, 20202:	Pres. Trump acquitted by the Senate in impeachment trial.
Feb. 7, 2020:	Dr. Li Wenliang dies.
Feb. 16, 2020:	The Westerdam is allowed to dock in Cambodia where one American is incorrectly found to test positive for COVID-19, setting off a disquieting chain of events.
Feb. 19, 2020:	Game Zero soccer match between Atalanta and Valencia is played in Milan before 45,792 fans.
Feb. 20, 2020:	Man in Lombardy tests positive after having been released from hospital.
Feb. 24, 2020:	The stock market reels on word of new cases appearing in Italy, Iran, and South Korea. The DJIA falls 1,031.61.
Feb. 27, 2020:	Pres. Trump appoints V.P. Pence to head the White House Coronavirus Task Force.
Mar. 2, 2020:	Pres. Trump holds his last rally at Bojangle's Stadium, Charlotte, NC.
	New York City gets its first confirmed case.
March 6, 2020:	Pres, Trump signs $8.3 billion coronavirus package.

Mar. 7, 2020:	Italian authorities decide to impose lockdown on northern parts of Italy. The news leaks and residents flea to the south.
	Stock market drops 2,013,67 points.
Mar. 8, 2020:	Northern lockdown takes effect in Italy amidst confusion and disregard for the mandate.
	Thousands participate in women's march in Spain.
Mar. 9, 2020:	Spain imposes national lockdown.
	Saudi Arabia promises to flood oil markets intensifying price war with Russia.
Mar. 11, 2020:	WHO declares global pandemic.
	Pres. Trump declares national health emergency from Oval Office.
Mar. 14, 2020:	Pres. Trump suspends travel to EU.
	CDC issues No-Sail Order
Mar. 22, 2020:	Bernie Sanders holds rally before thousands in San Diego.
Mar. 23, 2020:	England is placed on lockdown.
Mar. 27, 2020:	Pres. Trump signs the CARES Act.
Apr. 9, 2020:	CDC extends its March 14 No-Sail Order for another 100 days.
Apr. 16, 2020:	PPP funds exhausted

Preface

In January 2020, after eight months of furiously researching America's healthcare, I was finally ready to launch my new book, *The Case for Free Market Healthcare*. In early February, the manuscript was sent to the printer, and by March we were ready to go. *The Case* took all the experiences from twenty years of practicing medicine in the academic, military, and civilian sectors, the knowledge and insights from law school, and the work I had done in four years of service as state representative, and delivered them in the most comprehensive arguments for free-market principles and conservative healthcare policy I could assemble. I was convinced, and still am, that our policymakers and pundits are completely missing the boat on the issues plaguing our nation's healthcare delivery system and that it is time to cast a new, conservative light on the model our nation should have. The day of the roll-out was going to be exciting, and the opportunities to engage the public were going to be plentiful.

And then the world collapsed.

Within weeks, the stock market, which had been flirting with record highs almost daily, lost more than a third of its value. Americans went from being the most employed population in the nation's history, and probably the world, to one riddled with uncertainty and angst. The very fabrics of our society, our customs, natural courtesies, and the institutions we value were subjected to a massive assault, leaving many to ask whether it was better for us to abandon any or all of them. More directly related to *The Case*, questions about healthcare delivery options, the government's role in healthcare, our nation's readiness, and the government's manipulations of our abilities to receive it were playing out before my eyes with an urgency and fluidity I had never witnessed or even imagined. In essence, everything I had examined in *The Case* was being tested in a very public and rapid fashion. It was as if a laboratory had been purposely set up to place our healthcare delivery system under a microscope. Indeed, the Wuhan pandemic served as an advanced study on healthcare, the free market, and on the dangers of government involvement in medicine.

I quickly realized there could be no case for free-market healthcare without considering the lessons learned from this pandemic. There could be no *The Case for Free Market Healthcare* without *Coronalessons*. Thus the genesis of this book.

What is government's role in protecting the population from a massive pandemic such as the one America faced in 2020? Are the government's authorities plenary in such a situation, or are they limited? What's the purpose of government? Ought we abandon the principles and premises that gave rise to our country in exchange for ones that will keep us all safe? And are they really inalienable rights if the government can take them from us? These are the issues explored in *Coronalessons*.

Because they are intimately intertwined with healthcare and government's proper role in it, the questions posed here are inextricably related to those explored in *The Case*. In fact, some issues detailed in this book cannot be addressed without a close reliance on *The Case*, while others venture out onto new territories. For example, except in a historical context designed to explain the evolution of America's healthcare system, the state's emergency powers were little explored in *The Case*, but they make up the crux of *Corona-lessons*. Others, like rationing, are deeply discussed in *The Case*, but the context in which they were studied is far different from the ones evaluated in *Coronalessons*.

The writing of this book has been a task different from any other because it took place in real time. Conclusions were developed and arguments made only to be disassembled in light of insights gained from more recent events. Aside from its inefficiency, there is a great disadvantage in writing a book in this manner, namely the incompleteness of the data available through which to study the issues and proffer conclusions. But life plays itself out this way, so it is proper that *Coronalessons* should have played itself out this way, too. Besides, the insights gained from *Coronalessons* are so informative to the decisions we are making at this time that they must be engaged now, not later when its too late to direct our vessel to the proper shore.

The term "coronavirus" is too imprecise to refer to the respiratory infection that plagued the world between 2019 and 2020 since it actually denotes a group of viruses in the Coronaviridae family. The fact is that saying, "I have the coronavirus," really doesn't mean much beyond communicating that one is likely suffering from a virally induced, upper respiratory tract illness. So, with an eye for precision, throughout this text, I use the term "SARS-CoV-2" to refer to the virus causing the illness experienced during this pandemic. The condition, or the illness itself is referred to as "COVID-19," which is short for "Coronavirus Disease 2019," and the pandemic is the "Wuhan pandemic," denoting the place of its origin.

There are times in the book, mostly in the "Introduction," where I purposefully use the term "coronavirus." There, I am referring to the members of the family Coronaviridae. During the sections dealing with the course of the pandemic and our response to it, I occasionally use the term "coronavirus." In this context, I am generally staying true to the term used by the press or a particular politician. Suffice it to say here, that when I use the terms SARS-CoV-2, COVID-19, and Wuhan pandemic, I am specifically referring to the virus, illness, and pandemic respectively.

Coronalessons has a voluminous "Introduction," much larger than I normally write. The "Introduction" is not designed merely to set the stage for the material that follows. It does that, of course, but the bulk of the section is meant to inform a reader who may not be as familiar with virology and epidemiology about the bare knuckles knowledge and terminology used by epidemiologists, scientists, biologists, and doctors when discussing the various aspects of the pandemic. For perspective's sake, I also include a brief history of epidemics and pandemics that have affected humanity. For those readers with either little interest in the science behind pandemics or their histories, or with sufficient knowledge about them, skipping through these sections will not represent a major impediment towards understanding and following the rest of the material presented. However, even if one decides to skip over "The Virology of a Pandemic" through "Coronaviruses," I recommend picking the text up at "SARS-CoV-2" because it is there where I discuss many of the scientific developments specific to this virus, including potential treatments and testing.

I am indebted to my wife, Dr. Gina Arabitg, for everything! But here, I would like to thank her in particular for the incredible patience and support she has shown me as I furiously wrote one book and then just as fervently launched into another. She spent most of the shutdown dealing with the background clicking noise of my computer and my obsession over "coronaevents." I can't thank you enough, Gina, for your patience, your support, and your love. My two assistants have been super-heroines in this endeavor. Eugenia Freni has provided incredible insights about getting the message out. If you heard about this book, it was likely because of a suggestion Eugenia made. Her advice about the content of the book and its organization has been invaluable as well. Sophia Grand is the architect of the content in "Chapter 5: Trends and Correlations." The statistical analysis and graphwork is all hers. As it turns out, her contribution is one of the factors that make this work so unique. As always, Rod Thomson and Dr. Michael Patete have been steeples in this endeavor just like they were in *The Case*. Without their numerous phone calls to inform me of events that had just transpired or new insights gained, this book would be a mere shadow of itself. Additionally, Rod's economics expertise saved me from embarrassing myself more than I usually do. To Chris Angermann goes my gratitude on the compilation of the copyright page.

Because of the nature of the topic and the speed with which the material needed to be shared, this book is by necessity an unfinished work. There is much more to be gained from the events of the Wuhan pandemic and more still that need to play out. In order to get this information out to the public in record time, I have delivered it only in electronic form. It takes at least a couple of months to prepare this same material in print, thus I opted to bypass this delay. . . for now. I fully expect there to be an updated version and perhaps, as the material matures and gains stability, even a printed volume. I apologize for any grammatical errors there may still exist and the unpolished state of the citations. These remain not for a lack of attention to, or pride in, the quality of my work. Rather, it is the necessary price to be paid to get a large volume of relevant material to your screen quickly while its content is most relevant. I thank you for taking the time to consider the messages shared about this tumultuous time in our history and hope that it adds a little wisdom to what until now has been an insane, largely disruptive discussion.

Julio Gonzalez, M.D., J.D.
June 2020

Introduction

In December 2019, the world became subjected to a concerted and ruthless attack the likes of which it had seldom experienced. But the attacker, or the attackers' weapon, was no missile or rocket, nor was it an overwhelming military brigade or naval armada. Rather, this attacker was a particle so small that neither the naked eye nor a conventional light microscope could see it. In the truest sense of the word, this attacker was invisible. It was silent, imperceptible and stealth, but its effects have been nothing less than Herculean. As of the time of this writing, nearly 7,000,000 people have been ravaged by disease and nearly 400,500 lay dead. Countries have been decimated. Families have been lost. Businesses have been closed. The world's economy has been brought to its knees, and relations between men, and even nations, have been forever altered.

What was the catalyst of this most devastating agent?

A mere virus.

But this is no ordinary virus as its name heralds. It is a coronavirus, so named because of the series of protruding, crown-shaped proteins that serve as its grasping points for its prey.

Coronaviruses have laid siege on the human population at least six times before. And although the strain has produced some very mild members, it has also included two of the most aggressive contagions experienced in modern times, SARS-CoV-1, the virus responsible for Severe Acute Respiratory Syndrome (SARS) and our most recent nemesis, SARS-CoV-2, the virus responsible for Coronavirus

Infectious Disease-2019, (COVID-19). Like its more aggressive cousins, SARS-CoV-2 is fast, merciless and relentless. It is so efficient that within weeks its tentacles spread across the world and its effects were experienced in every corner of the globe. In fact, the only location on earth so remote and so desolate to escape its chilling grip is Antarctica where only a few scores of humans live separated from their nearest neighbors in Ushuaia Argentina by over 1100 miles.

As humanity is apt to do, it has survived this attack, colossal as it was, and we live on to continue to worship, produce, love, fight, and die. As is the case with any survivable experience, there are lessons to be learned. In this case countless of them.

Of course, the fight against this coronavirus has left us with numerous insights regarding virology, physiology, medicine, epidemiology, and disease, but in this particular case, the experience has taught us so much more. We have learned about international relations, national vulnerabilities, ethics, resource allocation, and population management. And most of all, we have learned about our relationship with our Creator.

Indeed, so vast and varied are the lessons learned from combating this virus, that the global experience will forever be referenced, nationally and internationally when fighting natural and man-made disasters.

This text aims to define some of these lessons while recognizing that it will not reflect the final word on any of these insights. In the pages that follow we will undertake an evaluation of the world's experience with the coronavirus pandemic while paying special attention to the actions of our home, the United States. We will review our collective experience with the illness, the virus's origin, its spread, and the many attempts at its containment. We will analyze where we have succeeded and failed. By necessity, the effort will take us into a highly technical world of epidemiology and population health. It is in that world that we begin our endeavor.

The Virology of A Pandemic

A virus is an entity existing somewhere between the living and the nonliving. It shares some properties with living organisms in that it is a carbon-based organism that reproduces and in it own way, feeds off others. It is nonliving because it cannot engage in any of its self-replicating activities on its own. It cannot feed. It cannot heal. In fact, so long as a virus fails to gain access to other organisms, specifically those it is designed to invade, it cannot engage in any activity at all.

A virus is also imperceptibly small, having diameters measured in nanometers, or billionths of a meter. A virus is about 100,000 times smaller than the diameter of a strand of hair and 1,000 times smaller than a bacterion, the smallest living organism. Viruses are so small that by comparison, the diameter of the average pore of a surgical mask is 16,900 times larger it is, or the size of 200 football fields relative to the size of a human being.

To be this small and continue to exist, a virus has to be specially designed to engage in only one mission: propagation. Its very nature is to exist and make more of itself. Essentially, a virus is nothing more than ultra-microscopic sac of genetic material (a blueprint) with an attached injection port. The sac itself, literally a microscopic bag of protein is called the capsid, which may itself be encapsulated for extra strength with either a capsule, or with a membrane material it steals from its victim. Some viruses have a long tail protruding from the capsid, imparting upon it the appearance of a mushroom or a tree. This "tail" is the attachment site that the virus uses to latch onto its target. Other viruses, such as the coronavirus upon which we direct most of our attention, do not possess a specific tail, but contain a number of molecules on their surfaces that server the same purpose. Regardless of the design, so stripped is the virus of extraneous resources that it is completely dependent on other organisms, what we call hosts, to manufacture more of itself.

But a virus cannot indiscriminately infiltrate just any host and take over its metabolism for its benefit. Instead, most strains of viruses are equipped with recognition molecules used to identify certain portions of a cell's surface and attach to it. Once the virus successfully attaches to its target cell, it can penetrate it and inject its contents into it. The injected material is genetic information that inserts itself into the cell's own genome turning the cell it into a virus making machine. These newly made viruses are subsequently released, and once outside the cell, these thousands of new viruses begin the process anew.

Viruses also differ from each other in the type of genetic material they inject into cells. For most viruses, this means packets of DNA, or RNA. DNA (deoxyribonucleic acid) are those long helical molecules organized into a double helix containing all the information a cell needs to live out its existence. When processed by the cell, DNA will direct its metabolism, the construction of its walls, the creation of its organelles, and the assembly of its power supply structures (mitochondria), among countless other activities.

Ultimately, the cell's DNA determines the proteins that are to be created within that cell. The specific set of proteins and the manner in which they are packed and processed define the cell. However, in order to create these proteins, the information in the DNA must first be transcribed into packets of RNA (ribonucleic acid). It is this RNA that then exits the nucleus into the cells watery body (its cytoplasm) where the information in the RNA is converted into the actual proteins.

A virus causes its effects by injecting its own DNA or RNA into the cellular victim. The injected material is then capable of taking over the cell's manufacturing system and fundamentally changing the cell's original purpose into a virus-replicating machine. The illnesses caused by the various strains of viruses depend on the specific qualities of each strain and the cells they are designed to infect. Some viruses do not infect humans because the cells they recognize are in other species such as bats, camels, cats, or certain birds. Within human beings, some viruses attack respiratory cells and are therefore the harbingers of colds and lung disease. Others attack the gastrointestinal track, causing nausea, vomiting, and diarrhea. Others cause heart problems, and others still have been blamed for causing diabetes, certain cancers, brain problems and skin diseases. Depending on the characteristics of a virus, virtually any illness or bodily condition may be inflicted. Similarly, those same characteristics inherent to the virus determine its aggressiveness, infectiousness, mode of transmission, lethality, and treatment.

Defenses

Despite the dreadfulness of a virus's modus operandi, neither the human body nor populations stand helplessly against its ruthless attack. The human body, like those of any advanced living organism, is equipped with an immune system that continuously surveils for signs of hostile invasion. The key detectors within the immune system are the plethora or antibodies that continuously travel throughout the body searching for the presence of invaders. These molecules are specifically designed to identify anything that appears to be foreign, particularly foreign protein molecules. If detected, they attach to the protein in locations called antigens; spots on foreign organisms recognizable to a host's antibodies. These antibody-antigen complexes then attach to the host's white blood cells allowing the invader to be destroyed.

As one can imagine, this process is continuously playing out. Organisms, be they bacterial, fungal, or viral, penetrate a body, and are spotted by the host's defenses. The invading organism is destroyed and its remnants disposed, sometimes so quietly that the host organism does not even display signs of disease or attack.

If however, the invader, in this case a virus, reaches its target cells, it can then set up its operations to reproduce, and at the very least cause illness, if not overwhelm the host and kill it.

It should be noted that antibodies do not necessarily randomly travel throughout the whole body. There are different types of antibodies with different tasks. IgG antibodies, the most commonly discussed, largely flow through the bloodstream and the body's interstitial fluids. They are generally not the first to respond to an invasion; that role falls upon IgM antibodies. For this reason, clinicians and scientists are able to get a clue regarding the recentness of an infection by looking at the relative concentrations of these immunoglobulins in a patient. This is often done in patients with hepatitis, for example, a viral disease affecting the liver. If a patient has a high IgG titer (concentration) in his blood and a low IgM titer, it means the exposure took place at least six months prior to the test as the body has had time to develop IgGs against the virus. Alternatively, those with high IgM titers and low IgG titers have only recently contracted the disease.

And there are other types of immunoglobulins. IgA antibodies tend to reside in the internal body linings like the respiratory tract, the gastrointestinal tract, and the urogenital tract. IgD antibodies reside on specific immune cells as do IgEs, the ones triggering allergic responses.

The body's response to foreign invaders such as viruses does not end with recognitions. Indeed, once antibodies specific to that invader recognize the foreign antigen, they are picked up by white blood cells, which then mount a counter-attack. This immune response is what gives the illness its signature characteristics such as fever, chills, nausea, vomiting, malaise, upper respiratory symptoms, and even diarrhea. The specific appearance of each illness is dependent on the specific characteristics of the response and the intracorporeal location of the attack.

There are also external factors that may help combat a disease. Chief amongst these are medications. Few can doubt the amazing benefits achieved by antibiotics in defeating infections. But antibiotics, although integral to defeating certain bacterial diseases, do not generally work against viruses. In rare circumstances pharmaceuticals have been developed that specifically work against certain viruses. For example, H1N1 was found to be susceptible to the antiviral medications amantadine and rimantidine,[2] and other medications have been found to be effective in the treatment of HIV/AIDS. These treatments however, have not been as effective in eradicating viral conditions as have their anti-bacterial counterparts. In fact, to this day, only one viral condition, hepatitis C, has been found to be curable with the use of antivirals (sofosbuvir/velpatasvir also known as EPCLUSA),[3] although recent claims are starting to be made with regards to HIV/AIDS.[4]

Because antivirals are generally more toxic than antibiotics and tend to not cure the infection, but rather just control it, vaccines have become the mainstay of protection and prevention against viral infections. Remember many viruses do not have an antiviral that work against them. Here, public health efforts have centered on imposing a heightened level of protection against infection prior to contracting the illness. Vaccines work by exposing an individual's body to particles that appear to be like the virus.[i] The body is then induced into producing antibodies against the virus. When the actual virus hits, the individual is already immune to it and can rapidly deter the attack.

Of course, vaccines are not 100% effective and some vaccines may actually cause infection of an otherwise healthy individual. Some patients cannot mount a strong immune response against a virus even after being vaccinated. Nevertheless, despite these shortcomings vaccines have demonstrated great success in the fight against viral spread.

The widespread use of vaccines against a specific virus can instill a second advantage: the development of herd immunity. Herd immunity is a situation where enough of the population has achieved heightened resistance against a contagion such that the population as a whole essentially achieves resistance. Exactly what that minimum percentage of the population needs to be in order to achieve herd immunity depends on the disease, its contagiousness, and its mechanism of spread. For many diseases, immunity percentages of 80%-85% are needed in order to achieve herd immunity. For others, resistance rates as low as 40% may be sufficient.

The process of developing a vaccine against a virus is not simple. The first strep in is to obtain the virus itself and grow it in mass quantities in media such as chicken eggs[5] . These viral particles are then purified and processed, forming the vaccine itself.[6] In the

---

[i] There is a detailed discussion on vaccine physiology and the history of their development in my book *The Case for Free Market Healthcare*.

United States, the proposed vaccine then has to undergo vigorous testing under the supervision of the Food and Drug Administration (FDA), a process that can take over a year to complete. Bear in mind that from the FDA's standpoint, approval of a vaccine should be more strenuous than approval for medications because vaccines are being administered to healthy people, not those that are sick and need to be treated. In the case of H1N1 in 2009, for example, a vaccine never became available for public distribution even though one was constructed by September 15, 2009.[ii]

There is one other intervention needing consideration here since it played a significant role in the discussions regarding the Wuhan pandemic: convalescent plasma transfusions. Here, blood products from patients who have already recovered from a viral infection are transfused into a patient infected with the virus. The logic is that the immunity the recovered patients have amassed through the development of antibodies to the virus could be passively conferred upon the sick patient. This technique has been infrequently done in other illnesses. As we will discuss below, it is an heroic intervention used in the treatment of deathly ill patients.[iii]

Epidemiological Considerations

Just as the characteristics of each particular strain of virus defines how it interacts with human cells and the diseases it causes, they also determine how the virus sweeps through a population. Like in any other communicable disease, viral illnesses share certain characteristics in the manner in which they spread through a population. Generally, the shape of the spread of the illness over time resembles that

[ii] See section on H1N1.

[iii] See section on responses.

of a bell, the so-called bell-shaped curve. Initially when few people have a disease, the incidence of the condition is quite low. However, very quickly the number of people infected each day increases precipitously to a peak (the top of the bell). Once that peak is reached and more people get exposed to the condition, fewer are available to suffer from it, and the number of new cases per day begins to drop until it tapers back down to zero new infections per day.

In the case of a new, or novel communicable disease there are usually very few initial cases. These initial cases are usually contracted from a common source. Subsequently, depending on how contagious the condition is, it is either able to spread rapidly, or fizzle away to nothing. A more aggressive condition will spread within a community or a specific geographical region so that its occurrence is widespread within that area. Such a phenomenon is known as an epidemic. Rarely, a communicable disease can be so aggressive and its spread so pervasive that it infiltrates throughout a large nation, a continent, or the world. Such situations are known as pandemics and are caused by immensely aggressive contagions.

Another commonly employed term referring to a massively pervasive illness is a plague. Technically, a plague refers to bacterial diseases, as opposed to viral conditions, and may actually refer to an illness affecting a specific individual. Historically, though, illnesses meriting the use of the term have been extremely aggressive and have ravaged whole populations at a time such that they may easily be characterized as epidemics or pandemics.

Initially, most epidemics were due to bacterial diseases. One of the earliest known epidemics was the Plague of Athens, which happened around 430 B.C. and killed about 100,000 people.[7] Perhaps the most famous epidemic was the Bubonic Plague of 541-542 A.D. It was a massive historical event where over 10% of the population perished.[8]

The disease was of such magnitude that it changed the course of history, as it marked the beginning of the descent of the Byzantine Empire. No less in scope was the Black Death spanning from 1346 through 1353 and spanning two continents. It is estimated that half of Europe's population was wiped out as result of this pandemic.[9]

Disease and epidemics defined much of the North American colonial experience as well. In fact, one theory regarding the disappearance of the Lost Roanoke Colony of 1585 is that an infection decimated the small European population.

In the seventeenth century, the principal communicable diseases that would ravage the populations in the North Americans colonies were tuberculosis, pneumonia, and typhoid fever, although there were many waves of malaria, yellow fever, and beriberi largely brought to North America through the importation of slaves.[10] Towards the eighteenth century, the offending agents tended to change, with local populations seeing greater outbreaks of smallpox. In 1702, for example, Boston was subjected to a wave of smallpox that killed 302 people out of a population of 7,000.[11] The outbreak was part of a much larger epidemic involving the St. Lawrence River Basin.[12] A few years later, yet another major outbreak took pace in Philadelphia,[13] and in 1793 a large outbreak of yellow fever gripped Philadelphia in 1793, killing over 5,000 people.[14]

Only after the implementation of an aggressive vaccination campaign in the latter half of the eighteenth century did the recurring epidemics of smallpox begin to abate, but not in time to prevent the catastrophic effects of these largely European diseases on the Native American population. The outbreaks were so devastating to the those whose presence in North America predated the arrival of the European, that approximately 90% of the indigenous population was erased as a result.[15]

With the development of antibiotics and the improved effectiveness in warding off bacterial diseases, the primary infections devastating vast swaths of human populations switched to viral ones as humanity traversed through the nineteenth century and entered the twentieth. The greater versatility and contagiousness of viruses coupled with the improvements in transportation that increased the mobility of human beings led to faster patterns of spread and much broader geographical footprints.

In 1889, influenza, a viral disease, took a deadly grip upon the world with a peak mortality rate just five weeks after the outbreak's onset in St. Petersburg, Russia.[16] A second influenza outbreak in 1918 had its impact magnified by the devastations of World War I resulting millions of deaths.[17] In 1957, the Asian flu caused by an H2N2 virus arose out of Singapore killing over a million people globally, 116,000 in the United States alone.[18] Largely due to the instability of the virus's genome, influenza's assault on human populations has continued, with each year bringing a different strain and requiring the creation of a new vaccine. Since 2010, the CDC has estimated there have been between 9 and 45 million cases of influenza per year with between 140,000 and 810,000 hospitalizations and between 12,000 and 61,000 deaths.[19]

Fig, Intro-1: CDC Estimate of U.S. Influenza Burden, by Season (2010-2019)

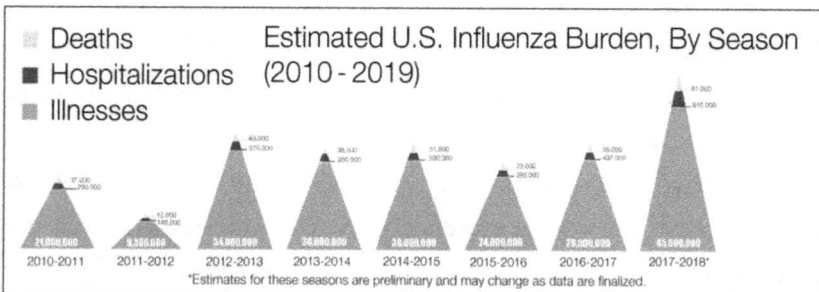

Source: "Influenza (Flu) Burden of Influenza," CDC, accessed Apr. 13, 2020, https://www.cdc.gov/flu/about/burden/index.html.

The 2002 Severe Acute Respiratory Syndrome (SARS) outbreak is likely the most relevant to the study of Coronavirus Infectious Disease-2019 (COVID-19). SARS was the first, highly contagious coronavirus in humans.[20] Ultimately given the scientific name SARS-CoV-1, the SARS virus, bears significant resemblances to SARS-CoV-2, the virus causing COVID-19. Like its successor, SARS-CoV-1 emanated from China and came from bats. However, SARS-CoV-1 seems to have jumped from bats to humans through civet cats whereas it is presently believed that SARS-CoV-2 directly spread to humans from a bat.[21]

Just like SARS-CoV-2, SARS-CoV-1's spread was explosive.[22] Within months, the number of SARS cases went from 0 to a full-fledged epidemic affecting at least 29 countries. Vexingly, its propensity to spread varied between patients, with some patients not appearing to spread the virus, while in others, the transmission was large and tagged "super spreading events."[23] As an example, a patient in Guangdong with SARS stayed one day in a hotel in Hong Kong. Fifteen guests were infected from that one brief exchange, who then traveled to other countries taking the virus with them.[24]

In 2009, the Swine flu pandemic struck, caused by a strain of coronavirus named H1N1. The disease began in Mexico and infected about one third of the world's population and left about half a million dead.[25] In the United States, it was first detected in California on April 15, 2009, in two children, aged 8 and 10 years.[26] Within days, testing on these two cases confirmed that the virus was the same one infecting patients in Mexico and Canada,[27] and although it was initially called swine flu because of its similarities to other viral conditions emanating from various types of swine, later investigations demonstrated the absence of any association with pigs resulting in the abandonment of that name for the one used today "the H1N1 virus."[28] On April 25, 2009, a cluster of H1N1 cases was identified in a New York High School prompting the United States to declare a national public health emergency.[29] Twenty-five percent of the supplies in CDC's Strategic National Stockpile (SNS), including 11 million regimens of antiviral drugs, over 39 million respiratory protection devices (masks and respirators), gowns, gloves and face shields were released.[30] As will become relevant later, they were largely left unrestocked.

The federal government also purchased 50 million courses of the antiviral agents oseltamivir and zanamivir, with the various states buying even more, and the FDA allowed for the off-label use of the two medications for the treatment of H1N1.[31] A travel advisory was issued for Americans traveling to Mexico. Advisories were also issued requesting Americans work from home, cover their coughs and sneezes, and avoid going to school or work if sick were also made.[32] However, despite 98% of suspected flu samples being positive for H1N1 by May 4, 2009,[33] and H1N1 causing an estimated 60.8 million cases in the United States, 274,304 hospitalizations, and 12,649 deaths,[34] no mobilization comparable to what was seen in COVID-19 was undertaken in response this or any pandemic.

A couple of other points regarding the H1N1 pandemic are worthy of notice. First the pandemic was so massive that over 0.007% of the world's population succumbed to it.[35] Also, in many ways the H1N1 pandemic was upside down with regards to its demographic characteristics. Contrary to most other illnesses of its kind, 80% of mortalities from H1N1 took place in those younger than 65.[36] One possible reason is that the virus causing the illness, (H1N1)pdm09, shared many characteristics with the influenza virus, to the point that it was ultimately categorized as an influenza A.[37] Consequently, more than one third of people older than 60 had already developed antibodies against (H1N1)pdm09, affording them some resistance, while children generally had no resistance.[38] Finally, vaccine development against H1N1 began in earnest on April 21, 2009 under the auspices of the CDC.[39] Although the complete gene sequence was released on April 24 of that year, a vaccine did not become available until September 15, 2009, about a month prior to the peak of the illness's second wave in October.[40]

A few other more recent pandemics are of great significance even though they did not share the same methods of spread. Perhaps most notable is the polio outbreak in the United States that began in 1916. Polio terrorized families as children became exposed to a virus that led to permanent paralysis. Not until the development of the Salk vaccine in 1954 would humanity effectively fight back against this vicious crippler to the point where it was nearly completely eradicated.[41]

Another pandemic, the Acquired Immunodeficiency Syndrome, or AIDS, saw its onset in the 1980s. It is cause to the Human Immunodeficiency Virus (HIV) present in chimpanzees. The disease is spread through the exchange of bodily fluids as with sexual contact or the sharing of dirty intravenous or hypodermic needles. Until very recently, AIDS had no known cure even though medications were developed that would prolong a victim's life.[42] To date, no vaccine has been developed, and it still has a grip on the intravenous-drug-sharing and homosexual populations.

West African Ebola is particularly frightful. Also caused by a coronavirus and centered about the Sudan and the Democratic Republic of Congo, this hemorrhagic condition has been recognized for decades. In December 2013, a case was reported in an 8-month-old boy who appeared to have contracted the condition from bats.[43] Within three months there were 49 confirmed cases and 29 deaths.[44]

The disease spread to Liberia and Sierra Leone where it wreaked havoc upon the population.[45] The Ebola outbreak continued its spread throughout Africa and Europe, eventually reaching the United States.[46] Without a cure and a mortality rate of nearly 40%,[47] the disease struck horror in all that contracted it. Eventually, the outbreak receded, but the virus is still present in Central Africa.

Finally, the Zika virus. This virus began in South and Central America in 2015. Carried by mosquitoes and in some cases, sexual activity, the disease made its way into the southernmost reaches of the United States. Its effects are significant in the unborn where it has been linked to anencephaly, or stunted brain development.[48] The Zika virus did have some bearing on the United States' response to the COVID-19 pandemic since its containment efforts further depleted the SNS.

These experiences teach at least one indisputable lesson. We can count on the appearance of novel viruses in the future, sometimes very aggressive ones. We should not be taken by surprise when the next one emerges.

Coronaviruses

Coronaviruses are medium-sized (between 80-150 nanometers in diameter), membrane-coated viruses covered with surface projections. The surface projections, which are crown-like in shape, are responsible the group's name.[49]

Coronaviruses contain RNA genes within them. The RNA inside each coronavirus directs the production of new viruses. It does this by creating one large protein, which is then cut by other proteins that are also made at the direction of the virus's RNA gene. The resulting proteins, along with the viral RNA that is also produced by the infected cell, spontaneously fall together while still inside the host's cell to form new viruses. These new viruses are then ejected from the cell, each one wrapping itself with a layer of cell membrane as it is extruded. In the process, the cell is destroyed.

The fact that the coronaviruses are lined with cell membrane accounts for their susceptibility to detergents and bleaches, as these chemicals destroy the fat-soluble cell membranes. Also, because they are sensitive to warm temperatures, coronaviruses tend to be seasonal, occurring more frequently during winter and spring in temperate climates.[50]

Coronaviruses initially did not attract much attention since they were thought only to be a secondary source of the common cold, the most common being rhinovirus. As a matter of fact, coronaviruses were estimated to be responsible for about 35% of colds.[51] That changed in 2002 with the appearance of SARS.

From an epidemiological standpoint, there does not appear to be any cross-protection between the different types of coronaviruses. If a person is vaccinated against one strain of coronavirus, he or she will not be immune to another,[52] so merely because one is immune to SARS does not make one immune to COVID-19. Additionally, immunity to any one coronavirus appears to be short lived, with reinfections occurring within months.[53]

Although coronavirus such as SARS and COVID-19 are classically associated with respiratory symptoms and disease, they have been detected in stool samples.[54] Whether there is an association with gastrointestinal symptoms such as diarrhea is more controversial. It should also be noted that nausea, vomiting, and diarrhea have been suggested to be associated with COVID-19 in addition to the well-recognized upper respiratory symptoms.[55]

SARS-CoV-2

Since our main text deals with events and responses to them, a few words about the biological understanding of Severe Acute Respiratory Syndrome Coronavirus-2 (SARS-CoV-2) is in order, the virus causing COVID-19. As previously noted, SARS-CoV-2 is a member of the coronavirus family. It shares many of the characteristics of SARS-CoV-1, the virus that caused SARS in 2002. Whether it escaped from a lab or was naturally transmitted in the Wuhan region, it seems to be based on other coronaviruses naturally found in the horseshoe bat in southern China.

Like its cousins, SARS-CoV-2 is a positive-RNA containing virus.[iv] Its capsid is surrounded by cell membrane material, which it picks up as it is extruded from the host cell. Also like other coronaviruses, SARS-CoV-2 uses its multiple, crown-shaped spike proteins to attach to its host cells, in this case the angiotensin-converting enzyme 2 receptor (ACE 2 receptor). In humans, the ACE 2 receptor molecule is an enzyme that binds angiotensin-2, which is a molecule in the bloodstream that helps maintain one's blood pressure. Receptors for angiotensin-2 are found in lung tissue, certain kidney cells, and in the gut.

Because of its affinity for ACE-2 receptors, SAR-CoV-2 tends to attack lung cells. The virus does this by using its spike proteins to attach to the ACE-2 receptors in pulmonary cells. Once attached, a protein called cathepsin-L is activated to fuse the virus to the cell. The virus is then able to release its RNA into the cell and take over the host's metabolic mechanisms. From the virus's RNA, the cell is

---

[iv] Here the term "positive" means that the RNA exists in a form that is ready to be transcribed (used to make new proteins) by the protein-making enzymes. "Negative" RNA is one that needs to first be translated into a positive strand before it can be used to make proteins.

able to translate a large polyprotein (a big protein made up of many smaller proteins) that is then cleaved by two proteases[v] derived from the virus's own genome. The split pieces then manufacture positive and negative RNA strands. The positive strands are packaged into new viruses, and the negative strands are used to form the membranes and spike proteins. All of these components are assembled inside a capsid to form new viruses, which are then released from the cell, taking some of the membrane with them as they go.[vi]

Naturally, determining whether a particular person has contracted SARS-CoV-2 is of great importance. For the individual, being able to tell whether he or she is infected guides his treatment and helps inform the patient, clinician, and loved ones about the patient's prognosis and projected clinical course. From a population health standpoint, knowing the prevalence of the SARS-CoV-2 infection is just as important. Data regarding the incidence and prevalence of an infection, as well as its regional distribution, allows policymakers and public health officials to take effective action in containing the spread of the virus. Areas with high concentrations of the disease can be isolated to prevent its spread, and individuals carrying the disease can be quarantined for the safety of those around them.

If we know that a certain individual is carrying a disease and is contagious, his or her providers can be protected from contracting the illness through the implementation of isolation methods and through the use of personal protective equipment (PPE) that would be too onerous or expensive to require from all members of a population.

---

[v] A protease is a protein whose purpose it is to cut other proteins. Some proteases are very specific about the location where another protein is cut.

[vi] It is because the SARS-CoV-2 is surrounded by plasma membrane that they are susceptible to disruption by alcohol and detergents.

Additionally, with population-based data, epidemiologists are able to track the progress of the illness and make determinations regarding the state of the pandemic. Accurate information regarding the spread of the disease can also inform the public and policymakers about the infectiousness of the virus and the vulnerability of the various subgroups of the population.

Understandably, the development of a test that could efficaciously detect the presence of the SARS-CoV-2 is paramount. Initial efforts revolved around the development of polymerase chain reaction (PCR) testing, a test that relies on the detection of the virus's genome. It appears that as of December 27, China had not yet developed testing specific to SARS-CoV-2. In fact, it is believed that China first identified the genetic sequence of the novel coronavirus on January 2, a step integral to the development of the most common testing methods. But China did not share the genomic sequence of SARS-CoV-2 until January 12, meaning the rest of the world could not begin working on tests designed to detect the virus's genetic material until that date.[56]

In the meantime, the World Health Organization (WHO) whose responsibility it is to inform the global community of potential health threats, first referred to a test created by European virologists as early as January 13,[57] but it was not until a January 21 press release regarding its recent visit to China that the WHO reported that "the Chinese Government released the primers and probes used in the test kit for the novel coronavirus to help other countries detect it."[58] It therefore appears that testing actually began in earnest in China in mid January, as this is when two European testing manufacturers, BGI and Co-Diagnostics, obtained clearances to release their tests.[59]

SARS-CoV-2 Testing

There are two general methods for testing for SARS-COV-2: chemical and serological. At this time, the chemical method is the more commonly applied method and revolves around the detection of viral genetic material. The technique, known as reverse transcriptase polymerase chain reaction, or RT-PCR, is often simply referred to as PCR, polymerase chain reaction. The test involves copying genetic material in a sample and then comparing it to the known genetic material in the virus. To develop this test, researchers must first have the virus's genetic material; otherwise, they would not know what they should be testing for. A positive test using this method makes it highly likely (greater than 90%) that the subject is actually infected with SARS-CoV-2. A negative test, one where viral material is not detected is not as useful, since it has substantial chance that the patient is still infected with SARS-CoV-2.

Another chemical test is a rapid-response test. This approach is different from PCR, but it is still a chemical detection test. Here, a test strip is impregnated with a chemical that can detect the specific virus, substance, or contagion. If a fluid sample, such as saliva, is allowed to come into contact with the test strip, a change in the strip, like in its color, will take place to allow the tester to know that the sought after substance is detected. The classic application of this technology is the home pregnancy test. Its advantages include not only the speed of the results and the test's potential for home use, but also the absence of swabs or pinpricks for sample collection, as it relies on a drop of saliva or sputum for testing. As of this writing, Sona Nanotech is developing one such test using lateral flow technology for COVID-19 in Canada in the hopes of being able to supply this test to the general public for home use.[60] It is slightly different from other rapid response testing in that it depends on the complex of the detecting chemical and the detected substance attaching to each other and traveling across a strip to create a visible stripe or a circle indicating its positivity. Although its COVID-19 test has been approved for use in other countries, the test is still undergoing review by the FDA for use in the United States.

Relatedly, the FDA authorized another at-home collection molecular test by LabCorp. Although the actual test is not performed at home, the collection can be, allowing the patient to swab himself or herself anywhere and deliver the sample to the lab for testing.[61] A variation of this approach is the rapid detection tests that be performed in a clinic or laboratory setting. This technique can test for the presence of multiple viruses concurrently and can have results within 2.5 hours.

The second method of testing is serology, or the testing of the immunoglobulins in a subject's blood. This method cannot tell a clinician or researcher whether someone is infected. Rather, it can tell whether the patient has been exposed to the virus. As we previously mentioned, a person who is exposed to a virus will mount an immune response. At first the response includes the production of IgM antibodies. Later on, the immune system switches to the production of IgG antibodies.

Serological testing is performed on a sample of the patient's blood, which can be as small as a drop of blood obtained through a pinprick. The detection of either IgM or IgG antibodies indicates a prior exposure, although it says nothing about the consequences of the exposure. For example, based on serology testing alone, one cannot tell whether the patient had a severe infection or a barely detectible reaction to the virus, but can conclude that the patient was either exposed to the virus, or to a vaccine against it. If broken into its IgM and IgG components, the test can give a rough idea about the timing of the exposure. If the patient has a high IgM titer but no IgG, the exposure was recent. If the IgM titer is low, and the IgG titer is high, then a more distant exposure took place.

Potential Treatments

Unlike in bacterial infections, there are generally no medications to kill viruses. Consequently, with rare exceptions such as HIV or hepatitis C, treatment for viral infections is only supportive, meaning that the caregiver treats the patient's symptoms until the patient is able to ward off the virus via his or her immune system. If the patient has fevers, the caregiver may treat the patient with acetaminophen (Tylenol) to bring the fever back down. If the patient has cold symptoms, cold medications or an antitussive may be used. Those with diarrhea, nausea, and vomiting may get placed on a clear liquid diet, or have an IV started in order to keep the patient hydrated.

Rarely, in severe respiratory viral infections, the lungs may shut down to the point where the patient is unable to breath on his own. Generally, this happens because the inflammatory response to the virus on the patient's part is so severe that the lungs get swollen, bogged down with fluid, and unable to exchange air for the patient. In these cases, the situation requires support from a ventilator, which pushes air into the patient's lungs, often with higher concentrations of oxygen and under pressure, in order to force the delivery of oxygen into the patient's body. Of course, in order to allow a ventilator to work, a tube is inserted into the patient's throat with an inflatable balloon that seals the airway allowing the high-pressure air to be delivered into the lungs.

The views on the role of ventilators in the treatment of COVID-19 patients have evolved. Initially, physicians were as aggressive in supporting the patient's breathing as they were with any other cause of respiratory failure. Later, evidence developed suggesting that the ventilators were actually causing more damage.[62] Physicians then became much more timid in the use of artificially delivered ventilation, which may explain why British physicians ultimately refrained from using a ventilator in the care of Prime Minister Boris Johnson.

Sometimes, in an effort to tamp down the immune response, the patient is given steroids, which have very strong anti-inflammatory effects. This is generally reserved for very advanced cases. For these patients, regardless of the virus causing such a massive response, the clinical situation is quite delicate. Just about any complication can take place in these most serious cases. The patient's kidneys may shut down where they stop creating urine and therefore stop maintaining the incredibly narrow salt balances required to sustain life. Those patients may be treated with diuretics, medications designed to stimulate the kidneys into working. Others may require dialysis where an external filter replaces the kidneys for the patient. The patient's blood pressures may drop, in which case he is supported with "pressors," medicines designed to elevate the patient's blood pressure. If a patient's liver stops functioning, the situation becomes even more treacherous since the liver is responsible for so much.

The patient may have a heart attack under all the stress. The pulmonary function may become so bad that the ventilator is unable to support the air exchange even at its highest setting. Or the patient may develop a super infection; an invasion by other organisms, usually bacterial, that serve to make his or her prognosis significantly worse.

SARS-CoV-2 is a particularly severe virus. Its contagiousness and aggressiveness, particularly in older patients, African-Americans, the weak, the infirmed, and men, is such that some patients are unable to ward off the virus, more so than is seen in milder contagions such as the common cold. Consequently, in addition to the many attempts at socially distancing individuals in order to prevent the spread of the disease, physicians and scientists have been searching for medicinal treatments that could help.

Early on, scientific impressions were formed that two related anti-malarials, chloroquine and hydroxychloroquine, were beneficial in the treatment of COVID-19. The first publicly disseminated clinical indication that hydroxychloroquine in combination with a commonly used antibiotic, azithromycin, could be helpful came from a randomly controlled study out of France involving 40 patients with early infections. All patients in the experimental group improved, except for one who was 86 years old and received the medicines in an "advanced form" of the disease.[63] In another study, patients were randomized to placebo treatment or to a 5-day treatment with 400 milligrams per day of hydroxychloroquine. The study was out of Wuhan, in its preliminary stages, and absent peer review, but the results were that the time to clinical recovery, body temperature recovery time, and cough remission time for those patients who received the anti-malarial medications were better than those who did not.[64]

But not all experiments on the efficacy of these two medications have been positive. One French study performed in patients with severe infection who were treated with hydroxychloroquine and azithromcin did not have favorable outcomes.[65] It was suggested that one reason for the poor results in this latter study is that the anti-malarial treatments lose their abilities to temper the patient's physiology as the infection worsens as the patient's ongoing deterioration starts to result from the overwhelming inflammatory reaction against the viral load. Alternatively, when applied early, because the overwhelming inflammatory response has not yet occurred, the reduction in the viral load due to the anti-malarial may allow the patient to more effectively combat the disease and recover.

In the laboratory, scientists also found data regarding the possible mechanisms of action for chloroquine and hydroxychloroquine. Laboratory observations indicate that either of these two medications (specifically chloroquine, the medications studied in this particular study) used in combination with remdersivir will increase a cell's internal pH and interfere with the penetration of the virus.[66]

Chloroquine and hydroxychloroquine hold particular promise because they are incredibly safe medications that have been used for over fifty years in the treatment of certain rheumatological disorders and for malarial prophylaxis. The medications are known to have some untoward effects, such as cardiac rhythm disorders and retinal abnormalities, but these are very rare and encountered at higher doses than those generally recommended for the treatment of early COVID-19 infections and their prevention.

These early experiences have been so promising that recommendations have been made not only for treatment, but also for prevention. In India, the National Task Force for COVID-19 recommended the use of hydroxychloroquine to prevent the acquisition of COVID-19 amongst its healthcare workers.[67] At the time of this writing, trials aimed at definitively answering the question of whether the routine use of chloroquine or hydroxychloroquine is efficacious in the prevention of COVID-19 infection are ongoing in Thailand, Spain, Washington, Minnesota, and New York,[68] so the final answer regarding the efficacy of these medications has not yet been formulated.

One retrospective review of the experience at America's VA Hospitals released in April[69] is worthy of mention as an example of how a poorly conducted study with misleading and scientifically unsound results may be used by the media to propagate fear in the public. The study compared no treatment, treatment with hydroxychloroquine, and a combination of hydroxychloroquine and azithromycin in patients hospitalized at the VA. It found that patients who went without treatment did significantly better than those treated with either hydroxychloroquine alone or in combination with azithromycin.

But the study suffered greatly from a lack of control and the absence of standardization of members of the study groups. All the researchers did was to go through the VA's records, identify anyone who was diagnosed with COVID-19, documented the medications used on those patients, and compare their results. This form of research is misleading because it does not take into account the severity of the people being treated. In a pure retrospective review such as this, it is very possible that the patients treated with the medications were sicker than those who were not. If a difference in outcome is detected, one can absolutely not conclude it was because the treatment regimen failed. It could be that all the reviewer detected was the difference in the severity of disease between the groups rather than an actual difference in the efficacy of the various therapeutic options. This lack of control is accentuated when the treatment is applied at different centers by different teams with uniformity institutions, as also took place in this study.

Indeed, there are numerous indications that the treated patients were sicker than the non-treated patients in the VA study, making comparisons between the groups meritless. Normally, such a study would hold such little weight as to not even be mentioned in an objective analysis of various treatment options. It is mentioned here because it was used by the media as an ill-founded, indefensible rallying cry against hydroxychloroquine.

Another study, published in *The Lancet* was a multinational registry analysis similar in methodology to the one performed by the VA, but involving 671 hospitals over six continents failed to show any benefits with the use of hydorxychloroquine or chloroquine with or without the addition of a macrolide, of which azythromycin is one.[70]

Much has also been said about the role of azithromycin, an antibiotic commonly used in the treatment of bacterial sinus infections and certain sexually transmitted diseases. Azithromycin belongs to a class of antibiotics called macrolides. By definition, it is not designed to treat viruses, but it has been shown to result in improved outcomes in the treatment patients with other non-bacterial conditions.[71] Similarly, some studies have found that azithromycin may have a potentiating effect on chloroquine or hydroxychoroquine when used in the treatment of COVID-19.[72] For the same reasons cited for the VA study, this study provides inadequate support in generating any conclusions. The study may even be more tarnished than the VA due to the great variability in data collection and medication administration (six continents and 671 hospitals) even though it does included extensive multivariate analyses.

Since azithromycin does not attack viruses, there must be another reason for its synergistic effects in the treatment of COVID-19. One may be that azithromycin actually has some effects in inhibiting the reproduction of viruses, as it may have in the case of Zika virus;[73] or it may be that azithromycin has some anti-inflammatory effects that may be protecting patients with

SARS-CoV-2 infections from mounting overwhelming inflammatory responses to the virus.[74] Regardless, of the mode of action, it has become commonplace to include azithromycin in the treatment of COVID-19 infections. Whether this favorable effect actually pans out to be real is still being actively investigated through the use of more meticulous studies designed to tease out these perceived benefits. But once again, there is enough experience regarding the safety of azithromycin, either used alone, or in combination with certain other medications, to make its application by a physician in the treatment of potentially life-threatening COVID-19 infections worthwhile.

Some physicians have also recommended the addition of zinc to a treatment regimen consisting of chloroquine or hydroxychloroquine in combination with azithromycin. Zinc is not really a medication. It is an essential mineral that humans must obtain through their diet and which has important functions in our maintenance. Specifically, zinc plays an important role in making sure that the immune system functions properly.[75] Consequently, if someone fails to obtain enough zinc in his her diet, the immune system may suffer. For this reason, some have recommended that zinc be employed as an adjunct in the prevention and treatment of COVID-19.[76] Again, this is a very safe intervention with unclear benefits in the setting of a rapidly-spreading, life-threatening disease.

Remdesivir is another medication that is holding promise for the treatment of COVID-19 infections. In fact, remdesvir has received an Emergency Use Authorization (EUA) from the FDA for use in hospitalized COVID-19 patients.[77] Remdesivir works by interfering with the proteins responsible for turning the information in RNA into their final products. These proteins, called RNA polymerases, bind to a strand of RNA in order to read each piece of information in the RNA, one at a time, and place the corresponding building block molecule to build the required protein.

Imagine RNA as being a long train of four different colored boxcars; say blue, green, white, and red. Next to the train and parallel to it is an empty street separated from the train by a median strip. There are men standing in the median strip directing the traffic of a series of trucks that will proceed in a specific sequence through the street and into the world. The color sequence of each trifecta of the train's boxcars determines the one type of truck that will pull up on the street next to each set of three boxcars.

In this example, the men directing traffic between the two conduits and therefore the assembly of the resulting caravan of trucks would be the RNA polymerases. The caravan of trucks (which would, by definition, be one third the number of boxcars) has specific jobs and destinations depending on their length, sequence, and the manner in which they are assembled.[vii] That sequence allows those caravans to go out into the world and perform specific functions. That series of trucks would be a protein with each truck representing an amino acid, the molecules that make up proteins.

In this example, remdesivir would is kryptonite for our assemblymen.

It would therefore make sense that a medication like remdesevir would work against SARS-CoV-2. Recall from the introduction that SARS-CoV-2 is an RNA containing virus, which uses a victim's cells own proteins (the cell's RNA polymerases) to make more of

---

[vii] Here's where the analogy breaks down because, in reality, there are post-sequencing changes that would take place to the trucks causing the caravan to take on certain shapes. Additionally, the trucks, as a unit, would be able to cleave, transport, or deform other caravans of trucks. Nevertheless, for our purpose, suffice it to say that those workers responsible for the translation of the train boxcar sequence and correlating them with specific sequences of trucks would be the RNA polymerases.

itself. Blocking the activities of those polymerases ought to stop the virus from being able to achieve its ends. But beware. If the medicine is too affective and blocks the patient's own polymerases, he or she may get horribly sick from the interruption of his or her necessary cellular activities.

The effectiveness of remdesivir was placed to the test in one study performed in the United States under the auspices of the company that manufactures the medication. Here, the medication was tested under a compassionate use basis for remdesivir. There were 53 patients treated who were hospitalized with confirmed SARS-CoV-2 infections and in need of supplemental oxygen.[viii] These very sick COVID-19 patients were treated with a ten-days course of remdesivir. Although the overwhelming number of patients improved with the treatment, seven of the 53 patients (13%) perished.[78] Missing from the study was any information regarding the viral loads the patients had and information regarding any concurrent treatments the patients may have received such as choroquine, hydroxychloroquine, or azithromycin. The study also suffered from a lack of a control group, so there is nothing with which to compare the outcomes of these patients, except for historical data on other patients that weren't part of this study. Also, fifty-three patients is a very small sample size, and despite the care in reporting and the impeccable reputation of the journal accepting it for publication, the study was performed under the auspices of the very company manufacturing it, making it more likely for favorable bias to infuse itself into the experiment.

Despite these shortcomings, these results coupled with the favorable experiences with the medication of many physicians treating

---

[viii] There were actually 61 patients treated, but because of irregularities in data collections and reporting, only 53 were ultimately included in the study.

COVID-19 patients, remdesivir has received an EUA from the FDA for the treatment of hospitalized COVID-19 patients while other treatment regimens have not.

Another treatment regimen showing great promise in its initial phase is convalescent plasma transfusion. Here, blood from a cured, but previously infected COVID-19 patient is processed and purified and infused into a sick patient with COVID-19. The logic here is that the sharing of the antibodies against the COVID-19 virus developed by the cured patient will confer resistance upon the sick patient, a state called passive resistance. One preliminary study out of China has demonstrated great success in the treatment of COVID-19 patients placed on ventilator (intubated). Here, five deathly ill patients were subjected to daily administrations of convalescent plasma. Each one of them was removed from the ventilator (extubated) and was breathing on his or her own.[79] At the time of the study's writing, three of those patients had been discharged from the hospital.[80]

In reality, none of these treatments has been proven to work against COVID-19 to the level we expect treatments to be, but it would be unreasonable to believe that anything could have been proven at this point. In *The Case for Free Market Healthcare*, I report the average cost of taking a medication from the laboratory to the marketplace is $1.2 billion, and the usual amount of time to complete the process is a little over 22 months.[81] Some of these costs and approval delays are the result of the myriad of regulatory requirements needed to take a medication through the FDA system, but some represent the requisite time to actually demonstrate the efficacy of some of these medications. The scientific proof of any intervention requires the treatment of scores of thousands of people, preferably with controls, and study subjects who are not treated with the medications for comparison. The mere mechanics of subjecting that many people with COVID-19 to these experimental treatments takes years of research. Consequently, it is not scientific proof we seek when responding to a newly appearing, massively threatening disease like COVID-19, but rather a scientifically sound, strong suggestion of efficacy in an undercurrent of safety. Although one may not have proof of an intervention's efficacy, it is sufficient to have strong evidence of the success of an intervention in light of an acceptable risk of harm with its application. In the cases of the each of the interventions discussed, the medical community has at least that.

Thus, at the time of this writing, there are some commonly employed, but yet not-scientifically-proven pharmacologic interventions in the battle against SARS-CoV-2. For prophylaxis, some are employing low doses of chloroquine or hydroxychloroquine. For the treatment of early disease, because younger patients and those without serious medical conditions are generally overcoming the virus on their own, only selected patients are being treatment. In general, older patients and those with coexisting medical conditions such as diabetes and obesity are being treated with either chloroquine or hydroxychloroquine and azithromycin, with some physicians adding zinc to the armamentarium. Those with severe disease are either treated with the above armamentarium, remdesivir, or both. And the most serious patients, such as ventilated patients in the intensive care unit may be treated with convalescent plasma therapy.

Vaccination is not a treatment, but it is among the most efficacious preventive measures known against viral infections. As noted previously, the purpose of a vaccine is to keep people from contracting the disease. This is particularly helpful for the containment and prevention of diseases where no known cure exists. We have already discussed the vaccination development process for SARS-CoV-1, the virus that causes SARS. In it, no vaccine was available for about five months despite the great interest at the time for developing one. For that virus, it took 20 months for the vaccines to even be tested in humans.[82] In the meantime, interest in vaccine development for SARS-CoV-1 subsided as the disease became less prevalent so no vaccine was ever brought to the market.[83]

The slow timeframe should be similar for SARS-CoV-2. According to Dr. Anthony Fauci, Director of the US National Institute of Allergy and Infectious Disease, optimistically, a vaccine against SARS-CoV-2 would likely not be available for over a year, and President Trump has mentioned his hope that a vaccine could be developed by the end of the year. Both these predictions are optimistic particularly when one considers that it has taken as much as fifteen to twenty years of work before the development of other vaccine,[84] but that doesn't mean the administration is incorrect in pushing for such a lofty goal. In fact, as a testament to his commitment for the rapid development of a vaccine against SARS-CoV-2, the President has launched Operation Warp Speed.[85]

Vaccine approval is tricky not because there is a risk of creating a vaccine that may be harmful to otherwise healthy humans, there is also the danger of "vaccine-induced enhancement." Under this scenario the person receiving the vaccine becomes more susceptible to infections from different viruses. Vaccine induced enhancement has occurred with vaccines against HIV, for example.[86]

With these considerations in mind, it is likely that no new vaccine will be available soon for the prevention of COVID-19. It is more likely that efforts regarding the physical mitigation of viral spread and the development of scientifically unproven, but generally helpful interventions will the mainstay of public health policy approach to combating SARS-CoV-2 in the foreseeable future.

The WHO

A few comments are necessary here about the WHO since it plays an integral role, at least it's supposed to, in the global response to a pandemic. Established on April 7, 1948, the WHO is the public health arm of the United Nations. Since its inception, the WHO has been the principal international agency in addressing global health issues and diseases. Throughout its history, the WHO has worked at the furthest reaches of the globe to provide relief for malaria, smallpox, HIV/AIDS, polio, tuberculosis, and water borne infectious disease among countless others. With a budget of over $4.4 billion,[87] it has been viewed as a symbol of all that is great about humanity, with people who selflessly travel, under threat of death from disease or human hostility to assist the poor, the destitute, the oppressed, and the sick.

From the beginning, the WHO was supposed to engage in its activities without political preference, and it was to show the same regard for borders as demonstrated by the diseases it was fighting. While the United Nations failed and faltered, the WHO continued to be held in great esteem because it was accomplishing the things the United Nations was supposed to be accomplishing, but didn't. But a branch of the United Nations the WHO ultimately is, and it seems to have been invaded by the same proclivities and political undercurrents its umbrella organization has been demonstrating. The United Nations has been demonstrating an increasingly anti-American tone over the past two decades. From its resolutions designed to frustrate the United States' efforts at promoting stability in the Middle East, to its indefensibly lax positions towards nations that routinely ignore the human condition, the United Nations has become an increasingly partisan organization. And thusly went the WHO.

In 2007, China was able to have one of its own, Dr. Margaret Chan, a Chinese Canadian out of Hong Kong indicted as the WHO's Director General. Dr. Chan served for ten years in the post. It was Dr. Chan who served as Director General when SARS broke out in Mainland China.

China's conduct regarding the SARS outbreak was remarkably similar to that of COVID-19. At the time, China was in the midst of preparations for the National People's Congress (NPC) in Beijing. As cases of SARS began spreading from its initial locale of Foshan in November 2002 to Beijing in January 2003, the Ministry of Health became aware of the outbreak and informed the WHO. Like in the present crisis, no containment actions were undertaken.[88] As the time for the NPC arrived, China's strategy was not one of disease containment, but rather of information containment.[89] Although WHO experts were invited into China, their visits were obstructed. Dr. Chan received a great deal of international criticism for the passive stance she took towards China during the outbreak including her lack of insistence for transparency.[90]

It is difficult to say what effects China's favorable treatment during the SARS epidemic by the WHO had on China's outlook towards the global agency, but as Chan's tenure came to an end, it played an aggressive role in the selection of her successor.[91] It was China's aim to arrange for the election of a second consecutive Director General sensitive to its interests. That person was Tedros Adhanom Ghebreyesus, an Egyptian microbiologist, the first non-physician head of the WHO in the organization's history.

Thus, when the COVID-19 pandemic broke out in Wuhan, it was not surprising that the WHO would take the same timid response towards China as it did during the SARS outbreak under Chan.

Indeed, Tedros's response to the COVID-19 virus has been pitiful. The WHO organization did nothing other than accept China's claims regarding the qualities of the virus and the extent of its spread at face value. When it became apparent that human-to-human transmission was a major factor in the spread of SARS-CoV-2, the WHO did not confront China about its misleading claims. It repeated them.

On January 22, after China was well on its way to covering up the events in Wuhan and had identified the virus's genome and suppressed its publication, Tedros had the audacity to state that China's efforts thus far had helped prevent the spread of the disease to other countries![92] One of the major reasons the United States and so many other nations were caught flatfooted in their response to the SAR-CoV-2 pandemic was because of the derelict actions of China and its support from the globe's most important health watchdog organization, the WHO. Regardless, as we shall see, the WHO's lackadaisical and suspect handling of the Wuhan pandemic was the source of strain with the United States, and more importantly the cause of a loss of standing among western nations.

This is not the first time the WHO has openly demonstrated its favoritism towards China. Taiwan, which considers itself an independent sovereign, but China insists is under its control, was prohibited from attending meetings in 2016 under Chinese insistence.[93] Even more obtrusively, the WHO organization denied two Taiwanese journalists a press pass so they would not even be allowed to cover a WHO meeting.[94] More recently, a WHO epidemiologist,

Dr. Bruce Aylward was asked whether the WHO would reconsider Taiwan's membership status, he claimed not to be able to hear the question, claiming he was having connection issues. The journalist called back and attempted to ask a question again, but was told they had already spoken about China and abruptly ended the interview.[95, ix] The brazenness of the disregard demonstrated by Dr. Aylward is stunning. The video link is cited for the reader's convenience.[96]

American Preparedness

Any great nation must be prepared to handle a foreseeable crisis. Such preparations must include a minimum level of subsistence; that is the ability to continue to operate independently of other nations. Even if a nation were to possess the strongest possible military and a robust economy, it may still be quickly brought to its knees if it is intimately reliant on another for its subsistence. Recall the Nazis' experience in the Battle of the Bulge where Allied Powers defeated their massively stocked opponents in no small part due to the latter's deficient fuel supplies. As soon as Hitler's tanks ran out of fuel, the persistent Allies were able counter their attack, and the war was over.

Following World War II, America entered the greatest epoch of economic growth in its history. The Post-War Economic Boom was bolstered by a combination of unparalleled population growth and unmatched innovation. Activities traditionally performed by hand were substituted by machines that were safe and compact enough to be installed in the home. Americans were young, happy to be done with the war, and raising families. They were all too willing to find

---

[ix] The brazenness of the disregard demonstrated by Dr. Aylward is stunning. The video link is cited for the reader's convenience.

automated ways of making their lives easier and their chores more efficient. Meanwhile, potential economic competitors like China were considered adversarial, as the war against fascism transitioned to a war against communism. American companies had the run of the market all to themselves. Between 1945 and 1975, the United States economy grew from a GDP of $228 billion to one of $1.68 trillion.[97] More specific to the 1950s, the United States GDP in 1951 was just short of $347 billion. By 1960, it had shot past $542 billion.

The period between 1946 and 1964 also saw a surge in American births. Between 1925 and 1945, for example, the United States had a birth rate of about 2.6 million per year. Between 1946 and 1964, the Baby Boom years, that rate increased to 44 million births per year.[98]

Faced with an onslaught of demand for products and no one else to quench it, manufacturing in the United States blossomed, but with the arrival of the 60s and 70s, things began to change. By this time, the Progressives were able to accelerate their hold on labor and manufacturing. Increasingly, laws were passed to bolster labor, workplace, and environmental protections, and America lost its lead as the least expensive option for manufacturing. Slowly, but relentlessly, the manufacturing sector egressed from the United States, and by 1973, the acclaimed sociologist Daniel Bell recognized that America was transitioning from an industrialized nation to a post-industrialized one.

As an example, in 1953, production from the manufacturing sector accounted for 28.1% of the GDP. By 2017, it accounted for only 11.6%.[99] Additionally, today, 80% of American jobs are in the service sector.[100] This tendency is not the product of some malfeasant plot against the United States, but rather it is merely the result of commerce pursuing economic efficiency. As the 70s transitioned into the 80s, countries once considered overtly hostile to the United States were no longer viewed as threats. As such, the United States sought to create trade partnerships with them. As it did so, companies realized they could manufacture products more cheaply if these were either entirely partially produced elsewhere.[101] Consequently, much of the manufacturing for American products moved offshore.

And where did the manufacturing segment go? A substantial portion went to China, although other partners arose such as Mexico and India also developed. Indeed after the turn of the century, China positioned itself as a prime manufacturer of car parts, toys, electronics, antibiotics and pain medications.[102] And although the cost savings have been very beneficial for American consumers, the trade-off is an increased reliance on the part of the United States on foreign manufacturers.

Much of that reliance has occurred in healthcare. Presently, China is responsible for supplying 90% of America's antibiotics and 13.4% of drugs and biologics by import lines.[103] Indeed, America has become so reliant on foreign sources for its pharmaceutical ingredients that about 80% of them come from foreign sources,[104] and most disturbingly, it has lost its ability to make many generic antibiotics such as penicillin![105]

America's reliance on foreign actors for healthcare products has other consequences as well. For example, the FDA has had difficulties ensuring the quality of pharmaceuticals imported into the United States. One contemporaneous example of this, ironically, has to do with the importation of N-95 masks. As SARS-CoV-2 invaded the United States, a predictable run on masks ensued. China is a major manufacturer of N-95 masks, but many of those that have been lately imported are failing to even remotely meet standards.[106]

Without the appropriate oversight, the United States has been unable to stop these faulty producers until after their products have infiltrated its markets.

The reason for a lack of productivity of American healthcare products is not solely the result of competition. As discussed in *The Case for Free Market Healthcare*, government-initiated interventions that predictably curtailed American production of pharmaceuticals and durable medical equipment also hurt. One of these is Medicare's intervention in the free market. In *The Case*, I reported the over 225 medications, most of them injectable generics, that are unavailable or difficult to obtain in the United States.[107] One of the reasons these medications are in short supply is because the Medicare Modernization Act of 2003 forced the reimbursement to pharmaceuticals for generic medications to drop as much as 90% relative to the price of the same medication prior to losing its patent. The only entities able to produce these medications at such artificially suppressed prices are foreign manufactures that could care less about the environment or the wellbeing of their workers. Added to this are the anti-competitive effects of group purchasing organizations (GPOs) that have been cornering the market for larger manufacturers. A statutory loophole allowing GPOs greater profitability have enhanced their stronghold on the market and serve as a selective funnel for products trying to reach consumers. Consequently, the American manufacturer's market for healthcare products has diminished to as few as three to six primary players for whole classes of inventories.[108]

But the nation's readiness does not only entail long-term manufacturing independence. It also implies the accumulation of materials and resources for times of crises or overwhelming demand. In the United States, such preparation includes the development and maintenance of the Strategic National Stockpile (SNS). The SNS dates back to the efforts of President Bill Clinton following his reading of *The Cobra Event* a novel about a bioterrorist attack on the United States.[109] As he asked questions stemming from the events in the novel, Clinton learned that although the federal government stockpiled antibiotics to be used for the treatment of military personnel, no similar cache existed for the general public. His inquiries led to the creation of a National Pharmaceutical Stockpile. As the program matured, it was expanded to include other types of medical supplies leading to the change in name.

As of 2016, the SNS included a multi-billion dollar inventory designed to ensure that medical supplies, medications, and equipment were available for the public in times of health emergencies.[110] Exactly how much is maintained in the SNS is difficult to say, as even the locations where these supplies are housed are secret. Suffice it to say that many of these materials are kept in 50-ton "12-hour Push Packages" designed to rapidly deliver materials to their destinations.[111] There is much evidence, however, that these stockpiles were partly depleted during the Obama Administration after the materials were used in response to H1N1 and Zika outbreaks.[112] Truth be told, the failure to restore the nation's stockpile rested with the Republican Congress as much as it did with the executive branch.

Regardless what the actual numbers may be, the nation's readiness essentially consists of the materials and personnel in the public square plus whatever the country may in storage. In the end, these were the resources the United States had when SARS-CoV-2 arrived. For better or for worse, as Defense Secretary Donald Rumsfeld once said, "[Y]ou go to war with the Army you have. . . not the Army you might want or wish to have at a later time."[113]

Chapter 1

The Beginning of a Global Crisis

As the official story goes, on December 10, 2019, Wei Giuxian began feeling ill. Wei was a seafood merchant in the Hua'nan Wholesale Market. Thinking she was suffering from a cold, she went to a nearby clinic. After being treated, she returned to work.[114] Over the next few days, she became increasingly ill, her symptoms taking her to the brink of death. Others would follow such that by December 21, about three dozen people showed symptoms similar to Wei's, all of them situated in or around Wuhan.

By December 27, health authorities in China began making a connections between the rash of infected patients and the Wuhan market.[115] Three days later, on December 30, patients began being transferred to Jinyitan. That same day, Dr. Ai Fen, a physician at a local medical clinic, received the results of a test she performed on a patient who had presented three days earlier. They indicated the presence of SARS coronavirus.[116] Aware of the effects the SARS virus had in 2002 on China, Dr. Ai alerted hospital authorities of the cluster of viral illness while ordering members of her department to don masks.[117] She was subsequently disciplined,[118] and in the span of two months, three doctors from Dr. Ai's department died.[119]

The information shared by Dr. Ai was eventually leaked to Dr. Li Wenliang who placed the finding on a WeChat messaging app where over 100 of his medical school classmates participated.[120] Amazingly, the response was negative, with at least one of his classmates telling him that he was sharing information that could be subject to censorship.[121] Li was formally reprimanded shortly thereafter and had to write a "self-criticism letter" where he admitted that his disclosure of the information "had a negative impact."[122] Li would die of COVID-19 on February 7. He was 33 years old.[123]

Table 1-1: Earliest Cases

Date	Name	City	Market Contact
Dec 8.	Chen	Wuhan	No
Dec. 10.	Wei Giuxian	Wuhan	Yes
Dec 12	Market Vendor	Wuhan	Yes
	His family of 3	Wuhan	Yes

Source: Jeremy Page, Wenxin Fan, and Natasha Khan, "How it All Started: China's Early Coronavirus Missteps," *The Wall Street Journal*, March 6, 2020, accessed March 19, 2020, https://www.wsj.com/articles/how-it-all-started-chinas-early-coronavirus-missteps-11583508932.

On December 31, China reported a cluster of cases emanating from the Hua'nan Wholesale Market to the WHO.[124] The next day, authorities closed the market,[125] but questions appeared regarding the origin of the SARS-CoV-2 virus. The original theory was that a person or groups of persons came into contact with an infected bat at the Hua'nan Wholesale Market providing the conduit for the virus to gain access to humans. But this theory is anything but solid. For starters, the first person infected by the Wuhan virus has not been definitively identified, so we don't even know whether patient zero was even at the market. Further, many of the originally identified patients denied having gone to the market,[126] and although the contention is that the virus originated in the horseshoe bat of southern China, at least one group of researchers has recognized that there were no bats at the Wua'nan Wholesale Market at the time of the appearance of the original case.[127]

More disturbingly, the Wua'nan Wholesale Market sits about 20 miles away from the Wuhan National Biosafety Laboratory, the only Biosafety Level 4 facility in China authorized to handle the world's most dangerous viruses.[i] So worried were Chinese authorities that the virus had actually emanated from work at the lab that they urgently summoned their pre-eminent bat virologist, Dr. Shi Zhengli on December 30, 2019, to study the samples from Wuhan patients.[128] Dr. Shi had been studying bat viruses for over sixteen years, earning the title of "bat woman." Her studies had included expeditions to remote caves in China in search of some of the most elusive bats in the world in the quest to collect and identify the viruses infecting them.[129]

At first, Shi worried that the new coronavirus had actually come from her lab at the virology institute,[130] so it was with a great deal of anxiety that she urgently reported to her lab with the mission of mapping the virus's genetic sequence.

In a rare interview Shi reported anxiously checking the results of the polymerase chain reaction testing of the samples collected from the Wuhan patients with the genetic recording of the viruses in her lab and finding that they materials did not match.[131] According to Shi, she concluded the virus had proceeded from the same "natural reservoir" as other bat viruses she had collected because they were 96% identical to the genetic material from the horseshoe bats she

---

[i] Ironically, an article dealing with the training in the Wuhan National Biosafety Laboratory and written by Chinese scientists was published in the CDC's website in 2019. Han Xia, Yi Huang, et al., "Biosafety Level 4 Laboratory User Training Program, China," Emerging Diseases CDC (blog), Vol. 25, No. 5, May 2019, accessed April 9, 2020, https://wwwnc.cdc.gov/eid/article/25/5/18-0220_article.

had studied.[132] Shortly after Shi identified the virus sequence, Chinese authorities silenced her.[133]

Through Shi's efforts On January 2, the Wuhan Institute of Virology successfully identified the new coronavirus inclusive of a mapped sequence. A similar virus identification took place at a medical research center in Shanghai, which notified the National Health Commission. Neither organization shared the information with the public,[134] nor did Chinese authorities confirm the presence of the new coronavirus they had already mapped. In fact, China would not admit the presence of a new virus until January 9, after *The Wall Street Journal* had independently reported its existence![135] It would not be until January 12 that Chinese authorities shared the genome with the rest of the world.[136]

On January 7, 2020, China, although admitting that the cluster of illnesses in Wuhan was associated with a novel coronavirus,[137] continued to insist that there were no signs of human-to-human transmission. According to Chinese sources, the cases represented a first-time zoonotic transmission, most likely from a bat.

But over the next few weeks, the evidence grew of the virus's interhuman transmissibility. Not only were the number of sick patients who had denied visiting the market growing, but the families of the sick were contracting the virus as well. And then there were the laboratory and clinical personnel who like Li and Ai's colleagues were catching the virus after caring for coronavirus patients. Despite the Chinese assertions, by January 24, the day Wuhan was scheduled to host the Chinese Lunar New Year banquet, the evidence of human-to-human transmission was incontrovertible.[138] Nevertheless, the banquet was a major event for Wuhan and for China with over 40,000 families expected to be in attendance from all over the world.[139] Despite the warnings and the imposition of strict social distancing measures,[140] Wuhan hosted the event as planned. Although the attendance was dramatically less than in prior years, the thousands of people in attendance over the six-day period intermingled and then dispersed.

China's reckless approach in these early days proved to be fatal. As it turns out, and Chinese authorities surely knew, SARS-CoV-2 was a highly contagious strain, able to leap from one human being to the next with great ease even before the virus had incorporated in the person sufficiently to cause any symptoms. The people who had accumulated at the Wuhan Lunar New Year banquet acted as shrapnel in a sort of biologic bomb, taking with them contagions to the greater parts of Asia and Europe. That event alone did more to rapidly disseminate the virus on a global scale than any other, and any degree of responsible oversight would have stopped it from happening.

In reference to China's early, catastrophic errors, Zuo-Feng Zhang, an epidemiologist at the University of California, Los Angeles, said, "If [China had taken] action six days earlier, there would have been fewer patients, and medical facilities would have been sufficient. We might have avoided the collapse of Wuhan's medical system."[141] In fact, a study from Southampton University estimates that if interventions of social distancing and mitigation had been started just one week earlier, there stood to be 66% fewer cases of COVID-19 in China alone, and a three-weeks head start would have prevented 95% of cases."[142]

Separate from China's concealment of the appearance of the virus and its potential role in its dispersement was its reluctance to acknowledge the potential for human-to-human transition. Repeatedly, the Wuhan Municipal Health Commission insisted that there was an absence of evidence indicating any human-to-human transmissibility of SARS-CoV-2. It did this despite being fully aware that such transmissions were indeed taking place.

Complicit with the actions of China were those of the WHO, which on January 8, 2020, after completing a visit to China, did not issue any travel advisories to the world regarding the immensely contagious nature of the virus and did not confront China on its unsubstantiated claim regarding the virus's interhuman transmissibility. Even on January 14, 2020, the WHO held a press conference where it only acknowledged the possibility of limited human-to-human transmission, lockstep with the overtly erroneous claims the Wuhan Branch of the National Health Commission delivered the same day.[143] Indeed, it would not be until January 20, 2020, that China would officially confirm the presence of human-to-human transmission.[144, 145] At its International Health Regulations Emergency Committee meeting on January 22-23 regarding the outbreak of the novel coronavirus, the committee found that the events in Wuhan did not constitute a Public Health Emergency of International Concern despite acknowledging that there were "exportations in the Republic of Korea, Japan, Thailand, and Singapore.[146] Only on January 27, over six weeks following the appearance of the initial known cases in Wuhan and nearly a month following the celebration of the Lunar New Year in Wuhan, did the WHO admit that the virus's spread was indeed a world health emergency.[147] Even still, Director General Dr. Tedros Adhanon Ghebreysus continued to lavish praise upon China regarding its handling of the SARS-CoV-2 outbreak, stating that China's actions "actually helped prevent the spread of the coronavirus to other countries."[148]

China's deceit coupled with questions regarding the safety of the Wuhan National Biosafety Laboratory[149] opened the door to even more questions. By mid-April, unnamed sources in the highest levels of the United States government were sharing their "increasing confidence that the COVID-19 outbreak likely originated in a Wuhan laboratory,"[150] with one source saying, "This may be the 'costliest government cover-up of all time.'"[151] The hypothesis grew that the virus originally did come from a bat, but that the virus actually infected one or more personnel at the Wuhan National Biosafety Laboratory and that one or more human hosts traveled to the Wuhan market where it propagated.[152] By late April, even the President of the United States was acknowledging the possibility that the possibility of Chinese negligence was being investigated.[153]

What's more, even the claim that the origin of the pandemic occurred in December has come into question. Some researchers now believe there may have been cases in China dating back to October. Supporting that contention is one study out of Stanford University finding the seroprevalence of SARS-CoV-2 (the percentage of people demonstrating evidence of having previously been exposed to the SARS-CoV-2) amongst people in Santa Clara County, California, by April 1 ranged between 2.49% and 4.16%, or 50-85 times more than the prevalence of confirmed cases.[154] Amazingly, the study did not break down the frequency of IgM and IgG positivity within those studied, which could have provide insights about the chronicity of the seroconversions. Another study out of Massachusetts found similar positive seroconversion rates[155] raising the question of whether those rates could even be possible if the pandemic had truly started in December.[156]

But China's cover-up efforts continued as they began claiming that the pandemic had actually started elsewhere. A tweet published on March 12 by Chinese Foreign Ministry Spokesman Zhao Lijian stated, "When did patient zero begin in US? How many people are infected? What are the names of the hospitals? It might be US army who brought the epidemic to Wuhan. Be transparent! Make public your data! US owes us an explanation!"[157]

When that attempt failed, the China Global Television Network then floated the idea that the COVID19 actually originated in Italy.[158] One Chinese article claimed, "Currently, we can find no clear evidence on the origin of the virus. It could be China, U.S., Italy or anywhere else."[159] And consider this exchange from February 28 at a press conference held by the WHO between Christian Lindmeier, Communications Officer for the WHO, "Shane" from China Central Television, Dr. Maria Van Kerkhove, an American epidemiologist consultant to the WHO, and Dr. Michael Ryan, Executive Director for the WHO's Health Emergencies Program:[160]

Lindmeier: Thank you. We have our colleagues from the Chinese agency. Please.

Shane: Shane from China Central Television. My question is about the virus origin. Right now there have been some opinions published by scientists saying they are not sure about the virus, whether it is really from China or from some other parts. Also there has been no clear evidence that this virus comes from China so my question is, are there any updates about the virus origin? Because there are some cases not related to travel history in China, and also the first cases reported in China does it necessarily mean that the virus itself came from China or it could be from somewhere else? Thank you.

Von Kerkhove: This is an area of active investigation right now, of looking at the zoonotic source of this outbreak, that is what is the animal source for the initial human cases and there's a lot of activity in this area of work. As you know, some of the initial cases identified in December from this cluster of pneumonia had mentioned this exposure at the seafood market but some early cases didn't have exposure at that market. So what's really important is to go back and look at those first cases, the first 50 cases or so and say, what are the exposure of those individuals and how did they differ. There were some investigations that took place at the market. There was some environmental sampling that was done at the market in Wuhan and in other area markets in Wuhan where they found evidence of virus in the market, in environmental samples so swabs of surfaces. There's a lot of area of work of looking at the virus in animals, in wildlife in the markets themselves but also in source farms where the animals came from into those markets. As far as we're aware from the mission itself and from beyond that we haven't seen any evidence of the virus in animals in Wuhan. There's one paper that mentions the pangolin and that there's some close association with the COVID-19 virus and that could be the intermediary host but that's not the full story so there's a lot of area of work that needs to be conducted to really identify the intermediate hosts so what are those animals that may have resulted in exposure to people who were infected there. We don't have a clear answer on that yet but it's an area of active investigation.

Ryan: I think it's also important in terms of looking at the emergence of any disease; disease can emerge anywhere. Coronaviruses are a global phenomenon; they exist on a global basis. It's an unlucky accident of history or nature that they emerge in a certain place and it's really important that we don't start to ascribe blame to geographic origin and that we look at this in terms of how we respond, how we contain and how we stop this virus. Congo is not responsible for the emergence of Ebola; Nigeria's not responsible for the emergence of Lassa fever and no-one is responsible for influenza pandemic. So it's really important that our narrative and our rhetoric is balanced. The discussion we need to have is, yes, we need to understand the origin of the virus so we can prevent it re-emerging, not in away of trying to find out who's at fault and what poor animal is at fault for the virus. The animals aren't at fault for this so I think we need to be careful in the language we use because the language of stigma and origin and who's to blame is something that's become an unfortunate part of the global narrative, which is not helpful.

Why was the WHO taking such great care to protect China? One naive explanation could be that it was legitimately concerned about racism. However, the effort at preventing racist aspersions has no role in the objective and scientific identification of a pandemic's origin. Indeed, the mere fact that any particular pandemic can emerge anywhere ought to suffice in cautioning against ethnic or nationalistic hostilities. If there were a true concern over undue prejudice, then that answer to "Shane" ought to have been that although the data was pointing at Wuhan as the place of origin for this particular pandemic, the next one could start anywhere. Instead of finger pointing, what was needed was the enhancement of measures designed to contain and defeat the virus. But this was not the position the WHO officials took at its press conference. Additionally, the mere act of preventing racisms would not explain Dr. Ryan's refusal to call out China for the death of Dr. Li, the Chinese physician who first brought attention of the human-to-human transmissibility of SARS-CoV-2 to his colleagues.[161] The fact is that had China acted differently towards Li and the virus, Li may still be alive today, and scores of thousands would likely have been saved. But again, the WHO did not acknowledge these overwhelmingly obvious conclusions.

Instead, the temerity and apologetic nature of the two WHO doctors' responses suggest secondary motivations behind their positions, and in the case of the WHO and China, these confounding factors undoubtedly exist. In 2020, Dr. Tedros was elected Director General of the WHO largely due to his support from China. This may help explain his unfounded praise of China's response to COVID-19 and the hostility aimed squarely at the United States upon being called out on it. "Please quarantine politicizing COVID," Tedros said. "We will have many body bags in front of us if we don't behave."[162] Tellingly, in an article published in The Atlantic, reporter Kathy Gilsinan observes, "The structure also gives WHO leaders like Tedros an incentive not to anger member states, and this is as true for China as it is of countries with significantly less financial clout."[163] If there ever were a series of events pointing to the life-threatening consequences of an inherent flaw in the WHO's structure, its handling of the initial spread of the Wuhan pandemic was it.

Regardless of the cause, the United States ultimately responded by halting its funding to the WHO, at least until an investigation is completed.[164] The move could potentially be a costly blow to the Organization as the United States contributes about $893 million of its $6 billion budget.[ii, 165, 166] Later, with tensions continuing to simmer, the President threatened to pull the United States out of the WHO altogether,[167] and eventually did. By comparison, China contributes $86 million to the WHO.[168]

[ii] Interestingly, the second largest contributor to the WHO is the Bill and Melinda Gates Foundation at $531 billion, greater than the United Kingdom. Mr. Gates has taken a strong interest in vaccine development and distribution. The WHO is highly influential in the machinations of the global administration of vaccines. Its partners, the Pan American Health Organization and the United Nations Children's Emergency Fund is responsible for approximately 7% of the worlds vaccine purchases, or $1.47 billion. Additionally, the Gates Foundation helped create the Global Alliance for Vaccines and Immunization, or GAVI, and has contributed over $750 million dollars to the organization.

Chapter 2

The Spread

Italy was caught by surprise.[169]

For a long time, it had been struggling financially and domestically. The decision to join the European Union (EU) had not produced the great results the Mediterranean nation had hoped for. Prices rose. The cost of living increased. And its industries struggled. In 2019, the Italian unemployment rate still hovered just short of 11% without any signs of fast, dramatic improvements. More ominously, its youth unemployment rate stood at 33%.[170] All the while its country aged. The younger generations were not reproducing at a rate sufficient to offset the country's aging demographics.

Meanwhile, the People's Republic of China (PRC), always working on increasing its sphere of influence, had been promoting an initiative it called One Belt one Road (OBOR), but whose name was later changed to the Belt and Road Initiative (BRI) over the ominous implications of its use of the word "one."[171] The program was essentially China's effort at engaging in the construction of infrastructure projects in foreign countries in exchange for arranging their financing and having its own companies build out the projects. The program, of course, would benefit China, both politically and financially, as it stood to improve its standing in the world stage, increase its revenue stream, and provide a source of employment for its citizens.

As twenty-first century wore on, the EU's posture towards the PRC morphed. At least in public, China was being described less as a threat and more as an economic partner. Perhaps China was no longer a country to be opposed, but one with which democratic nations should partner.

Caught in all this was Italy. It desperately wanted to improve its infrastructure, particularly in its wealthier northern provinces where a large portion of its commerce took place. For it, the prospect of China building roads, upgrading Italy's ports, and improving its infrastructure was appealing, and by 2019, Italy was prepared to have China do just that. Italy signed a Memorandum of Understanding with Beijing involving ten trade agreements that could infuse $22.4 billion to the nation[172] and bring Chinese workers to Tuscany and Lombardy. Italy was the first G7 nation to participate in the BRI.[173]

In December 2019 and into January 2020, when the Wuhan coronavirus outbreak was expanding inside China, there was continuous economic intercourse between China and Italy. In fact, Italy hosts the largest Chinese population in Europe.[174]

From a public relations standpoint, China's initial strategy regarding the SARS-CoV-2 outbreak was to conceal. In retrospect, it appears their hope was that the country could ride out the outbreak while the virus burned itself out. Towards that end, China did not ban international travel to and from Wuhan until January 23, 2020,[175] even though it had already restricted travel inside its borders. By that time, however, scores of thousands had traveled from the affected areas to destinations outside of China; and Italy was one of them.

With an average age of 46.5 years,[176] Italy has the fifth oldest population in the world.[177] It boasts the second highest concentration of senior citizens of any nation,[178] and their elderly tend to live with their families.[179] As such, Italy was particularly vulnerable to the destructive effects of an aggressive contagion like SARS-CoV-2.

But Italian officials had not yet appreciated the full tenacity of the virus. In January and into February, COVID-19 was viewed as a largely Chinese problem due to a combination of the unprecedented speed with which the outbreak grew, and more importantly, because of China's and the WHO's concerted efforts to conceal the extent of the suffering and destruction that gripped Wuhan and the Hubei Province. In one particularly onerous example, on February 4, Mayor Dario Nardella of Florence supported a video posted on YouTube by the Chinese Global Television Network (CGTN) showing numerous individuals hugging an ostensibly Chinese, blindfolded man standing next to a sign declaring, "I'm not a virus. I'm a human. Eradicate the prejudice."[180] The video description says that the mayor "has suggested residents hug Chinese people to encourage them in fight against the novel coronavirus."[181] The video was also supported by the Associazione Unione Giovani Italo Cinesi, a Chinese organization geared at improving relations between Italians and Chinese people.

Further accelerating the spread of the virus were the events related to an Italian Cinderella story involving a soccer team from a small town named Atalanta. Atalanta sits in Bergamo, an area within the northern part of Italy where commerce and intercourse with China was blossoming as a result of the BRI. Much to the glee of northern Italians, Atalanta was positioned to play Valencia on February 19 in Champions League play. "It was the biggest soccer game in Atalanta's history," said one report,[182] pitting an upstart team without a chance against powerhouse Valencia, in the most impassioned and beloved sport in Europe. The game was played at Milan's San Siro Stadium before an audience of about

45,792 fans, many of them from Bergamo, and about 2,500 Valencian fans. One Italian pulmonologist called the event "a biological bomb."[183]

A week later, Bergamo saw its first confirmed case, while in Valencia a Spanish journalist who had attended the match became the second person infected in Spain.[184] Fifteen members of the Valencia club were infected,[185] and at the time of this writing, Italy and Spain are the hardest hit countries in Europe, the former with 209,328 cases (3,462 cases per million) and 28,710 deaths (475 deaths per million).[186] Spain has 245,567 cases (5,252 cases per million) and 25,100 (537 deaths per million).

Once the infection began spreading, Italian authorities attempted to contain the virus within the hardest hit regions. Italy planned on shutting down Venice, Modena, Parma, Piacenza, Reggio Emilia, Rimini, Pesaro and Urbino, Alessandria, Asti, Novara, Verbano, Cusio, Ossola, Vercelli, Padua, and Treviso on March 8,[187] but news of the impending shutdown leaked the day prior to its implementation[188] allowing many to quickly move to the south and join their families.[189] The lockdown also suffered from confusion and lackadaisical enforcement.[190] The effort having failed, two days later, the government abandoned its initial plans and locked down the whole country.[191]

The situation got so bad in portions of Italy that stark rationing measures such as age restrictions on assisted ventilation were implemented.[192] Italy bought thousands of ventilators, but it still faced personnel shortages.[193] There simply weren't enough trained personnel to handle the onslaught of sick people. Most distressingly, when Italy asked to activate the European Union Mechanism of Civil Protection in an effort to obtain desperately needed medical equipment, no European Union country responded, . . . but China did![194]

Lombardy, the hardest hit area from which about two thirds of its deaths came,[195] first tried transferring its ICU patients to other regions.[196] For many who were not yet on life support, physicians found themselves deciding whom to intubate and whom not.[197] In fact, throughout the country, people were dying of non-COVID-19 conditions because there simply weren't enough hospital beds to handle them. Others reported waiting over an hour on the phone just to have someone respond by asking them to call back if their condition worsened, even if that condition was a heart attack.[198]

Most tragically, people were dying alone, a dynamic that was to be repeated in the United States. People were dropping off their loved ones in the emergency room and not seeing them again.[199] Another tragic error was the push to have patients moved to nursing homes in order to open up beds in the hospitals. Although investigations are still ongoing, it is suspected that this zeal to transfer patients to area nursing homes led to a high number of deaths within those facilities, many of which were never tested for COVID-19.[200] Estimates are that 40% of the deaths in Italy from COVID-19 occurred in nursing homes,[201] and over 17,500 deaths are either confirmed or suspected to have occurred in Spain's nursing homes,[202] a pattern of behavior and outcome that was repeated by Governor Andrew Cuomo in New York.

With Italy infected, the spread of the virus to the rest of Europe was facilitated. Particularly hard hit was Spain, a country that saw its first case on January 31 in the Canary Islands.[203] Like in Italy, many factors worked against Spain's ability to effectively respond to the healthcare crisis. Another of the PIGS countries[i], Spain suffered from an economy with decades of lackluster per-

---

[i] An acronym for the four weakest economies in Europe during the European debt crisis: Portugal, Italy, Greece, and Spain.

formance and a relative disregard for healthcare funding.[204] As a result, the virus quickly exhausted its intensive care unit beds.[205] Spain also suffered from a slow governmental response, an active nightlife, and a stubborn resistance to lockdowns.[206] And Spain also had a massive accumulation of people to help propagate the spread of the virus. On March 8, thousands of women marched in Madrid against gender inequality,[207] just one day prior to Spain imposing Europe's second national lockdown.[208]

Other countries followed suit as SARS-CoV-2 made its way throughout the continent. France was hit at a time when the government had cut the healthcare budget,[209] slashing numbers of medical staff and hospital beds. Due to the government cuts in a nation where the state runs the country's healthcare system, most nursing homes found themselves facing the virus without protective gear.

Predictably, as the numbers grew in France, hospitals quickly became overwhelmed. Insightfully, the French government equipped the nation's railway systems with portable intensive care unit facilities to move patients from harder hit areas to those with available intensive care unit beds.[210, 211] But it appears that France neglected its nursing homes. Because of insufficient use of contact and respiratory precautions in that nation's extended care facilities, asymptomatic staff carrying the virus inadvertently transmitted it to their frail, elderly, nursing home residents.[212] Making matters worse, overwhelmed hospitals in the hardest hit areas were refusing nursing home patients. More than 10,000 nursing home patients died from COVID-19 in France, among the highest rates in the world.[213]

In England, a lockdown was issued on March 23. But its response was hampered when its own Prime Minister, Boris Johnson, a key player in the facilitation of his country's Brexit strategy, was stuck with the virus. On March 26, Johnson tested positive for COVID-19. By April 5, he was admitted to the hospital and transferred to the intensive care unit two days later. Although his Foreign Secretary was deputized so that he could take over the prime minister's duties, it was difficult for him to substitute for Mr. Johnson.[214] England suffered because of it. With the eyes of the world on him, Johnson recovered from his infection. Details of his course and treatment are scarce, but it appears that his doctors worked desperately to avoid intubating the Prime Minister, using continuous positive airway pressure masks instead. That decision may have saved the Prime Minister's life.

Sweden took a decidedly different approach. Instead of locking down, the country asked those over 70 years of age to stay home while the rest of the economy, including its schools stayed open.[215] It also discouraged nonessential travel and gatherings of greater than 50.[216] Using this strategy, Sweden has encountered 22,088 cases (2,186 cases per million) with 2,088 deaths (264 deaths per million),[217] which is significantly higher per capita than its neighboring, Nordic countries; 9,407 cases (1,642 cases per million with 475 deaths (82 deaths per million) for Denmark[218] and 5,254 cases (948 cases per million with 230 deaths (42 deaths per million).[219] Whether Sweden's approach was worthwhile is up for debate. Like in other countries, more than half of Sweden's deaths occurred in nursing homes, and despite its efforts at not shutting down its economy, Sweden's unemployment rate still rose dramatically (from 6.5% to 11%).[220]

Swedish authorities argue that its strategy will pay off in the medium-to-long run as they are expecting the country to reach herd immunity by May. However, these officials define the herd immunity threshold as 50% whereby most others believe that herd immunity against SARS-CoV-2 will not take place until an immunity prevalence of 50% to 70% is reached.[221]

Although Europe and the United States were the hardest hit areas outside of China, the spread of the virus was no less dramatic in other parts of the globe. Like Italy, Iran entered into the BRI with China. For Iran, the relationship with China served as a buffer against the aggressive posture of the United States, and so, there was extensive intermingling between Chinese visitors and native Iranians. According to Iranian authorities, its assault from the coronavirus began in Qom, a city where the Chinese Railway Engineering Corporation was building a $2.7 billion rail line.[222] Iran closed its flights to Beijing on February 1, even before it encountered its first reported case. But by May 1, Iran was suffering from 96,640 cases and 6,091 deaths. Iran's daily cases peaked at 3,186 on March 30, and its daily deaths at 158 on April 4, but its ordeal still placed it ninth in the list of most severely affected nations.[223]

Iran wasn't alone in suffering from its nearness to China. On February 15, when Iran had still not confirmed its first case, Singapore had 72 cases,[224] at the time the third highest outside of Mainland China.[225] But Singapore, just over 2,000 miles away from Wuhan, deployed an aggressive policy of tracking, testing, and quarantine to cut down on its infections. Anyone who tested positive for SARS-CoV-2 was quarantined in a hospital, and travelers from China were banned.[226] Most ominously, those failing to maintain distances of greater than one meter, or assembled in groups of greater than 10 were subject to incarceration.[227] Despite its initial success and its use by many as an example for its successful coronavirus deterrent strategies, Singapore experienced a swift uptick in cases of COVID-19 later on. On April 10, the daily cases rate in Singapore suddenly increased by 120. Since then scores of cases continued to appear, peaking on April 20 at 1,426.[228] As of May 2, the trend had still not dropped below 528 cases per day[229] such that it is now, once again, the fourth most infected nation in southeast Asia after China, India, and Pakistan.

Despite the rising caseload, Singapore, has faired much better in preventing COVID-19-related deaths. With the exception of two days in April where two deaths occurred, only one death occurred in Singapore per day from COVID-19 as of May 2.[230] In fact, Singapore's overall COVID-19 death rate stands at an amazingly low 3 per million people with and infection death rate is 0.85 per thousand cases,[231] numbers that are among the lowest in the world.

A possible explanation for Singapore's success is the relative youth of its population, with approximately half aged 25-54 years and a median age of 35.4 years.[232] Singapore owes its relative youth to a large immigrant population living largely in "dormitories" where the virus has been able to sweep through while causing only mild symptoms upon its victims.[233]

Perhaps the greatest success story in warding off the COVID-19 infection is in Hong Kong. A mere 570 miles south of Wuhan, Hong Kong in early May still only had a remarkably low 1,041 cases (139 per million) with a mere 4 deaths (0.5 deaths per million).[234] This, in a country that was not only disadvantaged by its geographic proximity to China, but also by the promptness of its exposure. Indeed, by February 15, Hong Kong had already reported 56 cases and one death.[235] But in Hong Kong, perhaps unlike any other country, the reaction may not have been as government led as it was organic.[236] Hong Kong's residents had already gone through a similar experience in 2003 with SARS. At that time, it suffered 1,700 cases with almost 300 dead.[237] The suffering and the fear of a repeat occurrence had trained them, so when Hong Kong's residents heard of the events in Mainland China, they took action. Without a directive, the people of Hong Kong spontaneously undertook the necessary precautions. They were donning masks, maintaining separation, and liberally using hand sanitizers.[238] By the time the government began calling for cooperation with a lockdown, the people of Hong Kong were already undertaking it. Additionally, within a week of recording its first case, the government of Hong Kong shut down its borders.[239] Thus an evaluation of the total case curve shows that whereas the cases started logarithmically climbing on March 18, by April 12, it leveled off at 1005 with only 36 new cases reported between then and May 5.[240]

But by all measures, the same pressures and angst affecting people elsewhere about a return to normalcy have affected those in Hong Kong. Despite their first-hand experience with SARS, people longed to go back to work, and when they did, a second wave began, which was successfully shut down by quick and decisive government action.[241] It closed down bars, gyms, and sports facilities. It cut down on seating capacity, and it implemented strict quarantine measures confirmed by electronic tracking bracelets.[242] Yes, Hong Kong achieved great success, but it came at a stark price to the limited freedoms enjoyed by its people.

India is in a different situation.[ii] With a median population of 28.7 years and 41.56% of its population between 25 and 54 years of age, India has seen 90,648 cases and suffered only one death per million for a total of 2,871 deaths from COVID-19 as of May 17. What is remarkable about India is that it has only suffered 69 cases per million.[243] In comparison, the United States has suffered 4,602 cases per million and Canada has suffered 2,041 cases per million by May 17.[244] Like Singapore, India's low death rate can easily be explained by its youth, but the same factor does not ex-

---

[ii] Because of a later surge in its numbers, India's statistics were revisited on May 17.

plain its dramatically low infection rate. Although there is yet no definitive answer as to why there have been so few cases in India, a number of possible explanations are worth exploring. First, India has engaged in an aggressive social distancing campaign inclusive of an aggressive 21-day lockdown that some have criticized as draconian,[245] but this cannot be the sole reason for its success since many other countries that have faired much worse have done the same. It is possible that India's low numbers could be due to discrepancies and shortcomings in India's counting methods, as their accuracy has been questioned.[246] India is in short supply of RT-PCR testing[247] and thus has not been able to engage in the levels of surveillance and confirmation that Singapore and South Korea have, for example. Most recently, there have been concerns raised about the increasing daily case rate in India encountered during the first half of May. Although the spikes may be due to an actual increase in the number of new cases, it is also possible that India is undergoing a game of statistical catch-up as older cases are just now being reported for the first time.[248]

But there are at least two factors in dealing the COVID-19 pandemic that make India unique. First India has been aggressively employing hydroxychloroquine as a prophylactic agent. In late March, India's National Task Force for COVID-19 recommended the use of hydroxychloroquine as a preventive method for COVID-19 for its healthcare workers.[249] Additionally, the Indian Council of Medical Research has recommended that asymptomatic contacts of people with confirmed cases also be treated with hydroxychloroquine at a recommended dose of an 800 mg on the first day of prophylaxis followed by 400 mg tablets once a week.[250] So aggressive has India's position on hydroxychloroquine been that at one point it banned the exportation of the medication to save its stock for its own citizens.[251] The move was subsequently reversed at the insistence of the United States.[252]

As of this writing, there is no information on how many have received hydroxychloroquine and how they have faired. Additionally, a proposed study to evaluate the effectiveness of the medication at preventing COVID-19 in Mumbai's slums has been temporarily scrapped,[253] so no formal study will be forthcoming anytime soon.

India also has a universal bacille Calmette-Guerin (BCG) vaccination policy.[254] The BCG vaccine is administered for the prevention of tuberculosis. It is not employed in the United States because of the low risk of tuberculosis infection here.[255] Yet, there are some indications that the BCG vaccine may provide "trained immunity" against SARS-CoV-2.[256] Trained immunity is a situation where a vaccine against one infectious agent provides an enhanced ability for the host to ward off other infections. BCG is such a vaccine because, although it is designed to ward off tuberculosis, it has been found to improve "all-cause" infant mortality and protect against certain allergic diseases including asthma.[257] Although the favorable India experience provides a potential lead for future investigations, the fact is that BCG vaccinations are administered in countries with warmer climates, the same areas where coronaviruses are thought not to fair as well, thus complicating the interpretation of any associations between BCG vaccination programs and COVID-19 prevention.

South Korea has also been touted as a country demonstrating success at warding off COVID-19. With an overall infection rate of 57 cases per 1 million people and a death rate of 1 per million,[258] South Korea's numbers are definitely impressive. But once again, the relative youth of South Korea's population with 44.6% of its population being aged 25-54, and a median age of 43.2 years,[259] provides protection against a high death rate. More importantly, like in India, South Korea has been able to keep the prevalence of the infection rate down, but it has done so without a lockdown. South Korea was one of those countries where the virus arrived early. On February 15, it was reporting the second highest number of infections in the world at 28 cases.[260] Only China had more cases. With the rapidity of the spread in China, the prospects for that country were looking dire. According to Park Neung-hoo, South Korea's health and welfare minister, the country weighed the option of a shutdown, but rejected it in favor of a program of aggressive testing and surveillance.[261] South Korea quickly ramped up its testing methods inclusive of drive-thru testing and supplemented it with electronic communications technology.[262] Communication technology was integral since it allowed authorities to identify potential contacts with infected individuals through mobile phone data, credit card usage, and closed circuit television. What's more, cooperation from affected people was voluntary.[263] It is also worthy of note that South Korea does engage in universal BCG vaccination program.[264] What role the BCG vaccination is playing at keeping South Korea's infection rates low, if any is a subject requiring further analysis.

Two non-European and non-North American countries that do not have a mandatory BCG vaccination program are Australia and New Zealand.[265] Each has done remarkably well. Australia, has maintained a relatively low per capita infection of 267 persons per 1 million and a per capita death rate of 4 in 1 million.[266] Australia relied on social distancing and closing its borders, both entering and exiting, as its primary methods of warding off the pandemic.[267] Social gatherings of more than two people were prohibited as was leaving one's home for other than essential reasons.[268] But perhaps the most important aspect for Australia's response was its promptness. Australia restricted flights from China on January 23, even before the United States did.[269] By January 31, Australia had begun mandatory quarantines for anyone entering the country from China, and by March 15, it was requiring all travelers entering the country, inhabitants or not, to self-isolate for 14 days.[270]

Neighboring New Zealand has also had success in beating back the pandemic.[271] New Zealand was also able to implement a prompt isolation program. For example, New Zealand restricted access to China on February 3, prior to recording its first COVID-19 case, and then widened its restrictions to include Iran by February 28.[272] Like Australia, New Zealand's daily incidence curves are on the downswing, suggesting that it may getting over the virus's initial wave while amassing a 258 per million case rate and a 4 per million death rate.

On the other side of the globe, Latin America had been relatively quiet, causing many to hope that it would be spared the full brunt of the virus's fury. But in March, the tide began to change. Brazil, which had reported its first case on February 25 and only had cases on March 4,[273] saw its numbers dramatically increase in March. By March 17, Brazil had its first death,[274] and then things turned dramatically worse. Within days, Brazil's new daily case rate increased to over 3,000 and deaths numbered over 400 per day.[275] At the time of this writing, Brazil has 97,100 cases (457 cases per million) and 6,762 death (deaths per million).[276] However, Brazil's testing practices are dismal. No one believes the numbers are accurate, and one study estimates the actual number of cases could be as high as 1.6 million on May 3.[277]

But Brazil's numbers don't come close to describing the dire conditions on the ground. Most of Brazii's cases are located in Sao

Paulo and Manaus, the latter a hub for North American and European tourists going on safaris. Deaths are occurring so rapidly in Manaus and its resources so overwhelmed that its victims are being buried in mass graves.[278] Manaus is woefully undersupplied with hospital beds and even fewer ICU resources. Making matters worse, the Brazilian government under the leadership of President Jair Bolsonaro is virtually denying the scope and intensity of the pandemic. The President, for example describes the virus as a "little flu,"[279] shakes hands with the multitudes, and does not wear a mask.[280] What little stay-at-home directives and isolation pleas are enacted by state and local governments, all the while being undermined by the President who urges businesses to reopen![281]

Clearly, the devastation we will witness in Brazil, at least in its hot spots will rival practically the worst humanitarian crises. This is not to say that its neighboring nations are protected from the onslaught. Peru, a Latin American country with limited resources that neighbors Brazil has seen 42,536 cases and 4,987 deaths as of this writing.[282] It is striking that Peru was showing no confirmed cases until March 5.[283] Argentina, which saw its first case on March 2,[284] now has 4,681 cases and 237 deaths.[285] And finally, Ecuador, presently reports 31,881 cases with 1,569 deaths,[286] when its first case was confirmed on February 29.[287]

This global review of SARS-CoV-2 spread throughout the world clearly indicates the complete disregard the virus has for distances, or political borders. It is also clear, that it was equally not going to honor the wealth or relative isolation of the richest nation in the world, the United States of America. Ironically enough, as will be described below, SARS-CoV-2 likely craves wealth.

Chapter 3

Ships

Before discussing America's experience with the Wuhan pandemic, there is one segment we must still investigate: ships. When an infectious disease hits a sailing vessel, the results can be devastating. Most commonly, the illness ripping through the crew and passengers is gastrointestinal, with large portions of the ship's population being struck with nausea, vomiting, and diarrhea. This is why ships commonly enact strict handwashing policies, particularly in common eating areas such as the mess halls or the ship's restaurants. Combating an outbreak on board ship is usually a matter of containment by isolating the affected passengers or sailors. We have all heard tales of individuals being restricted to their cabins or being unable to disembark at a port-of-call because they were sick. Ostensibly these are the reasons why.

Airborne illnesses are much more difficult to contain since such diseases can be transmitted through the air as well as surfaces. Here, containment becomes less effective. Just the air the passengers are breathing is enough to spread a germ or a virus, and in many spaces, a ship's air is exchanged very slowly. Additionally, the ship's ventilation system can blow air from one space to the next, allowing for airborne organisms to be transported from one area of the ship to another.

Maritime vessels carry the added hazard of being mobile. As such, they can transport hundreds, if not thousands of people, to previously untouched areas, allowing the seeds for new clusters to spread. At every major port, there are health officials well aware of the dangers a disease-laden maritime vessel carries for the spread of potentially life-threatening conditions to the local population. These officials have the authority to not allow crew and passengers to disembark and to refuse docking rights to vessels altogether.

The concern over disease spread is ever-present in the maritime industry and peppers the provisions of maritime law, but when the contagion is SARS-CoV-2, with its high lethality and contagiousness, the stakes reach even higher proportions and the effects can be catastrophic.

The *Diamond Princess* set sail from Yokohama, Japan, on January 20, 2020,[288] with 3,711 souls on board.[289] Included in its muster was one passenger who had developed respiratory symptoms the day prior to departure. On January 25, the patient with respiratory symptoms disembarked from the ship in Hong Kong,[290] and on February 1, she was found to be positive for COVID-19.[291]

Upon entering Japanese waters, the *Diamond Princess* was immediately quarantined.[292] On February 3, the ship returned to its final destination in Yokohama with no one being allowed off the ship.[293] By February 5, there were 10 confirmed cases and by the time the passengers were allowed to disembark on February 23, there were 691 cases.[294]

The conditions on board the *Diamond Princess* served as a laboratory where disease progression could be observed and studied. Initially, the passengers were subjected to a shipboard quarantine, meaning they were free to mingle with other passengers as they wished. Subsequently, the ship tightened its restrictions such that those with known infections were confined to their cabin.[295] As it turns out, the enhanced isolation helped to significantly diminish the contagiousness of the virus.

Ultimately, SARS-CoV-2 infected over 700 people from the *Diamond Princess*, giving it the dubious distinction of being, for weeks, the largest outbreak in the world.[296] All told, seven people died from their ship-borne infections, every one of them 70 years of age or older.[297] Subsequent studies demonstrated 18% of the infections were asymptomatic,[298] and the infection fatality rate was 0.5%.[299]

The unfolding drama aboard the *Diamond Princess* sent shock waves throughout the cruise industry. Holland America's *Westerdam's* experience was a classic example, not only of the heightened protections the maritime industry encountered but also of how events can go horribly wrong. With 1,455 passengers and 802 crewmembers, the *Westerdam* set sail on February 1, 2020, from Hong Kong on a 14-days travel itinerary.[300] This was the same day and the same city where the passenger who had tested positive for COVID-19 disembarked from the *Diamond Princess*.

The *Westerdam* made its first destination on time in Kaohsiung, Taiwan, on February 4. After successfully disembarking, the ship was turned away at Taipei, Taiwan, its next destination. Other ports followed, with declines rolling in from Japan, the Philippines, Guam, and Thailand.[301] It would not be until February 16, 2020, with the ship's assurances that none on board was sick that authorities in Sihanoukville, Cambodia, allowed the ship to dock.[302] For Cambodia, accepting the *Westerdam* was an opportunity for its sinophilic prime minister to tout its closeness with China and to publicly minimize the pandemic. So enthusiastic was his interest in publicly welcoming the otherwise unwelcomed ship that Prime Minister Hun Sen personally greeted the departing passengers dockside.[303] As the passengers disembarked, an 83-year-old, American woman made her way off the ship and onto a flight to Malaysia. But upon arriving at Kuala Lumpur, she failed the thermal screening, and along with her husband, was immediately detained.[304] The couple was taken to a hospital for treatment where her husband was eventually diagnosed with pneumonia and presumptively treated for COVID-19.[305] In the meantime, the American woman tested positive for COVID-19, not once, but twice, causing disembarkation at the *Westerdam* to immediately cease with 233 passengers and 747 crew members still on board.[306]

Amazingly, the American woman was eventually deemed to have experienced false-positive tests since everyone else on board the *Westerdam* tested negative[307] and subsequent tests on her were also consistently negative. The series of events, although harrowing for some, turned out to be all for naught.

Closer to home, the *Grand Princess* left San Francisco with 1,179 souls on board and a planned, two-voyage excursion.[308] The first leg would take the passengers to Mexico before returning to San Francisco. The second trip was bound for Hawaii.

The ship began its first leg uneventfully returning to San Francisco after its four planned stops in Mexico. While the ship picked up more passengers for the second leg, most of the crew and passengers present in the first part of the voyage remained. Finally, on February 21, the ship departed with a total of 2,422 souls on board.[309]

On March 4, while the *Grand Princess* was at sea, California authorities reported that two passengers who had been on the first voyage were diagnosed with COVID-19. The following day, the captain ordered the ship to immediately return to California and initiated in-cabin quarantines of passengers and crewmembers with respiratory symptoms.[310] When the ship docked all persons were transferred to a land-based facility in Oakland to continue their quarantines.

Unlike in the *Diamond Princess*, passengers on the *Grand Princess* were allowed to decline testing so that not all on board were tested.[311] Consequently, an accurate estimate of the outbreak's spread and death rate could not be made. Suffice it to say that sixteen percent of those aboard were positive,[312] and three persons died, including one of the original patients. All three deaths occurred in individuals 60 years of age or older.[313]

Meanwhile, Holland America's *Zaandam* departed from Buenos Aires on March 31 for a 31-days cruise exploring Latin America. The ship departed with 1,827 souls on board.[314] Early on, the ship was able to make port calls in Uruguay, the Falkland Islands, and Punta Arenas in the Pacific. That's when the passengers learned that Argentina, their next port had closed its borders, so they would not be able to dock there.[315] By March 21, some of the passengers began displaying coughing symptoms and others had flu-like symptoms. By the end of the day, the captain ordered in-cabin quarantines for all passengers.[316] As the ship made its way north to its ultimate destination of Port Everglades in Fort Lauderdale, indications began trickling in that the passengers' departure was going to be impeded there as well.[317]

On March 27, with 138 people sick on board, two of them critically, the crew began pleading with Panamanian officials to allow them to cross the Panama Canal despite prohibitions against passages for "sick ships."[318] Conditions aboard ship soured as passengers with medical conditions worried, and Mexico refused acceptance to two critically ill patients.[319] The ship was joined by another Holland America ship, the Rotterdam to which some of the passengers were transferred. The pair was eventually allowed passage across the Canal under cover of night and the ship darkened.[320]

As time passed, the ships edged closer to Florida where matters seemed to be at a stalemate with Broward County officials. Apparently, the hold up was that Florida Governor Ron DeSantis was unwilling to accept the ship. The impasse broke when President Trump called Governor DeSantis to ask that the ship be allowed to dock.[321]

On April 2, with four dead passengers, the ships did dock at Port Everglades. The passengers slowly disembarked and were shuttled to vehicles taking them to their ultimate destinations. Although the *Zaandam* had departed at a time when no prohibitions to sailing had been issued, by the time of their arrival, the CDC's no-sail order had been in place for over two weeks.[322]

But the Wuhan pandemic didn't just disrupt leisure travel. America's war vessels also faced their own challenges. On March 8, the aircraft carrier *USS Theodore Roosevelt* visited Vietnam as part of a 25-years celebration of relations between the two countries.[323] Shortly thereafter, three cases of COVID-19 were detected aboard ship.

The ideal remedy would have been immediate disembarkation of those on board with quarantines when ashore. Alternatively, cabin quarantines would be undertaken. But unlike cruise ships, a war vessel is virtually devoid of passengers, and each sailor is vital to the conduct of the ship's mission. Compounding the issue, there are very few cabins on a navy ship, and these are usually reserved for the highest-ranking officers. Middle-ranking officers, at the very best, share small, enclosed, two-man staterooms, and lower-ranking officers sleep in six to twelve men spaces. Making infection containment matters worse, the ship's enlisted personnel sleep in open sleeping bays often housing 70 sailors at times, and some cots are retracted during working hours so the spaces may double as workspaces. Areas such as the engine rooms, hangar bays, aircraft control towers, and common spaces are generally tight, openly shared spaces where dozens of men and women subsist in very constricted quarters.

Following the report of the initial three cases, the outbreak aboard the *Roosevelt* quickly spread over the next few days infecting over 100 crewmembers. Captain Brett Crozier quickly made plans to pull into port and quarantine his crew for at least fourteen days. The move was drastic, to be sure, but thought the Captain, the *Roosevelt* was not at war, and allowing the virus to continue to spread was only going to further negatively impact the ship's readiness. Unfortunately, the nearest port, Guam, did not have either sufficient space or beds to accommodate a quarantine of over 4,000 persons.[324]

Frustrated, the Captain wrote a memo to his superiors requesting "all available resources to find NAVADMIN and CDC compliant quarantine rooms for my entire crew as soon as possible."[325] The communication was quite detailed and cited the ongoing maritime industry's experience with COVID-19, and in particular, the experience aboard the *Diamond Princess*.

Unfortunately for Crozier, he sent the memorandum to multiple recipients. Within twenty-four hours, the letter was leaked to the press,[326] bringing undue attention to his ship and to the navy. His letter was used to embarrass the military's chain of command and to cast aspersion upon the press's favorite target, the President of the United States. Crozier's letter was also met with great disdain from navy officials, not the least of which was Acting Navy Secretary Thomas Modly who called the captain "too naïve or too stupid" to remain in command of one of America's aircraft carriers. He then made a profanity-laden accusation of betrayal against the captain. Within days of his diatribe, Modly resigned from his position.[327]

Crozier, a seemingly very popular captain, was also quickly removed from command, not because of the email but for sending it to so many that it was leaked. And if matters had not been bad enough for the navy with the loss of a captain and the Acting Navy Secretary, they took a dramatic turn for the worse on April 9, just two days after Crozier's resignation, when Aviation Ordnanceman

Chief Petty Officer Charles Robert Thacker[328] was found unresponsive aboard ship[329] and emergently transferred to U.S. Naval Hospital Guam.[330] He died on April 13.[331]

As part of Crozier's last acts while in command, the *Roosevelt* docked in Guam and unloaded many of its sailors. All members of the crew were tested for SARS-CoV-2 amounting to at least 4098 tests. Eight hundred forty initially came back positive,[332] and over a thousand ultimately turned positive.[333] By this time, of course, the Chinese and others picked up on the American fleet's disabilities. Sensing weakness, China engaged in aggressive naval exercises and even sank a Vietnamese fishing boat in the South China Sea, a location where the United States has served as a strong check on China's presence and power.[334] And to leverage its advantage and perhaps ridicule the United States, Chinese military leaders then went on to claim that despite having "tens of thousands of the soldiers and their family members" interacting with local residents,[335] not a single member of the Chinese military had become infected with coronavirus, and that the virus had actually improved Chinese combat readiness,[336] a claim that was propagated, without query, by CNN.[337]

The *USS Theodor Roosevelt* was not alone among American military ships crippled by SARS-CoV-2. The *USS Nimitz, USS Ronald Reagan*, and the *USS Carl Vinson* were amongst American aircraft carriers contracting the illness.[338] And in the Caribbean, the *USS Kidd* experienced an outbreak affecting over a dozen sailors.[339] Interestingly, as of May 15, despite the impression that the outbreak aboard the *Roosevelt* had been contained and the scrubbing down of the ship itself, five sailors who had previously been quarantined and had twice tested negative were taken off the ship with apparent recurrences. As of this writing, the *Roosevelt* is still docked in Guam.[340]

Chapter 4

COVID-19 Reaches the United States

By early January, the CDC had learned of the outbreak in Wuhan. With China minimizing its scale and insisting that human-to-human transmission was either not occurring, or very rare, the CDC, like most other health agencies, believed that the risk from the virus was low. Nevertheless, on January 6, 2020, it issued a Level 1 Travel Health Notice regarding Wuhan, China,[341] its lowest advisory, meaning that travelers were to take usual precautions when traveling there.

The United States' first case materialized on January 15, 2020, when a young man returned from his trip to visit his family in China.[342] Although he had spent time in Wuhan, he did not visit the Hua'nan Wholesale Seafood Market, nor did he recall having come into contact with any ill persons in China.[343] Nevertheless, on January 19, 2020, he presented to an urgent care clinic in Snohomish County, Washington, after reading public health warnings about the outbreak. At the time of his presentation, he had been harboring a two-day history of nausea and vomiting, a dry cough, but no shortness of breath or chest pain.[344, 345] Specimens from the patient were sent to the CDC for testing, which were able to confirm the presence of SARS-CoV-2 the next day.[346] The patient was immediately admitted to an airborne isolation unit at Providence Regional Medical

Center,[347] and by January 17, 2020, the CDC and the Department of Homeland Security began screening travelers from Wuhan China at San Francisco, JFK, and Los Angeles airports.[348]

On hospital day 6, due to his persistent and severe symptomatology, the treating team initiated compassionate use therapy with remdesivir.[349] He improved over the ensuing forty-eight hours and was able to come off supplemental oxygen. He was eventually sent home.[350]

The Initial Response

On January 21, the CDC reported the case to the public, alerted clinicians to be on the lookout for persons with a travel history to Wuhan, and activated its Emergency Operations Center.[351] Two weeks later, the federal government began arranging chartered flights to bring Americans back home from Wuhan.[352]

Also on January 21, the CDC placed travel restrictions on other countries and initiated screening of passengers traveling from Wuhan by Customs and Border Protection. Despite these restrictions, about 4,000 people who had been in Wuhan entered the United States through Los Angeles, San Francisco, and New York.[353]

America would see its second case announced on January 24 when a woman who had traveled to Wuhan to care for her sick father was diagnosed with the illness.[354] Similar to the first case, the Illinoisan did not exhibit any symptoms while traveling, but developed them upon her return to the United States.[355] In a stroke of great prudence, President Trump issued the first federal quarantine order in over 50 years on January 31 when he required people returning from China's Hubei province to be isolated for fourteen days prior to entry.[356] The order coincided with the suspension of entry into the United States of a foreign national who posed a risk of transmission of the corona-virus.[357]

SARS-CoV-2 struck the American people at a remarkably partisan time. To understand the nation's reaction to the coronavirus, oddly enough, one needs to understand its relationship with its President, Donald J. Trump. The press had harbored an irascible disdain for President Trump dating back to the moment he announced his candidacy. Interestingly, before announcing his run, Trump was treated very kindly by the press. He was bombastic, confrontational, and unpredictable, but it was precisely because of these qualities that the press loved him and his opinions so highly sought.

But the moment Trump descended down those golden escalators in Trump Towers, everything changed. From the beginning, the media painted him out to be an unqualified candidate for the Office of the Presidency of the United States. They mocked him as he traveled through the country in his Trump plane despite his consistent command of audiences numbering in the tens of thousands. They made fun of him when he said he was being wiretapped, calling him paranoid, even though he was being illegally surveilled by the FBI.[i] Particularly hostile to him were CNN and MSNBC who routinely begged that he be the Republican nominee because, in their view, there was no way he could defeat Hillary Clinton. Long are the examples of media pundits and commentators affirming that Trump could never be elected.

But Donald J. Trump did win in 2016. Although he did not prevail in the popular vote, he amassed a resounding, 307-to-227 majority in the Electoral College. The dismay over the Clinton defeat was palpable amongst the Left, with the candidate herself refusing to appear before her supporters for a conciliatory speech.

[i] Technically, he was being surveilled by the FBI.

Almost on command, the efforts from the press and the Democratic Party turned to invalidating the new President's election. First, they balked at his failure to win the popular vote. Then, they attempted to get the Republican electors to defect at the Electoral College, bolstered by a cooperative media that jovially reported the possibility of a "reverse outcome." In fact, Change.org actually collected 43 million signatures in support of a reversal in the Electoral College.[358] After all, the Left would argue, the successful election of Donald Trump had been an error, and it was up to the Trump electors to rectify the aberrancy by electing Hillary Clinton despite what the voters may have said at the voting booth. Ironically, when the fateful day came, more Clinton electors defected to the new President than Trump electors defected to Hillary.[359]

And when President Trump finally did get inaugurated, the press immediately moved into impeachment mode. On January 20, 2017, *The Washington Post* headline read, "The Campaign to Impeach Trump Has Begun,"[360] with a similarly entitled article published by Time on the same day.[361] But the never-Trumpers realized that even under the most ideal circumstances, impeachment would take time. After all, the President would first have to do something wrong and narratives would need to be fabricated.

So the press and the never-Trumpers turned to a more immediate agenda. They built the narrative that President Trump had not really won the election because he had lost the popular vote. President Trump won, according to the new Democrat and press narrative, because the Russians had assisted him in winning!

Thus began the Russian interference narrative that eventually led to the Robert Mueller investigation. And after $32 million,[362] 22 months, 19 lawyers, 40 FBI investigators, 2,800 subpoenas, 500 search warrants, and 500 witnesses nothing of substance was found.[363] Despite the many accusations and innuendoes, no laws were broken and no evidence that the Trump candidacy had coordinated with the Russian government was ever found. The whole thing was a hoax driven by the disgruntled Democrat leadership and their threatened inside-the-beltway autocrats.

Then, finally, towards the end of 2019, the opportunity for impeachment arrived, not through a Russian conspiracy, but through an anonymous report by an informant who claimed the President had engaged in an illegal, quid pro quo arrangement with the President of Ukraine in a telephone call on July 25, 2019. According to the whistleblower who did not witness the call, President Trump sought the assistance of the Ukrainian President in an investigation of former Vice President and then-presidential candidate Joe Biden regarding his dealings with a Ukrainian gas company aimed at having his son, Hunter Biden, appointed to a well-compensated position in its Board of Directors.

But the veracity of the comments was quickly dismissed when President Trump released the transcripts of the conversation. Although many suggested the President's conduct was inappropriate, layer upon layer of evidence demonstrated there was no quid pro quo. The dismissal of the allegation's validity was further enhanced by testimony from the Ukrainian President detailing his lack of participation in, or even awareness of, any quid or quo.

Still, the press and the Democrats persisted, arguing, among other things, that the President's assertions of his due process rights in a sham impeachment process represented an abuse of power and an obstruction of Congress, an allegation contrary to the most basic precepts of judicial rights.[ii] Regardless of the meritless nature of

---

[ii] The absurdity of this argument is heightened by its dismissal of those basic constitutional premises regarding witness rights, presumptions of innocence, and burdens of proof.

the accusations against the President, the impeachment proceedings continued well into December. When the articles of impeachment were finally drawn up and passed by a partisan vote in the House of Representatives in late December, Nancy Pelosi, the Speaker of the House of Representatives, unnecessarily held them in her chamber, hoping to bolster the chances of a conviction in the Senate. Thus the weeks passed and January arrived with a divided and resentful nation waiting for a trial destined for failure to begin. The Senate would not even begin its proceedings until January 16, 2020, nor conclude the trial until February 5, 2020.

The timing of the events and the press's obsession with them is important. In December, while Pelosi was holding her impeachment proceedings, the virus began making its way through Wuhan, and China concocted its scheme to suppress it. Once again, the accusations against the President were orders below what was envisioned as appropriate for impeachment. Yet, while China schemed, the House and the press recklessly pushed their agenda. And in January, as the cover-up continued and America was in the grips of a particularly strong flu season, the nation's leaders were consumed with the progress of a trial.

In fact, the only people who seemed to be paying attention were the President, who ordered the discontinuation of Chinese travel, and Arkansas Senator Tom Cotton who called for an investigation on the origins of this still very foreign and distant virus in China. Another person who claims to have been paying attention was Dr. Rick Bright, a whistleblower, who in a *60 Minutes* interview claimed that as the Director of the Biomedical Advanced Research and Development Authority, he had been sounding the alarm since January and had been furiously working, against the administration's resistance, to stock up on PPE.[364]

Regardless, a watchful press and a responsible Congress would have easily seen the signs of the impending crises and reported on them. Had Congress and the press done their jobs, of course, America's experience with SARS-CoV-2 could have been markedly different. But instead, we had a whole political class made up of leaders and reporters obsessing over the impeachment of the President. As a result, in their intoxication with the smell of the President's political blood, they took their eyes off the ball, and China continued undisturbed while it promoted its misguided agenda.

Indeed, the slumber in which America found itself was such that on January 28, despite the increasingly bright signs emanating from the eastern hemisphere, Secretary of the Department of Health and Human Services Alex Azar said, "Americans should know this is a potentially very serious public health threat, but Americans should not worry for their own safety."[365]

And Azar was not alone. That same day, the Director of the CDC's National Center for Immunization and Respiratory Disease, Dr. Nancy Messonier said, "We have no evidence of human-to-human transmission in the United States."[366] Even Dr. Anthony Fauci, in an interview with Newsmax on January 21, said the coronavirus "is not a major threat to the people of the United States, and this is not something that the citizens of the United States should be worried about right now."[367]

The delirium continued as the country entered into February. Secretary Azar said on January 31, "The risk of infection for Americans remains low,"[368] despite having issued a Public Health Emergency for the United States that same day. As late as February 24, Speaker Pelosi was publicly walking the streets of San Francisco to quell the fears of visiting her district in the midst of the Wuhan pandemic. "You should come to Chinatown," Pelosi was quoted to have said that day,

"Precautions have been taken by our city. We know that there is concern about tourism all throughout the world, but we think it's very safe to be in Chinatown. I hope that others will come."[369] President Trump continued his rallies, where tens of thousands would assemble as he celebrated the debacle of the impeachment efforts against him and prepared for his reelection campaign. It would not be until March 2 when President Trump would hold his last campaign rally at Bojangle's Stadium in Charlotte, North Carolina.

Clearly, the nation, particularly it's leaders, was not paying attention, obsessed with the proceedings over a crisis they themselves had created.

Those in opposition to the claim that President Trump took the Wuhan pandemic seriously from the beginning say that the President called it a hoax, a charge that has been often repeated in the press. In point of fact, the President did not call the pandemic a hoax. Quite the opposite. At his February 28, rally in Charleston, South Carolina, the President actually said the following regarding the Wuhan pandemic:

> *5:14: Now, the Democrats are politicizing the coronavirus. You know that, right? The coronavirus. They're politicizing it. We did one of the great jobs. . . you say, "How's President Trump doing?" You say, "Oh. Not good. Not good." They have no clue. They don't have any clue. They can't even count their votes in Iowa. They can't count their votes! One of my people came up to me and said, "Mr. President, they tried to beat you on Russia, Russia, Russia, and that didn't work out too well. They couldn't do it. They tried the impeachment hoax. That was on a perfect conversation. They tried anything. They tried over and over. They've been doing it since you got in. It's all turning. They lost. It's all turning."*
>
> *Think of it. Think of it. And this is their new hoax. But you know. We did something that's been pretty amazing. We're 15 people in this massive country and because of the fact that we*

went early. . . we went early. . . we could have had a lot more than that. We're doing great. Our country is doing great. We're so unified. The Republican Party has never ever been unified like it is now. There has never been a movement in the history of our country like we have now. Never been a movement.

So a statistic that we want to talk about. . . go ahead. . . say 'U.S.A.' It's okay. U.S.A.

So. A number that nobody heard of that I heard of recently and I was shocked to hear it. Thirty-five thousand people on average die each year from the flu. Did anyone know that? Thirty-five thousand. That's a lot of people. It could go to a hundred thousand. It could be twenty seven thousand. They say usually a minimum of twenty-seven. It goes up to a hundred thousand people a year die, and so far, we have lost nobody to coronavirus in the United States. Nobody. And it doesn't mean we won't, and we are totally prepared. It doesn't mean we won't. But think of it. You hear thirty-five and forty thousand people, and we've lost nobody. And you wonder; the press is in hysteria mode.

CNN fake news and their camera just went off. The camera just went off! Turn it back on. . . [eggs the crowd against the press and speaks about an assortment of other issues]."

12:10: We are. . . magnificently organized with the best professionals in the world. We're prepared for the absolute worst. You have to be prepared for the worst, but hopefully it will all amount to very little. That's why I tell you when he have the flu at the thirty-five thousand and, this one, is uhh. . .we have to take it very very seriously. . . That's why we're doing. . . We are preparing for the worst.

My administration has taken the most aggressive action in modern history to prevent the spread of this illness in the United States. We are ready. Totally ready.

On January 31st, I ordered the suspension of foreign nationals to have recently been in China from entering the United States. An action which the Democrats loudly criticized and protested and now, everybody is complementing me, saying,

"Thank you very much. You're a hundred percent correct." Could have been a whole different story.

But I say, let's get this right. A virus starts in China. Bleeds its way into various countries all around the world. Doesn't spread widely at all in the United States because of the early actions myself and my administration took against a lot of others wishes, and the Democrats' single talking point, and you see it, is that it's Donald Trump's fault. Right? It's Donald Trump's fault.

Nah. Just things that happen, but you know what? This does show you. Things happen. Who would have thought of this? Two weeks ago, who would have thought this would be going on? Four weeks ago, you wouldn't . . .But things happen. But in life, and you have to be prepared, and you have to be flexible, and you have to be able to go out and get it. And my guys say we have the best professionals in the world. The best in the world. And we are so ready. At the same time that I initiated the first federally mandated quarantine in over fifty years, we had to quarantine some people. They weren't happy. They weren't happy about it. I wanna tell you, there are a lot of people that are not so happy. But I wanna tell you that after two weeks they got happy. You know who got happy? The people around them got happy. That's who got happy.

I also created a White House Virus Task Force, it's a big thing, a virus task force. I requested $2.5 billion to ensure we have the resources we need. The Democrat said, "That's terrible. He's doing the wrong thing. He needs eight and a half billion not two and a half billion." I've never had that before. I ask for two and a half. They wanna give me eight and a half. So I said, "I'll take it." Does that make me a better. . . I'll take it. I'll take it: Never had that before. I never had it. "We want two and a half billion. That's plenty." ""We demand you take eight and half. He doesn't know what he's doing. We want eight and a half." These people are crazy.

We must understand that border security is also health security. We've all seen the wall has gone up like magic. Gone up like magic. [speaks about the wall]

We will do everything in our power to keep the infection and those carrying the infection from entering our country. We have no choice. Whether it's the virus that we're talking about or many other public health threats, the Democrat policy of open borders is a direct threat to the health and wellbeing of all Americans. Now, you see it with the coronavirus. You see it. You see it with the coronavirus. You know. You see that. When you have this virus, or any other virus, or any other problem coming in. . . It's not the only thing that comes in through the border, and we're setting records now at the border. We're setting records. And now, just using this. So important, right? So important.[iii]

At the very least, it is clear from the President's words that he was preoccupied about the virus. Any person devoting twelve minutes and forty-five seconds to a topic in a campaign speech is definitely giving the issue its worth. He spoke of having set up a task force, about slowing down migration from China, about the nation's border being a health border, about the national security threats from the virus, and about funding for efforts against the coronavirus. And he spoke about being ready and taking the virus "very very seriously." In fact, in the whole nearly thirteen minute discussion, he used the word "hoax" once, and it was in the context of how his political opponents were politicizing the coronavirus to use it against him in the same manner that so many issues had been previously used against him. Going from that, particularly in light of everything he said around that comment, to claiming the President thought the pandemic was a hoax is a far stretch, but it is one that the press has been happy to eagerly take.

[iii] Donald J. Trump in "Live: President Trump in North Charleston, SC," YouTube, Feb. 28, 2020, 5:14-16:59, accessed May 18, 2020, https://www.youtube.com/watch?v=no0MnomPzLw&t=1020s.

As President Trump mentioned in his speech, on January 31, he had shut down travel from China. The reaction to the President's action was swift and turbulent. In a later-deleted tweet, the liberal news service, Vox, tweeted, "Is this really going to be a pandemic?"[370] Further, when President Trump announced on the same day that he was adding six African countries to the travel ban, Speaker Pelosi said in a statement,

> *The Trump Administration's expansion of its outrageous, un-American travel ban threatens our security, our values and the rule of law. The sweeping rule, barring more than 350 million individuals from predominantly African nations from traveling to the United States, is discrimination disguised as policy . . . With this latest callous decision, the President has doubled down on his cruelty and further undermined our global leadership, our Constitution and our proud heritage as a nation of immigrants.*[iv]

The Speaker also announced she would be bringing a bill for the NO BAN Act to the House of Representatives aiming to "prohibit religious discrimination in our immigration system and limit the President's ability to impose such biased and bigoted restrictions. We will never allow hatred or bigotry to define our nation or destroy our values."[371] The next day, presidential candidate Joe Biden tweeted, "We are in the midst of a crisis with the coronavirus. We need to lead the way with science — not Donald Trump's record of hysteria, xenophobia, and fear-mongering. He is the worst possible person to lead our country through a global health emergency."[372]

Even more, healthcare-centric commenters, who should have been cognizant of the colossal threat SARS-CoV-2 was posing, took

[iv] Nancy Pelosi in "Pelosi Statement on President Trump's Expanded Travel Ban," Nancy Pelosi Speaker of the House Newsroom (blog), Jan. 31, 2020, accessed Apr. 30, 2020, https://www.speaker.gov/newsroom/13120-2.

the opportunity to attack the President for his decision. STAT, a website claiming to deliver "fast, deep and tough-minded journalism about health, medicine, life sciences and the fast-moving business of making medicines,"[373] said the decision to discontinue travel with China, "was preceded by calls for similar policies from conservative lawmakers and far-right supporters of the president. Public health experts, however, warn that the move could do more harm than good."[374] And Dr. Michael T. Osterholm, epidemiologist and director of the Center for Infectious Disease Research and Policy at the University of Minnesota is reported to have called the President's decision "more of an emotional or political reaction."[375]

Not to be left outside of the cacophony, the mainstream media lent their voice to the leftist, hypercritical choir. In an opinion piece published in *The New York Times* entitled "The Racism at the Heart of Trump's 'Travel Ban,'" Jamelle Bouie wrote,[v]

> *Although immigration policy deals with the external boundaries of the United States, the elevation of whiteness has internal consequences as well. Not because the president intends to distribute benefits and favors on the basis of race — although there are elements of that in his administration's behavior — but because it sends a larger signal about who matters in this society. Every time Trump and other members of his administration make the decision to stratify and racialize, they are also making a statement about who receives a voice and who deserves respect.*

After publishing an article explaining how the coronavirus was exacerbating racist tendencies throughout the world,[376] on February 7, CNN published an analysis of the possible negative ramifications stemming from the Trump travel restrictions. But even here,

---

[v] Jamelle Bouie, "The Racism at the Heart of Trump's 'Travel Ban,'" *The New York Times* (blog), Feb. 4, 2020, accessed Apr. 30, 2020, https://www.nytimes.com/2020/02/04/opinion/trump-travel-ban-nigeria.html.

CNN could not help itself as it quoted Eric Carter, an associate professor of geography and global health at Macalester College in Saint Paul, Minnesota as saying, "Historically a lot of these border security measures have used public health as a pretext for discrimination. It's very easy to see how a public health rationale would be used to limit immigration for whatever reason. And I'm not saying that that's actually occurring, but it well could in this particular political climate, not just in the US, but internationally."[377]

In retrospect, as we review those actions that worked in containing the spread of the virus and those that did not, it becomes obvious that the President's decision towards China was exactly what was needed, and if he is to be criticized, it is for not being even stronger and more prompt. Yet, in light of these insights, there has been no widespread acknowledgment from the press regarding the prudence of the President's actions, and certainly no retractions on the criticisms cast upon him.

Trump Declares War on COVID-19

The five weeks following the President's imposition of travel restrictions and a federal quarantine were relatively quiet from an infectious disease policy standpoint. The press continued myopically covering an impeachment trial that had no future, and Congress remained paralyzed, as half its chambers were hamstrung with the trial. There was nothing that could be accomplished by the legislative branch during this time, and no one was reporting that there was anything of substance to accomplish.

Following the President's exoneration, attention remained fixated on the fallout of the trial. On the Left, the coverage centered on Republicans' recklessness for not convicting the President, and on the Right, the accusations centered on the audacity of allowing trumped-up charges against the President to proceed. As the press slowly transitioned away from impeachment there was still minimal coverage of the outbreak. Instead, the attention focused on the presidential race. Meanwhile, the virus continued its spread, silently at first, as asymptomatic people infected asymptomatic people.

The investors were the ones who first focused attention on events overseas. Up to this point, the American economy had been churning at record levels. The Dow Jones Industrial Average (DJIA) was flirting with the 30,000 mark, reaching 29,551.42 on February 12. The unemployment reached a remarkable 3.5% and America's gross domestic product (GDP) was growing at rates spanning between 2.1 and 3.2 percent.

But a surge of cases in Iran, Italy, and South Korea appearing over the weekend of February 21st sent the global number of cases of COVID-19 past 79,000, with more than 2,000 of them occurring outside of China. By Monday, the low-grade anxiety investors had been harboring over the events in China blossomed into outright fear as they exited higher risk positions in search of whatever safe harbors they could find. In one day, the DJIA fell 1,031.61 points. The ten-year Treasury note also declined to record lows, and gold prices increased to $1,672.40 an ounce, a seven-year high. What the media had ignored, and the politicians missed, the markets perceived. Suddenly, Washington awoke.

By the end of the day, President Trump was asking Congress for $2.5 billion in emergency funding to aid in vaccine research, develop therapeutic drugs, and purchase PPE.[378] The

Democrats responded by wanting more, which neither the Republicans nor the President opposed. While Congress wrangled with the President's proposal, President Trump created the Coronavirus White House Task Force (CWHTF) headed by Vice President Mike Pence. The following were its members:

U.S. Global AIDS Coordinator Dr. Deborah Birx,
Surgeon General Jerome Adams
HHS Secretary Alex Azar
U.S. Deputy Secretary of State Stephen Biegun
Assistant to the President Robert Blair
HUD Secretary Ben Carson
Acting US Deputy Secretary of Homeland Security Ken Cuccinelli
Directory of the Office of Science and Technology,
    Kelvin Droegemeier
Director of the National Institute of Allergy and Infectious
    Diseases Anthony Fauci
Assistant to the President Joe Grogan
U.S. Commissioner of Food and Drugs Stephen Hahn
Executive Director Office of Management and Budget Kan Derek
Director of the National Economic Council Larry Kudlow
White House Deputy Chief of Staff Chris Liddell
Secretary of the Treasury Steve Mnuchin
National Security Adviser Robert O'Brien
Deputy National Security Advisor Matthew Pottinger
CDC Director Robert R. Redfield
Under Secretary of Transportation for Policy in the Department
    of Transportation Joel Scabat
CNS Administrator Seema Verma
Secretary of Veteran Affairs Robert Wilkie

Amazingly, for the first time in Trump's presidency, Congress expeditiously cooperated. Within days, Congress passed a major funding package. President Trump signed the $8.3 billion measure to help fight the coronavirus less than two weeks after his initial ask,[379] and the markets responded by dropping a whopping 2,013.76 points the next day.

On March 11, as the number of global cases continued to rise, and five days after the enactment of the aid package, the WHO organization finally declared the SARS-CoV-2 outbreak a pandemic. That evening President Trump responded with an announcement from the Oval Office where he announced that he would be "marshaling the full power of the federal government and the private sector to protect the American people." The President announced a suspension of travel from Europe, except for the United Kingdom, for the next thirty days. The insurance industry would be waiving all copayments for the treatment of coronavirus infections, and nursing homes were asked to suspend all medically unnecessary visits. Also during this speech, the President said he was going to take emergency action to provide financial relief so that "working Americans can stay home without fear of financial hardship,"[380] and concurrently instructed the Small Business Administration (SBA) "to exercise available authority to provide capital and liquidity to firms affected by the coronavirus."[381] The SBA was going to begin providing economic loans in affected states and territories, and the President asked that Congress increase funding by another $50 billion for disaster loans while providing immediate payroll tax relief.[382] Below is a summary of the actions the President announced in his March 11 speech:

- All travel from Europe was suspended for the next thirty days, except for travel from the United Kingdom;
- The insurance industry would be waiving all copayments for the treatment of coronavirus infections;
- Nursing homes were asked to suspend all medically unnecessary visits;

- All Americans were asked to avoid all nonessential travel particularly in crowded areas;

- The Administration would be issuing guidance on social distancing and avoidance of large gatherings;

- The federal government would be undertaking emergency action to provide emergency relief to ensure that working American could stay home without fear of financial hardship;

- The Small Business Administration (SBA) was instructed to exercise available authority to provide capital and liquidity to firms affected by the coronavirus;

- The SBA was going to begin providing economic loans in affected states and territories;

- Congress was asked to increase funding for economic loans by another $50 billion and to provide immediate payroll tax relief for all Americans; and

- All Americans were asked to place partisanship aside while combating the virus.

Of course, the President was immediately criticized. For starters, the European travel ban needed clarification. The way the President had phrased it during the speech, it appeared that all travel from Europe was to cease. In fact, the White House had to issue a clarification indicating that the ban would only apply to foreign nationals who had been in Europe during the two weeks prior to coming to the United States.[383] Further, although Americans returning from Europe would be allowed back in the United States, their entry would be restricted to one of thirteen American airports.[384] The White House also clarified that the travel restrictions would not be applying to trade from Europe. Additionally, the President had to answer why the travel ban did not include the United Kingdom.

Although he initially explained that the exclusion was because England had not yet experienced the problems with COVID-19 that the rest of Europe had, three days later, President Trump suspended travel from the United Kingdom as well. [385]

The war against the SARS-CoV-2 was now on in the United States. What no one imagined was the incredible toll it would take on Americans and on their way of life.

The Federal Government's Strategies

The federal approach centered on mitigation and treatment. On the mitigation side, the government was intent on implementing those restrictions that would minimize the spread of the virus. The CDC recommended that individuals remain at least six feet from one another, that they avoid gathering in groups, and that they avoid crowded places and mass gatherings.[386] The recommendations particularly applied to those who were at higher risk from the disease including older adults, those suffering from severe illness, asthmatics, and people with HIV.[387]

In short, people were being encouraged to stay at home, and if an individual had merely come into close contact with someone who had COVID-19, the recommendation was for that person to quarantine for fourteen days.[388] The hope was not only to keep people from getting sick but also to "flatten the curve." It was believed that if at the very least, the total number of people who got sick could be minimized or delayed, then the drain on the hospitals and other healthcare delivery facilities could be diminished to a more manageable number. Of course, a zealous effort at "social distancing" as it became commonly called, would require people to stop going to work, a move that would surely choke the economy. As we will see, the government would eventually have to take steps to allow for that to happen.

The second arm of the government's approach was treatment. Of course, at the time of the pandemic's spread, no helpful or curative treatments beyond the supportive care measures usually administered to viral infection patients had been demonstrated. Thus, the primary armamentaria for the treatment of patients with COVID-19 were material and personnel. So how much materials and personnel would the country need? For this, epidemiologists could rely on the course of the virus across the globe.

On March 11, the day the WHO had declared a pandemic and the President addressed the nation, Italy already had 12,462 cases with 827 deaths, Spain had 2,277 cases with 55 deaths, and Iran had 9,000 cases with 354 deaths, and these were all countries that had not seen a case of coronavirus mere weeks earlier. With all the travelers from Europe and China that had entered the United States, it was obvious that Americans were going to get hit hard, much harder than the mere 1,301 cases and 38 deaths they were already encountering. Still, the question remained, how many?

In February, the CDC had held a meeting where the results of four different models regarding the scope of spread, potential fatalities, and resource allocations attributable to SARS-CoV-2 were presented. The meeting was either closed to the public or garnered so little attention that the press was not present. Nevertheless, in March, *The New York Times* obtained some of the information presented at the meeting as confirmed by at least one attendee.[389] According to the modelers, the number of people in the United States that would become infected with SARS-CoV-2 ranged between 160 million and 214 million, and the estimates were that between 1.7 million to 2.2 million people in the United States would die.[390]

Some of the estimates included a figure of 2.2 million American deaths.[391] If these predictions were correct, the United States was going to be subject to an infectious disease event of gargantuan proportions. Under such a massive strain everything would be overwhelmed. There would not be enough hospital beds, equipment, intensive care unit beds, ventilators, masks, gloves, or gowns to protect those caring for the sick. Naturally, faced with the prospects of such a colossal event, the question arose about the SNS and its readiness. It seems the authorities found no consolation there.

"The shelves were empty," President Trump has lamented on more than one occasion.[392] The reality was, as we noted in our Introduction, that the SNS had been depleting its supplies under the strain of budget cuts from successive administrations, but even with an idealized inventory, the SNS was never meant to meet massive demands from all fifty states at the same time.[393] Although mitigation efforts designed to flatten the curve would certainly help to allay the strain on the American healthcare system, the answer to the supply question was that the United States would have to quickly and massively ramp up production.

With no time in his hands, the President turned to his recently appointed CWHTF for answers. Among the first moves it took was to create a messaging campaign called "15 Days to Flatten the Curve." The intent was to make an all-out effort to have the people of the United States self-isolate.

While that was taking place, it was clear that industry needed to rapidly increase the procurement and production of certain materials.

But which ones?

The United States was short on everything, and it needed all of it, now! For example, there were the shortages of masks and PPEs.

Without it, the nation's healthcare workers were going to be exposed. If healthcare workers got sick, the whole system would shut down. Additionally, if healthcare workers themselves began spreading the disease, the consequences would be unimaginable! Next, there were medications, IV fluids, and most pressingly, ventilators. Estimates were that the nation's hospitals had a total of 160,000 ventilators[394] with 12,700 more in the SNS,[395] but some were predicting that the United States would need as many as 810,000 ventilators by the end of May![396]

And even if the materials became available, how would they get to the places where they were needed? For this, the government relied on the Federal Emergency Management Agency or FEMA. Under the auspices of the U.S. Department of Homeland Security, FEMA had a great deal of experience responding to natural disasters, mostly in the form of hurricanes, earthquakes, and tornadoes. This time, however, FEMA was being asked to potentially attend to the whole country *at the same time*! FEMA, in turn, developed a COVID-19 Supply Chain Task Force (SCTF) designed to deliver critically needed supplies to locations where they were most needed.

But delivering supplies would be impossible if there were no supplies to deliver, and no government entity existed that would be able to create the necessary equipment in such a short time. The participation of the private sector would be required, and for this, President Trump was uniquely qualified.

Unquestionably, executing the kind of mobilization that would supply a massive stream of medical equipment, some of it intricately technical would be herculean, to say the least. Just in the case of ventilators, the United States had fewer than a dozen companies capable of making them.[397]

The President's initial approach was simply to ask. Very quickly, the White House contacted major American manufacturers to see if they could ramp up production for equipment many would not normally produce. From Ford, the Administration asked for ventilators. From Apple, facemask shields, and from companies like Hanes, Fruit of the Loom, and My Pillow, they asked for PPE. Generally, the manufacturers complied, but there were exceptions. President Trump could not come to terms with General Motors regarding his request that the auto manufacturing company produce more ventilators.

Here, there was another weapon the President deployed: the Defense Production Act (DPA).[398] And do so he did. Within a week General Motors came to terms with the United States for the rapid production of large quantities of ventilators.

Another controversy ensued when news came to light that 3M was exporting a substantial number of masks to Canada and Latin America instead of directing them to the American people. At an impasse with the manufacturer, President Trump issued an executive order under the DPA on Thursday, April 2, authorizing the Secretary of Homeland Security to "use any and all authority available under the Act to acquire, from any appropriate subsidiary or affiliate of 3M Company, the number of N-95 respirators that the Administration determines to be appropriate."[399] By Monday, April 6, the company arrived at an agreement with the Administration whereby it would continue to export facemasks to Canada and Latin America while producing 55.5 million masks per month for America's healthcare workers in addition to the 35 million the company was already producing for use inside the United States.[400]

All told, the mobilization efforts realized by President Trump and his administration were nothing less than spectacular. Less than a month after the effort began, the White House was reporting it had arranged for the production of 50,000 ventilators over 100 days from Ford and GE Healthcare, 165 million N-95 masks, 1 million face shields from Apple, new PPE production from MyPillow, Brooks Brothers, Hanes, Fruit of the Loom, Jockey, Ralph Lauren, and Bacardi, Pernod Ricard, Jack Daniels, La Crosse, and Anheuser Busch began producing more hand sanitizers.[401] There were also supply donations from Salesforce, Marathon Petroleum, Tesla, Google, Walmart, Home Depot among others, and enhanced shipment services from UPS.

Table 3-1: Private Sector Mobilization Volumes Reported by White House: April 14.

Supplies	In Thousands
N-95 masks	3,820
Surgical masks	3,260
Face Shield	5,500
Surgical gowns	4,700
Gloves	30,300
Coveralls	212
Medical Station Beds	8.6
Ventilators	11
Hydroxychloroquine tablets	28,000

Source: "President Donald J. Trump Has Led a Historic Mobilization to Combat the Coronavirus," The White House (blog), Apr. 14, 2020, accessed May 2, 2020, https://www.whitehouse.gov/briefings-statements/president-donald-j-trump-led-historic-mobilization-combat-coronavirus/.

But by April, testing was still an issue. At the time of the President's Oval Office announcement, the United States was woefully short on testing supplies just like it was on other medical equipment and resources. The most important test, and the most desperately needed, was RT-PCR testing. As described in the Introduction, this test allows clinicians and scientists to know who was infected. But producing it was a much more difficult enterprise. For starters, its use requires FDA approval, which, as I cover in detail in *The Case for Free Market Healthcare*, is a protracted and expensive process. Additionally, unlike masks, or even ventilators, the creation of a functional test is not merely about building the testing machine. A functional testing unit also requires multiple swabs, collection tubes, medium to place inside the collection tube so the biological material within it does not degrade, and the testing reagent. Further, like the weakest link in a chain, the deployment of the test is limited by the distribution of the least numerous of its components.

The government had indeed been working on the creation of the test since January 31 when Secretary Azar declared a public health emergency. In order to bypass many of the delays normally encountered by the FDA's approval process, on February 3, the CDC sought an EUA for coronavirus testing.[402] That authorization was granted the following day,[403] allowing manufacturing and distribution of the test to begin immediately. But performance issues were identified temporarily halting production. The CDC had to remanufacture its tests before re-releasing it, costing the United States precious time.

Even still, clinicians were not completely flying blind when diagnosing COVID-19. The characteristics of the population where the patient was being treated certainly played a role. Thus, in communities where thousands were presenting with flulike symptoms, physicians were more likely to conclude the patients had contracted SARS-CoV-2. In those communities where those presentations were rare, physicians would more aggressively look for other sources. Additionally, in sicker patients where CT scan evaluation was indicated, the virus was creating a strongly suggestive imaging pattern described as "ground-glass and consolidative pulmonary opacities with bilateral and peripheral lung distribution"[404] that would clue clinicians to the diagnosis. With this type of information coupled with a typical clinical course, physicians were sufficiently confident engaging even in specific interventions such as the administration of hydroxychloroquine or remdesevir.

As to the use of coronavirus testing in the implementation of a robust and aggressive social isolation policy, the harsh reality was that the opportunity to use the results in such a manner had already past. Nevertheless, testing was and continues to be important. An understanding of how the disease spreads throughout a population is certainly integral to future containment efforts. Additionally, tests help in making quarantining decisions regarding not only those who could be asymptomatically shedding the virus, but in managing the status of their contacts as well. Also, testing plays a crucial role in the management of patients undergoing non-essential surgeries.

Regardless, the President and his team faced the daunting task of ramping up testing from the point of non-existence to performing millions of tests per month in the span of a few months. Once again, a President with immense business acumen and a nearly limitless network of industry leaders proved invaluable. And once again, the coordinated efforts of private enterprise and government became the ideal model for achievement.

Initial tests like the ones developed by the CDC quickly came online. However, they were slow to perform. Even in a well-supplied area, patients and clinicians could expect a turnaround time of three to five days.

Others followed in obtaining authorization for laboratory-based, RT-PCR testing, but their numbers and their turnaround times were insufficient to sustain national testing efforts numbering in the millions. To meet this goal, home testing would be ideal, but at the very least point-of-care testing, those that could be performed at the doctor's office, would be required. Towards that end, on March 20, Cepheid became the first manufacturer to be awarded an EUA by the FDA for a point-of-care test. But the company estimated that there were only 5,000 systems in use throughout the country that could potentially crank out results in about 45 minutes.[405] On March 27, the FDA granted an EUA to Abbott laboratories for its point-of-care test, which had already obtained authorization for a laboratory-based test.[406] The test was called a "game changer," by Former FDA Commissioner, Dr. Scott Gottlieb.[407] Abbott's test could provide positive results in as little as five minutes and negative results in as little as 13 minutes.[408] Abbott was hopeful its machines could run 50,000 tests a day! Combined with its laboratory-based test, Abbott hoped to run 5,000,000 tests a month.[409] And in another development, on April 10, the FDA approved a saliva-based test in addition to the usual nasal swabs.[410]

In the meantime, the President's team obtained commitments from U.S. Cotton to manufacture over 10 million polyester Q-tip swabs per month to be used in support of home-based testing.[411] Oak Ridge National Laboratory ramped up production for 40 million tubes a month.[412] For finger-pricks employed in serology testing, commitments were made for the manufacture of 17 million lancets and an equal number of alcohol swabs.[413]

The rapid mobilization by the White House and industry allowed the United States testing efforts to grow from 4 tests performed by the CDC on January 18, 2020,[414] to a whopping

8,314,419 tests on May 8.[415] Although the number of tests performed in the United States is now greater than those of the next four highest test-conducting nations combined, it still ranks 39th in its rate of per capita testing.[416] In all fairness, many of those nations ranked above the United States are much smaller, making per capita mobilization much easier.

As the testing resources came online, the plan was to have those tests distributed to the various states for implementation. Beginning in March, the President routinely held conference calls with the governors to serve as a facilitator for the distribution and supplies. With FEMA's assistance testing supplies were delivered to the various states according to their needs. But as the private sector became even more involved and capable of handling demands, it started ramping private testing capabilities outside of what the state resources were providing. Almost overnight, Americans had multiple resources through which to seek testing to the point that in some locations, drive-thru collection stations were implemented.

The Governors React

Despite the massive application of funds and resources, the response to the Wuhan Pandemic needed mobilization, and on this front, the President, policymakers, and public health officials found themselves in a very tenuous situation. Never in the history of the United States had a national mobilization against a natural threat been undertaken. Yes, the United States had seen pandemics before. It had already combated the Spanish flu, smallpox, AIDS, SARS, and polio, to name a few, but it had never tried to convince the American people, *all the American people*, to stop what they were doing and stay at home. It was a herculean venture, to be sure, but the President was told that if Americans didn't do it, 2.2 million Americans were going to die. As we will explore later, the models were off, but it was the information the President had to go with, and President Trump was bent on not allowing 2.2 million Americans to die.

The first hurdle to getting the American people to stay at home was a constitutional one. The federal government was not expressly given the authority to suppress the movements of the people, even under unusual circumstances. Yes, Congress could suspend the Wirt of Habeas Corpus, but such power was limited to times when public safety demanded it, or "in Cases of Rebellion or Invasion,"[417] and even then, it was not the President who could do it, but rather Congress.[vi] And although the federal government was to guarantee the states its protection against "Invasion,"[418] no one could argue in good faith that the Framers were referring to invasion from a virus.

Additionally, Congress is not allowed to interfere with interstate commerce and force people to stay at home to combat a virus. Nor does Congress have any direct authority over nursing homes or other healthcare providers, unless these worked directly for the federal government. It quickly became evident that many of the measures the epidemiologists were recommending fell squarely upon the states to accomplish, and states were not mere departments of the federal government.

To be sure, state involvement had many inherent advantages. The impact of the virus's spread would have regional variations, and the states were in the best position to differentially apply mitigation strategies throughout the various portions of the country.

[vi] During the Civil War, Abraham Lincoln suspended the Writ of Habeas Corpus, but he was challenged. Congress, in order to avoid a constitutional crisis, suspended the writ.

Also, only the states possessed the necessary infrastructure to move materials and money to their ultimate destinations. But each state had its inherent philosophical differences and some like New York, Washington, and California had drawn bright battle lines against the President on numerous issues. If American lives were going to be saved, political differences would have to be placed aside, at least partially.

As the President began rolling out his response, some states took actions early and independently of the federal government. On March 11, as President Trump was preparing to deliver his speech from the Oval Office, California Governor Gavin Newsom issued a recommendation that gatherings of 250 or more people be cancelled and that "social distancing" measures be implemented.[419] Although the recommendation did not have any legally binding authority, the California Department of Public Health, through its Public Health Officer, followed on March 19 with a stay-at-home order "except as needed to maintain continuity of operations of the federal critical infrastructure sectors as outlined [by the Cybersecurity and Infrastructure Security Agency.]"[420] On March 20, the Governor himself issued a stay-at-home-except-for-essential-needs order. Interestingly, Newsom's order[421] did not make mention of any churches or church-related activities.

Other states followed suit until all, except for the Dakotas, Nebraska, and Iowa issued similar order, with Arkansas, Wyoming, Utah, and Oklahoma declaring partial stay-at-home orders instead. [422]

Additionally, states declared major emergencies making them eligible for disaster funding, beginning with New York on March 20 and ending with Wyoming on April 11. With Wyoming's declaration, 50 states found themselves concurrently under a disaster declaration for the first time in American history.[423]

Relatedly, the extents of the stay-at-home orders and the zeal with which they were enforced have varied between states. Amongst the most draconian is Michigan where Governor Gretchen Whitmer, a Democrat, declared a prohibition on sales of non-essential products. Amazingly, essential products were defined as those "necessary to maintain the safety, sanitation, and basic operation of residences."[424] Thus, the sale of American flags, seeds, gardening supplies, and even infant seats were discontinued![vii] In addition to bans on all public gatherings, the Governor's order included a prohibition on visiting friends or family.[425] Governor Whitmer's measures were so strict that on April 15, a mass protest consisting of over 15,000 automobiles descended upon the capitol causing gridlock in the streets of the capitol.[426]

Other governors even tampered with voting rights and election outcomes. In Wisconsin, the day before the primary election, Governor Tony Evers issued an executive order suspending in-person voting.[427] His order was overturned by the Wisconsin Supreme Court, and the elections ultimately proceeded.[428]

The actions of the various governors throughout the nation brought up a myriad of questions regarding their necessity and appropriateness. In New York, a prohibition on the dispensation of hydroxychloroquine or chloroquine by New York pharmacists "except when written as prescribed for an FDA-approved indication; or as part of a state-approved clinical trial related to COVID-19. . . . " was issued by Governor Andrew Cuomo.[429] In Nevada, Governor Steve Sisolak, reacting to a tragic accident where an Arizona couple drank fish-tank cleaner containing chloroquine phosphate that killed the man and sent the woman to the intensive care unit,[430] ordered

---

[vii] The Governor quickly clarified that her declaration did not include infant seats.

the use of chloroquine and hydroxychloroquine be restricted to only patients with certain non-COVID-19 diagnoses.[431] In Michigan, Governor Whitmer's administration sent a letter to licensed pharmacists informing them that they may face "further investigation" if medications were prescribed without "proof of the medical necessity and the condition for which the patient is being treated."[432] And throughout the nation, Leftist governors took the opportunity to release prisoners, even violent ones, from their jails.[433]

Other governors were more permissive with their orders. Governor Ron DeSantis of Florida did not issue a stay-at-home order until April 1, 2020.[434] Before that, though, the Governor had issued orders regarding the closure of Broward and Palm Beach Counties,[435] closures of state bars and gyms,[436] closures of restaurants and beaches,[437] closures of Dade County public access facilities,[438] and discontinuation of non-essential elective medical procedures.[439] Despite this surgical approach to mitigation, the press placed pressure on the Governor over the absence of a statewide stay-at-home order, suggesting that nothing but a carpet-bombing approach would do. Although neither the President nor his advisors expressed as much, Governor Desantis was becoming a drain on the President, as the press was daily asking him about the Florida Governor's tardiness in issuing such an order.

Governor DeSantis did ultimately issue an all-encompassing, state-wide order on April 1, quieting the press, but in fact, it didn't add much to the compendium of restrictions he had already imposed. What's more, DeSantis was very careful in specifically tailoring his stay-at-home order to limit activities in a specific manner without overextending its authority. His Order first instructed senior citizens and persons with underlying medical conditions to stay at home and "take all measures to limit the risk of exposure to

COVID-19."[440] It then defined essential (permitted) services and activities to include "religious services conducted in churches, synagogues, and houses of worship," caring for one's pets, and caring or otherwise assisting a loved one or friend.[441] In retrospect, his targeted techniques at isolating specific sectors of the population were amongst the sagest in the nation.

Clusters

Just about any gathering could be the source for the development of a new cluster of cases, and many did indeed crop up. In Albany, Georgia, two funerals, one held on February 29 and another a week later, set the stage for the invasion of the Wuhan pandemic into a small and rural community a world away.[442] By March 22, the virus had spread throughout the city of 90,000 inclusive of 600 confirmed cases and 24 deaths.[443] Needless to say, area hospitals were overwhelmed. The local economy was shut down and much suffering ensued.

By far, the biggest cluster in the United States was New York. The first reported case to hit New York occurred on March 1 in a healthcare worker who developed mild respiratory symptoms following her return from a trip to Iran.[444] The next day, an attorney from New Rochelle, a suburb 20 miles south of New York City, became the second case, and within days, nine people who came in contact with him tested positive.[445] By March 15, the State of New York posted 942 cases and 5 deaths.[446]

Neither the City nor the State of New York stood idly by in the face of the pandemic's assault. On March 6, Mayor Bill de Blasio urged residents to stay home, and the next day Governor Cuomo declared a state of emergency,[447] the first state to do so. The city also canceled its annual St. Patrick's Day Parade, and public schools were shut down on March 15.[448] By mid-March, New York State was essentially in full shutdown mode. However, despite these measures, the number of cases rapidly increased. By March 25, the state was seeing over 1,000 new cases appear *each day*![449]

The attorney's New Rochelle was hit particularly hard from the beginning. In early March, while New York City was still sporting 36 cases, New Rochelle already had 108 cases, many of them tied to the Young Israel Synagogue, the place where the New Rochelle attorney worshiped.[450]

Governor Cuomo recognized the potentially explosive situation and took decisive action by closing schools, enforcing quarantines, and shutting down the local market. In fact, Cuomo created a containment zone around New Rochelle and solicited the assistance of the National Guard to enforce it. But his efforts would be futile. A mere month later, New York would be infested with over 200,000 cases, and by early May, the state was riddled with more than 327,000 cases and nearly 21,000 deaths.[451]

What happened to New York was emblematic of the struggles of large urban areas with highly concentrated populations and extensive travel. For New York, the intense onslaught of cases and failed containment efforts meant hospitals were overwhelmed and resources were pushed to the brink of collapse.

Although New York was by far the worst cluster in the United States, it was by no means the only one. New Jersey, Seattle, New Orleans, San Francisco, Boston, Detroit, Albany, among many others, were all particularly hard hit. For the President and his team, it was a hectic race between the virus's spread and their ability to deliver the support they needed. And for the most part, the President delivered. When it came to ventilators, Governor Cuomo insisted that New York was going to need 40,000 ventilators, and it only had 12,000. The President pointed out that despite Cuomo's hysterical rants, there were thousands of unused ventilators stockpiled in New York. Cuomo faced some level of embarrassment when he was forced to admit that there were enough ventilators, but he was saving them. But New York never ran out of ventilators.[452] New Jersey never ran out of ventilators, nor did Michigan, or Pennsylvania, or any other state,[453] allowing the President to boast, "Nobody that needed a ventilator in this country didn't get one," while holding up news articles to support his contention.[454]

A similar contention was made about hospital beds, and the President responded by moving the nation's two hospital ships, the *USNS Mercy* and the *USNS Comfort* to Los Angeles and New York, respectively. Additionally, temporary hospitals were built in New York (the Jacob K. Javits Convention Center, Stony Brook University, and State University of New York College), New Jersey, New Orleans, and Detroit. Interestingly, despite the fervent demand by government officials for these facilities, they were scarcely used. The Javits Center ended up treating about 1,000 patients while the others were mothballed for future use.[455] The temporary hospital in Detroit treated less than fifty patients at the time of this writing. In New Jersey, two hospitals have treated less than 500 patients, and in New Orleans the hospital is populated by about 100 patients.[456]

The real clusters were the nursing homes. With its predilection for the elderly and the weak, the nation's nursing homes were the natural target for SARS-CoV-2. Indeed, the first cluster in the United States was a nursing home in Seattle.[457]

By February 26, Ash Wednesday, there was already a spike in upper respiratory cases at Life Care Center of Kirkland. Curiously, on that day, the facility held a Mardi Gras party. The next week, a spike of coronavirus cases left at least 35 dead and gave the Center the dubious distinction of being the largest cluster in the United States.[458] But Life Care Center of Kirkland was not alone. In Washington, 58% of its 1,019 deaths thus far have taken place in long-term care facilities.[459]

The Washington experience is actually not the worst performance amongst the 38 states reporting such data. In Oregon, 59% of COVID-19 deaths took place in extended care facilities, 60% in Massachusetts, 72% in New Hampshire, and 73% in Rhode Island.[460] Not to be left behind, in California 38% of COVID-19 deaths took place in nursing homes as did 42% in Colorado, 45% in Mississippi, 46% in Connecticut, 53% in Maryland, 53% in New Jersey, and 56% in Maine.[461] Overall, about 38% of all deaths in the United States have taken place in nursing homes, for a raw figure of 29,974 fatalities distributed amongst 33 states.[462]

New York's experiencing was particularly harrowing as it pointed to the ineptitude of its government leaders. According to the Kaiser Family Foundation, as of May 8, New York State had experienced 5,215 deaths in extended care facilities or 20% of all COVID-19 deaths.[463] Even more astonishing, New York's nursing home deaths account for one-fifth of all such deaths in the whole country!

New York is an example of what not to do with regard to nursing homes in one's state. First, New York has not been forthcoming in reporting the number of nursing home deaths. The state took weeks to report its first such deaths[464] and failed to include approximately 1,600 deaths from nursing home patients who had died in hospitals.[465] Adding to the deceit, some New York nursing homes have been reluctant to report their own deaths for fear of getting negative publicity.[466] But perhaps the worst aspect in the management of nursing homes stems from Governor Cuomo's actions. Governor Cuomo has been reluctant to supply nursing homes with PPE because the institutions are privately owned.[467] Even more offensively, in order to open up New York hospitals, on March 25, the New York Department of health *ordered* nursing homes to accept COVID-19 patients.[468] In an advisory that has been at least temporarily deleted from the New York Department of Health's website, the Department directed that "No resident shall be denied re-admission or admission to the NH solely based on a confirmed or suspected diagnosis of COVID-19."[469] The order served as a death sentence to all the other residents in those facilities. Imagine, a facility full of the frailest, most elderly of our citizens being forced to accept patients with known COVID-19 infections regardless of what it would do the elderly residents already living there! Adding to the insult, the same directive also stated, "NHs are prohibited from requiring a hospitalized resident who is determined medically stable to be tested for COVID-19 prior to admission or readmission."[470] So, not only is the nursing home forced to accept the COVID-19 patient, it is not even allowed to know that he or she is actually infected.

From a policy standpoint, there are a number of fatal problems with this directive. How is the nursing home supposed to know which newly admitted patient to isolate? Is the nursing home expected to deploy scarce PPE on all its patients?

Cuomo was supplied with a hospital ship and a number of temporary hospitals, which remained nearly empty, if not completely so. Instead of forcing nursing homes to admit potentially sick patients, hospitalized COVID-19 patients destined for nursing homes could have been sent to the Javits Center instead, or any of the empty military hospitals.[471]

The claim from state officials was that nursing home patients were outside of what was meant to be cared for in those facilities.[472]

Here too, the onus falls squarely on Cuomo, as the President frequently asked him whether he needed any type of support. There is no question that if Governor Cuomo had requested the President convert the temporary military hospitals into either destinations for nursing-home-bound patients with COVID-19 or hospitals serving as the primary receiving station for non-COVID-19 patients, the issue would have been addressed, but he never suggested it, and people died. The final insult is that New York already had experiences in Italy, Spain, and France available for their review. They should have known that repeating Europe's errors was going to lead to the same deadly results.

By contrast, Florida, a state with a higher population than New York, but with about one-tenth the number of cases and one-fifteenth the number of deaths, also performed much better in preventing nursing home deaths. Florida enacted much more effective policies at preventing exposure to its most vulnerable. For starters, in Florida, all hospitalized patients destined for nursing were *required* to be tested for COVID-19 and have negative results. Hospitals, therefore, held such medically stabilized patients in their facilities until such time that their tests came back negative. If a patient had a positive test, he or she would not go to the nursing home, but more likely would continue to be treated in the hospital. Additionally, the state ordered a prohibition on all visitations to nursing homes, except for "[f]amily members, friends, and visiting residents in end-of-life situations."[473] Also, persons with active COVID-19 infections, persons who have had contacts with known COVID-19 patients, and persons who have traveled through an airport or been on a cruise ship within fourteen days of seeking entry would not be allowed access to the nursing home.[474] The state's Department of Health website also provided advice and recommended checklists for nursing homes to follow in caring for their patients.[475] Thus far, 27% of the state's deaths occurred in nursing homes,[476] and if this is slightly higher than New York, it is because of the significantly lower total deaths, rather than a flaw in Florida's handling of the challenges associated with caring for these patients.

In Nevada, as of April 30, a mere 19% of cases have been associated with nursing homes,[477] with 155 out of 175 nursing home cases in Northern Nevada coming from two nursing homes and 19 out of 22 deaths came from one.[478] Interestingly, state officials did not impose any requirements upon its nursing homes. Instead, it sent out a technical bulletin laying out the CDC recommendations for extended care facilities and asked (not required) that all health care providers sign the document.[479] Despite the simplicity of this measure and its non-binding nature, Nevada still achieved one of the lowest nursing-home infection-related death rates in the nation. And even though one could make observations regarding Nevada's lower population density as an explanation, such comments are applicable to the state's total number of cases, not the rate of death amongst its nursing home patients relative to its total death rates. The only explanation for this result is the care undertaken on the ground to prevent this deadly virus from entering extended-care facilities.

One more item that must be discussed is the extreme isolation of nursing home patients dying from COVID-19. Except in situations like Florida where accommodations were encouraged for end-of-life situations, throughout the nation, examples abound of family members staring through windows while their loved ones slowly exited this present existence. The cell phone became the primary form of communication for these patients, either with the benefit of a window or not, until they slipped out of consciousness.

There was no hug. No handholding. No whispering final words of gratitude into their ears. There was only isolation and silence. And for the families, regret. Truly, one of the most tragic aspects of this disease is the manner in which we have mishandled the preservation of one's dignity in dying and the interference with priceless support and care loved ones deliver to the dying during their final moments on earth.

The Markets and the Economy

As previously noted, the markets were the first to appreciate the great threat posed by SARS-CoV-2. On February 24, after almost hitting 30,000 points, the DJIA dropped 1,031.64 in response to a surge of cases in Iran, Italy, and South Korea. Almost immediately, government officials sprung into action and worked out an $8.3 billion deal to fight the coronavirus, which the President signed on Friday, March 6. Despite these efforts, on Monday, March 9, the Dow still dropped 2,013.76 points to 23,851.02. But the punches against the American economy would not stop there. Saudi Arabia, in a continuing price war with Russia, escalated matters by promising to flood the oil markets. Immediately, oil prices tumbled by 30% to less than $30 a barrel.[480] The implications for the American economy was ominous as American frackers require a price of about $35 per gallon in order to compete. Even the sustainability of America's energy independence was placed at risk by SARS-CoV-2.

When the President delivered his speech officially declaring a national emergency and discontinuing travel from Europe, the markets predictably reacted with another tailspin of 2,352.60 points to close at 21,200.62. The stage was now set for the destabilization of the American economy in a manner unseen since the Great Depression.

American businesses either spontaneously shut down or were forced to cease operations by state and local directives. Movie theaters sat empty. Restaurants were closed. Department stores were forced into hibernation. Americans were literally forced to go into their homes and stay there. By March 22, more than one half of all Americans were subject to a lockdown order.[481] But the bills still kept coming, left to be unpaid. People were laid off or furloughed.

In less than a month, the United States went from having the lowest unemployment rate in its recorded history to having a record 3.3 million Americans filing for unemployment in one week. Consider that the week prior, with the economy already slowing, the number of first-time unemployment filings was a relatively paltry 282,000![482] Consider also that in February, the American economy was, by far, the strongest and most stable in the world, having marked "over 100-consecutive months of record-setting job growth."[483]

The situation was unsustainable. Without relief, the American economy wasn't just going to weaken; it was going to implode into a complete state of collapse. On March 23, the Dow hit bottom at 18,591.93. It was a heart-wrenching development. In the span of a month, the stock market had lost about a third of its value, or about $13 trillion.[484] All the gains realized during the Trump presidency were erased.

Once again both chambers of Congress and the White House worked at creating some sort of stopgap solution. What they produced, known as the Coronavirus Aid, Relief and Economic Security Act, or the CARES Act was signed by the President on March 27, and was the largest stimulus bill in American history.[485] Among other provisions, the new law included $377 billion in federally guaranteed loans for small businesses,[486] a provision to expand unemployment checks by $600 per week,[487] and an unprecedented program whereby each individual earning less than $75,000 per year would receive $1,200 directly from the federal government.[488]

Regardless of the gargantuan nature of the bailout, the market was unimpressed. Although stocks had risen above their low of March 23, they dropped nearly one thousand points the day following the signing of the bill. The lackadaisical response surprised some, but it was actually somewhat predictable. The United States was not having a money issue as had been seen in other times of economic contractions. This was a problem with uncertainty and a lack of confidence in the future. Throwing money at the problem, some analysts observed, was not going to solve the problems afflicting either Main Street or Wall Street.

Despite this, the CARES Act did provide welcomed relief for small businesses. Particularly popular was the Paycheck Protection Program (PPP), a measure that would lend businesses up to two and a half times their combined payroll, rent, and utilities, which would then be forgiven if at least 75% of the money loaned was spent solely on those items over the ensuing two months.[489] The PPP was so popular that despite some problems in execution, the money was distributed by mid-April.[490]

With no end in sight for the Wuhan pandemic, jobless claims continued to soar. To make matters worse, on March 29, the lockdown was extended for another 30 days. America was making progress in flattening the curve, the CWHTF said, but an effective effort was going to take longer. The United States prepared for another month of intensive social distancing while another 5.25 million jobless claims were filed. And while the total number of unemployed reached 20 million,[491] Congress prepared to act again. This time, Congress added another $484 billion to the CARES Act, most of which to replenish the PPP, although there were allocations aimed at providing relief for hospitals.[492] Small businesses once again lined up to receive the support they needed to keep their employees on their payrolls and their doors open.

The Federal Reserve undertook other efforts, but its actions were a lot more discrete and generally unnoticed by the public. First, in a series of interest rate cuts, the Fed cut short-term lending rate to near zero by March 15. Additionally, it cut the rates at which banks borrow by 1.5% and dropped the bank reserve requirement for banks to lend to zero.[493] This latter regulatory relaxation was particularly important because it freed up money in banks for lending.[494] Additionally, the Fed announced that it was going to start buying commercial paper, or guarantees for the payment of debts, and it also announced that it was going to buy up to $600 billion in loans made under the PPP while extending credits to banks that loaned money under the program. In all, without an act from Congress or any debate in the public square, the Fed moved about $6 trillion in liquidity into the American economy.[495]

But the economy still kept losing. On May 8, the April unemployment figures were out and the numbers were catastrophic. A single month erased a decade's worth of gains.[496] The unemployment rate rose to 14.7% making at least 33 million eligible Americans unemployed.[497] It became apparent that no amount of money was going to correct what was ailing the country. What was really needed was for businesses to open back up.

The Assault on Religion

The COVID-19 power grab also represented an opportunity to attack religion and religious worship. All over the country, particularly in more liberal jurisdictions, the people's abilities to

worship and assemble for worship were infringed. Many governments expressly prohibited residents from gathering in places of
worship while others did so through the omission of exemptions
or protections for religious worship. One particularly visible example took place in Florida prior to the implementation of Governor DeSantis's Executive Order regarding essential activities when
Sheriff Chad Chronister of Hillsborough County (Tampa) arrested Reverend Rodney Howard-Browne for attempting to hold two
church services on a Sunday in defiance of a county stay-at-home
order.[498] Although *The New York Times* was quick to point out that
the sheriff was a Republican,[499] he actually acted pursuant to an
executive order instituted by a unanimous vote of the county commission, the majority of which was Democrat, and about which
The New York Times was silent.[500] The Order, which took effect on
March 26, listed a litany of activities that were to be considered essential, ranging from gardening to laundry services, but it did not
include religious services. Yet the Hillsborough order exempted
religious personnel from the restrictions,[501] which the pastor certainly was. Thus, although the pastor was engaged in a prohibited
activity according to the order, the sheriff arguably did not have
the authority to arrest the pastor under the auspices of that same
order; yet he did.

In Greenville, Mississippi, among other places, the restrictions
were so onerous that even when the Temple Baptist Church attempted to hold services in a drive-in manner so that attendees would
remain in their cars for the services, they were still prohibited from
participating. As worshipers arrived, the police threatened to fine individuals up to $500.00.[502] It took a judicial ruling to put a stop
to the oppressive policing activity,[503] but the police said it would
continue to enforce the order.[504] The act was so offensive to religious

liberties and worship that it caught the attention of United States Attorney General William Barr who submitted a Statement of Interest in federal district court.[505]

In Louisville, Kentucky, a similar measure was implemented affecting the Fire Christian Church. This case was even more egregious as the church had been holding drive-in services for weeks, but was being forced to stop right before Easter. The church, with the help of the Liberty Counsel, sued the mayor of Louisville. The church prevailed in court with a biting rebuke from the judge:

> *On Holy Thursday, an American mayor criminalized the communal celebration of Easter.*
>
> *That sentence is one that this Court never expected to see outside the pages of a dystopian novel, or perhaps the pages of The Onion. But two days ago, citing the need for social distancing during the current pandemic, Louisville's Mayor Greg Fischer ordered Christians not to attend Sunday services, even if they remained in their cars to worship –and even though it's Easter.*
>
> *The Mayor's decision is stunning. And it is, "beyond all reason," unconstitutional.* [viii]

Governors were not immune from the authoritarian behavior. On March 17, Governor Ralph Northam told Virginians to avoid gatherings of more than ten people. Excluded from that restriction were essential services including "manufacturers, distribution centers, airports, bus and train stations, medical facilities, grocery stores, or pharmacies."[506] Conspicuously absent from this list were church gatherings and assemblies at places of worship. A similar statewide order was issued by Governor Gretchen Whitmer prohibiting all indoor accumulations of greater than 50 persons

---

[viii] Fire Christian Center, Inc. v. Greg Fischer, et al., Civil Action No. 3:20-CV-264-JRW. 3, Apr. 11, 2020.

punishable as a misdemeanor.[507] Only in the face of intense public outcry did the Governor issue a clarification stating that a place of religious worship was not subject to penalty.[508]

The deleterious consequences of omitting expressed protections for religious services in gubernatorial executive orders were by the Department of Justice (DOJ) in a letter he wrote cautioning Governor Newsom against his apparent neglect to this most important facet of our common existence. Explaining that government could not impose restrictions upon religious activities that did equally apply to nonreligious ones, the letter pointed out that religious gatherings could not be singled out even in times of emergency.[509] Specifically, the letter challenged the Governor to explain how church gatherings were different from gatherings of workers supporting the entertainment industries, studios, schools, restaurants, factories, offices, shopping malls, swap meets, and others so long as they were in compliance with social distancing requirements.[510]

In contrast, Florida Governor Ron Desantis's Order included "[a]ttending religious services conducted in churches, synagogues, and houses of worship as permitted "essential activities."[511] Following the implementation of his order, not a single arrest was made for worshipping in the State of Florida. Just as interestingly, all over the state, churches and synagogues either voluntarily closed their doors or found alternative ways of worshipping so that there was also no public nor professional outcry regarding the conduct of Florida's worshippers in the face of the pandemic.

The experience really did exemplify the hostility the Left has towards worship in America. Let us not forget that the single most "essential service" on earth is the contrite and reverential worship of God. Also bear in mind that the nation's very foundation was based on the vision of a society built under God where individuals were allowed to worship free of government persecution. In their response, the Left has demonstrated the little regard it has for the spiritual component of man's existence.

But the Left's concern regarding the potential spread of disease is well taken. In that vein, there was a case where the insistence on communally worshiping by a pastor may have contributed to his demise. In, Chesterfield Virginia, Pastor Gerald O. Glenn, Bishop of the New Deliverance Evangelistic Church, continued to hold services at his church despite Governor Northam's executive order to the contrary. The criticisms launched against him were formidable and scornful to whom Glenn responded, "I firmly believe that God is larger than this dreaded virus."[512] Although he was right, Bishop Glenn passed away from COVID-19 on April 11, 2020.[513]

Many have used Pastor Glenn's case as an example of what can happen when a church leader ignores science and places others, as well as himself, in danger. However, to Christians, particularly those familiar with the history of the early church, one who dies in an effort to better worship Christ is a martyr to be exalted and admired, even when that death is the result of an infection like leprosy or the plague. Such is the width of the schism dividing the religious from the secular in our country.

Models

As events unfolded, some sort of method by which an estimate could be made of the magnitude of the pandemic became important. Such predictions would allow policymakers and first responders to prepare for what was about to come. How many ICU beds were going to be needed and where? How many doctors? How many nurses? What would be the demands for masks and PPE? Each of these factors became paramount as the various states began to brace themselves for the unknown.

Additionally, Americans wanted to know how many people were about to get sick and how many were going to die. By mid-March, projectors were providing answers to these questions. In the United States, if we assumed no mitigation efforts were undertaken ("if nothing were done. . .") and an infectiousness quotient of 2.4 for the SARS-CoV-2., 286 million cases would take place with 2.2 million deaths.[514] The estimation sent shockwaves across the nation. If true, the calamity that was about to befall America was going to be overwhelming, literally! The prediction was so dire that it changed the President's attitude from one of confidence that the nation would get through this without too much sacrifice to deciding that the nation's economy needed to be shut down.

But the prediction was wrong, and it should have been dismissed by those advising the President of the United States. Here's why.

By April 1, the time the President began discussing the predictions, it was already easy to conclude that *even if Americans did nothing to circumvent the spread of SARS-CoV-2*, 2.2 million people *could not have died from the virus*. The first clue stemmed from a cursory look at the virus's behavior. At the time the President was allowed by his advisors to use the 2 million deaths figure, SARS-CoV-2 had already been in circulation for over three months with access to the far reaches of the globe. At that point, the number of cases. . . not deaths. . . but cases, *in the whole world*, was 976,249. With that information in hand, it was inconceivable for anyone to seriously argue that there would be over twice as many <u>deaths</u> in the United States than there were <u>cases</u> in the whole world!

But there was a more defective flaw to the estimate provided to the President. To recognize this, one has to understand the formula used by most epidemiologists in making their predictions: the Susceptible, Infected, and Recovered (SIR) model.[ix] Certain assumptions are made in the SIR model that makes it wholly inapplicable to what the United States was about to experience. First, the formula assumes that the spread of disease is dependent on the number of contacts between infected immigrants to a population interacting with the susceptible members of that population. Depending on the number of susceptible individuals and the infectiousness of the contagion, a certain number of members of the host population will predictably become infected. The formula tries to estimate that number. The formula also assumes that some of the infected would die (fatalities) and others would recover. And finally, once an infected individual recovers, the formula assumes he or she is healed and immune to the disease.

Like in any other complex mathematical description of reality, the SIR model requires that the investigator make some assumptions regarding the numbers in the population and the infectiousness of the contagious agent. Although the selection of the various numbers to be assumed as true is debatable, their proper selection is only that, debatable. But the SIR model also assumes that every member of the population is equally susceptible to the disease. Of course, we know this is not true. Elderly people are more susceptible than young ones. Immunocompromised patients are less resistant than ones with healthy immune systems, and people living in more densely populated areas tend to be more susceptible to the disease. But the impossibility of the calculation, and indeed the incompatibility of the formula with the American population is that

---

[ix] There are a few variations to this model such as the SEIR that adds exposure rates. The comments made here apply to most of these variations in calculating predictions.

the model assumes that every member of the population has an equal chance of coming into contact with every other member of the population. In other words, in the SIR model, a person living in New York is assumed to have an equal chance of coming into contact with his butcher down the street as he does with a shoe salesman in Wyoming. This assumption is so preposterous as to invalidate the whole prediction, yet it was accepted in creating the predictions that the President of the United States was to go with.

In the meantime, Dr. James Lawler a medical doctor and infectious disease expert from the University of Nebraska, in a presentation to members of the American Hospital Association on February 26, 2020, estimated 96 million Americans would become infected with 4.6 million hospitalizations and 480,000 deaths.[515] The exact manner by which Dr. Lawler arrived at his numbers could not be ascertained by the author, but he predicted less than a quarter the number of deaths arrived at by the SIRS model, a number much closer to the actual American experience.

Then there's the University of Washington's Institute for Health Metrics and Evaluation (IHME), also called the Murray model, which projected 81,766 fatalities over four months. The IHME model is "informed by the shape that other COVID-19 outbreaks are taking."[516] Because the IHME Model "is designed to specifically address the planning needs of hospital administrators,"[517] it is not geared to generate a worst-case scenario, but rather a more specific estimation of peak cases and other utilization measures. Unlike the SIR model, the IHME did not assume random mixing of the population.[518] Rather, the IHME approaches the question of predicting deaths from the opposite direction; namely, it predicts fatalities using the number of deaths that have occurred rather than by predicting the number of cases and then using that number to predict the number of deaths. This death-based method is an experiential model,[519] and therefore, according to its proponents, less likely to arrive at unusually high predictions. Thus, the IHME arrived at 81,766 deaths, as opposed to 2.2 million.

These estimates are important to more than just bracing the American public for impact. They also drive policy decisions regarding the necessity of shutting down an economy and resource allocations. For example, while some estimates were predicting that the United States would need as many as 810,000 ventilators by the end of May 2020, one study placed the need for ventilators, at peak usage, at only 19,481.[520] Obviously, the President of the United States would react much differently when being told that 810,000 ventilators were needed throughout the country than when less than 20,000 would do the job. That the President's team would run with numbers that were so unbelievably high was not only a disservice to the President but more importantly, to the American people.

The Media Hype

I arrived at Englewood Community Hospital a little before eight o'clock in the evening of April 13. My visit was the last of three hospitals where I was to round. As was a new reality of how we conducted healthcare, I got out of my truck, donned my lab coat and mask, and entered the building through the emergency room side-entrance to be screened.

Inside, I was greeted by a young, masked, certified registered nurse assistant. Her job that night was not to attend to patients but to screen persons as they tried to enter the building, placed there so she may earn some work hours instead of being furloughed or laid off. The policy was that no visitors would be allowed entry into the hospital with rare exceptions, so essentially, her job was to screen doctors, nurses, and other staff-members desiring to access the building.

"Hello, Dr. Gonzalez," she said through a masked smile and proceeded to ask me the four key questions. "Do you have a cough?"

"No," I said mechanically.

"Any fevers?"

"No."

"Have you traveled recently?"

"No,"

"Have you come into contact with anyone who has traveled into a high-risk area?"

I shrugged, as I routinely did when asked this question. "I have no idea."

"Yeah, I know," she said as she whipped out her touchless thermometer. "That one's stupid." She flipped the thermometer towards my forehead as I leaned in. A moment later, the electronic beep. "Ninety-seven point seven, Dr. Gonzalez. You can go in."

Thanking her, I made my way to the locked door behind her and waved my ID at it, the clicking sound signaling its approval. I opened the door and stepped through.

Before me was a long hospital corridor lined with doors on either side, except this hallway, like so many hospital corridors I had come across recently, was empty. There was no one scurrying between rooms. There were no physicians gathering to discuss some vexing laboratory finding or X-ray. And no families keeping guard outside their loved ones' rooms. In short, the hospital was desolate.

I made my way past the nurse's station and to my patients' rooms. I had two patients to see that evening, each a fracture patient. Each was wearing a mask in an otherwise uninhabited room.

After visiting with them, my next step was to document my findings. For that, I went to the physician's lounge. It had a number of computers, sodas, and snacks, and most importantly, it was bound to be empty, ensuring that I would not be interrupted while writing my notes and entering my orders.

As the doctor's lounge door gave way to my ID, I was met by the blast of the televisions set. I was too tired to find the channel changer to either turn it down, or turn it off, so I decided I would do my best to ignore it. Besides, I was only going to be there for a few minutes. I grabbed my soda from the refrigerator, sat down, and logged into the computer. Only then did I notice it was CNN playing and that a bespectacled Anderson Cooper was delivering his monologue.

You would have thought President Trump had been dragged away in straps by the way Cooper described him. According to Cooper, the President had lost his marbles that night.

Intrigued, I swiveled away from the computer and watched. To hear Cooper say it, the President's conduct at that evening's daily COVID-19 press conference was nothing less than floridly unprofessional. Both his colleagues and he said the President had become "unhinged." That he had entered into a diatribe. They described him as angry when taking questions and irritable. They also reported that a video that the President had played, which CNN was not going to air because, according to Cooper, it was "propaganda," misstated facts and "tried to rewrite history."[521] According to Jim Acosta, who was interviewed by Cooper on the matter, the video "looked something out of Beijing or Pyongyang."[522]

On the 30-minute commute home, I worried about the President. Based on what I heard and seen on CNN, the President's behavior *had* to be offensive. Obviously, thought I, the President had finally had it.

When I got home, I found my wife waiting for me with my family. The first words out of her mouth were, "You missed Trump. He was awesome!"

I was stunned. How could he have been *awesome*??

I told them what I had heard and how surprised I was to hear their report. To this, all three responded that the President had done fine. It was the press that had been repulsive.

So I did what any non-interested physician with patients in three hospitals would do. I reviewed the video. My first impression was that the President's performance was nothing like CNN's portrayal. It appears the White House entered the meeting with the intent of dispelling a false narrative being delivered by the press and the Democrats that the President had been slow to respond to the pandemic.

The meeting opened with a few words from the President, who at two minutes and thirty-seven seconds, handed the microphone to Dr. Fauci.

As it turns out, the day prior, Fauci had appeared on CNN with Jake Tapper in *State of the Union*. At one point, Tapper articulated the growing narrative that lives would have been saved if "social distancing, physical distancing, stay-at-home measures, had started the third week February instead of mid-March," and whether Fauci thought this was true.

In real time, Dr. Fauci's answer was not inappropriate. He said,

You know Jake, again, it's the "What would have? What could have?" It's very difficult to go back and say that. I mean, obviously, you could logically say that if you had a process that was ongoing and you started mitigation earlier, you could have saved lives. Obviously. No one is going to deny that, but what goes into those kinds of decisions is complicated. But you're right. Obviously, if we had, right from the very beginning, shut everything down, it may have been a little bit different, but there was a lot of pushback about shutting things down back then.

That comment, as innocuously delivered by Fauci, was all the fodder the Left needed to unleash a false narrative against the President. Specifically, the observation that if mitigation had started much earlier, some people may have lived that ended up dying. First, the premise ignores the myriad of factors that go into making such a monumental decision. The President of the United States cannot just shut down a nation. There are constitutional issues involved. There are lives that will be impacted and even lost from engaging in such a plan.

On February 21, the third week of February to which Tapper alludes, there were 35 cases of COVID-19 in the United States and zero deaths. So, essentially, Tapper's question to Fauci was based on the absurd premise that the President of the United States should have engaged in a full effort to shut down the American economy when there were 15 people in a country of 331,000,000 suffering from an illness that had not yet caused any loss of life in the country. Imagine the response to a president who attempted to paralyze the nation under such statistics. Imagine the number of times a president would have brought the people's livelihoods to their knees under similar situations when, in fact, no health crisis was to develop. The very question was absurd, yet it was being treated as a serious inquiry by the press.

The day following the Tapper interview, a headline for an article in Vox Media was "Fauci Acknowledged a Delay in the US Coronavirus Response." Coincidentally or not, that same day President Trump retweeted a tweet that included a call to fire Fauci.[523]

Meanwhile, on April 10, *The New York Times* published an article entitled, "He Could Have Seen What Was Coming: Behind Trump's Failure on the Virus," claiming that the President had been warned about the potential of a pandemic and had done little about it.[524] And in *Business Insider*, the title for an article published on April 12 read, "Trump Reportedly Squandered 3 Crucial Weeks to Mitigate the Coronavirus Outbreak after a CDC Official's Blunt Warnings Spooked the Stock Market."[525]

Thus, we arrive at April 13. Based on the full-fledged assault that was materializing from the Left and aided by the press, the President had to respond, and the most appropriate person to clarify, other than the President, was Dr. Anthony Fauci himself.

So, two minutes and thirty-seven seconds into the briefing, Dr. Fauci made some brief comments as to the progression of the illness and how he believed that the incidence of cases was starting to level off. He then summarized his meeting with the Congressional Black Caucus regarding the issue of health disparities regarding COVID-19 in the African American community. And then he spoke about his comments with Tapper:

> *The other point I wanted to make is that I had, uh, an interview yesterday, that I was asked a hypothetical question, and hypothetical questions can sometimes get you into some difficulties because it's "What would have or could have?" The nature of the hypothetical question was if in fact we had mitigated earlier, could lives have been saved? And the answer to my question was, as I always do and I'm doing right now, to be perfectly honestly say, 'Yes." I mean obviously if. . you. . . mitigation helps, I've been up here many times telling you that mitigation works. So if mitigation works and you instigate it, and you initiate it earlier, you will probably have saved more lives. If you initiate it later, you probably would have lost more lives. You initiate it at a certain time.*

That was taken as a way that maybe somehow something was at fault here. So let me tell you from my experience, and I can only speak from my own experience, is that we have been talking before any meetings that we had about the pros and the cons, the effectiveness or not, of strong mitigations. So discussions were going on mostly among the medical people, about what that would mean. The first and only time that Dr. Birx and I went in and formally made a recommendation to the President, to actually have a quote shutdown in the sense of, not really shutdown, but to really have strong mitigation, we discussed it. Obviously there would be concern by some that in fact that might have some negative consequences. Nonetheless, the President listened to the recommendation and went to the mitigation. The next second time that I went with Dr. Birx into the President and said, 'Fifteen days are not enough. We need to go thirty days." Obviously, there were people who had a problem with that because of the potential secondary effects. Nonetheless, at that time, the President went with the health recommendations, and we extended it another thirty days. So, I can only tell you what I know and what my recommendations were, but clearly as happens all the time, there were interpretations of that response to a hypothetical question that I just thought that it would be very nice for me to clarify because I didn't have the chance to clarify. Thank you."

And with that, the narrative the press was trying to build about the President being irresponsible, or insensitive to the concerns of his experts imploded. Those in the White House Briefing Room immediately recognized the damage that had been perpetrated to their agenda and immediately tried to rehabilitate their witness and resuscitate their accusations. Their first question was about the timing of Fauci's recommendations. Because perhaps Dr. Fauci first approached the President about mitigation on January 31, and what he was referring to was the Chinese travel restrictions. If that were true, then the case could still be made that the President had stalled for six weeks, not just since the third week of February. But here again, Fauci's answer was devastating,

> *The travel restrictions is separate. That was whether or not we wanted to go into a mitigation stage of fifteen days of mitigation. The travel was another recommendation. When we went in and said, "We probably should be doing that," and the answer was yes. And then another time was, "We should do it with Europe," and the answer was yes. And the next time "We should do it with the UK," and the answer was yes."*

And of course, the last gasp of hope at some impropriety, some cover-up that would replicate Watergate. "Are you doing this voluntarily or did the President [. . ., inaudible]?"

This is where Dr. Fauci became offended. "No, I'm doing it. . . everything I do is voluntary. Please," he said with a disgusted look, "Don't even imply that." And Fauci walked away from the podium while maintaining a disgruntled stare at the reporter who had just questioned his veracity.

The President then methodically, but clearly on defense, provided the press with a timeline of the appearance of the virus, and his actions in response. His response had to be delivered in a defensive style because what the press had engaged in during the previous twenty-four hours was an assault on his judgment and the seriousness of his considerations regarding the protections the federal government could provide the American people. The President delivered his defense meticulously, calmly, and precisely. Yet the media called his defense a diatribe. As if somehow the President did not have the right to defend himself.

Astutely, the President then played a video, documenting the press's prior disapproval of his early actions where he was called a racist for having implemented them and showing the progress his team and he had made in combating the virus. That informative clip, openly designed to express an opinion, a defense of the President, lasted two minutes and thirty-seven seconds, and the press corps did not appreciate it.

Immediately, the focus turned to the potential for impropriety behind the video. Who made the video? How long did it take to produce this video? Was this a campaign video?

In one fell swoop, the President had destroyed the press's narrative that it had so meticulously built against him over the prior week. There was no cover-up. There was no fooling around. The President listened to his advisers. He led. His actions were reasonable, and more importantly, prompt, about as prompt as they could have been in light of the circumstances he was handed.

At that moment, the press recognized the President had won, again. It understood that April 13, 2020, was the day the President had defeated and eviscerated their latest false narrative aimed at taking him down in time for his reelection. They had failed, just as they had with the Russian collusion narrative, the Mueller investigation, and impeachment; victims of their own hateful narratives and fabricated accusations.

And they were furious, which explains what I saw on CNN when I entered the physicians' lounge. At the time I entered the conversation, the left-wing media was engaged in the only measure available to them: discrediting the President of the United States and making him look unstable before anyone who would listen.

The events of the 13th illustrate the immense hostility the press has harbored against the President. Not only does this type of open misrepresentation undermine the press's integrity, but if effective, it undermines the authority of the President of the United States at a moment in our history when it is most needed.

Let's look back to March 11. President Trump declares a national emergency and closes travel from Europe. At this point, there was still no concerted anti-Trump narrative from the press. The President then began holding daily press conferences with the CWHTF. Every day, the President personally appeared at the White House pressroom to discuss the latest developments on what he called "The War on the Coronavirus." For the public, such transparency and direct interaction with the President was unheard of. For the President and his public relations people, to have the leader of the free world out in front, interacting with the press, taking questions, and reporting all the things he was doing to save lives was genial. But it was so irritating to the press because the President, its archenemy, was using them to deliver his message! To a press so hateful to the President, such an arrangement could not be allowed to stand. They needed to come up with a potentially destructive message. But there was none. They had been asleep at the wheel, fixating on impeachment and whatever other implication of impropriety they could generate. And now, when the news suddenly became real, they were too drunk in the recklessness to react.

It was actually Nancy Pelosi who finally came up with the new narrative. "The President's denial at the beginning was deadly," she was quoted as saying on March 29, "As the President fiddles, people are dying."[526] Suddenly, the press had its marching orders. The President delayed in his response.

The very next day, Marik von Rennenkampff wrote, "America, in short, is in the midst of a first-world health care catastrophe. And Trump bears much of the blame."[527] Days later, David Remnick, editor at *The New Yorker*, remarked," Trump's delay would be 'paid in human lives.'"[528] On April 7, David Frum, a known Democrat partisan, came out with an accusatory article entitled "This Is

Trump's Fault; The President Is Failing, and Americans Are Paying for His Failures."[529] Indeed, the speed with which the stories began appearing and the monotony of their tone bespoke of their orchestrated nature. It truly was as if someone was telling the members of the mainstream media what the narrative should be and that the time had arrived for them to deliver it. Never mind that their new message was full of inconsistencies, rank hypocrisy, and unfairness to the President.

First, to the inconsistencies. How could the media attack the President of the United States for reacting too weakly when they themselves were minimizing the virus? On March 7, 2020, CNN Health ran an article claiming that the coronavirus mutations were "much ado about nothing."[530] On February 10, *The New York Times* published an article where it expressed the concern that Trump's alleged "extreme fear of germs, disdain for scientific and bureaucratic expertise, and suspicion of foreigners could be a dangerous mix."[531] Vox Media tweeted that the coronavirus was "[not] going to be a deadly pandemic,"[532] while *The Huffington Post* ridiculed Republican Senator Tom Cotton for advising Americans in China to "Get out-now," calling his reaction "a meltdown."[533]

Next, the hypocrisy. On January 28, Secretary of the Department of Health and Human Services Alex Azar said, "Americans should know this is a potentially very serious public health threat, but Americans should not worry for their own safety,"[534] while the Director of the CDC's National Center for Immunization and Respiratory Disease, Dr. Nancy Messonier said, "We have no evidence of human-to-human transmission in the United States."[535] Even Dr. Anthony Fauci, in an interview with Newsmax on January 21, said the coronavirus "is not a major threat to the people of the United States, and this is not something that the citizens of the United

States should be worried about right now."[536] And in case one claims these quotes to be inapplicable because they took place so early, recall that on February 24, Speaker Pelosi encouraging all to come to San Francisco, as we discussed earlier in this chapter.

And finally to the unfairness. The President was correct in his April 13, 2020, speech. It is absolutely unreasonable to hold a president accountable for not having instituted a full mitigation response to a disease at a time when the country knew of 35 confirmed cases and no deaths. To do so would have been an extreme overreaction and resulted in dire consequences to the United States, the American people, and its economy.

This particular virus took a mere three months to go from a distant unknown to a full-fledged disaster. To say that the President ought to have foreseen the ravaging consequences of the virus upon the American people in February is to have ascribed to him supernatural powers that neither he nor his advisors possess. The fact is that the President generally acted with appropriate speed and diligence. On January 31, less than two weeks after the entry of the first case of SARS-CoV-2 into the United States, the President implemented travel restrictions from China, and on March 11, the same day the World Health Organization called the outbreak a global pandemic, President Trump declared a national emergency and shut down travel from Europe. He then mobilized the production of ventilators in anticipation of the exhaustion of the nation's supply and then diligently moved to the production of equipment, the procurement of medications, and the construction of hospitals with the mobilization of associated personnel. Finally, he mobilized the nation's testing capacity to levels that had not previously been seen. Although there is always room for critiques and suggestions for improvement, none of his actions merited the vitriolic response from the press.

But the press failed in more ways than merely the manner in which it covered the President. It failed in the manner in which it covered substantive issues related to the Wuhan pandemic. One example is its coverage of chloroquine and hydroxychloroquine. As we covered previously, information began trickling as early as January that these two antimalarial medications could have a positive role in the treatment and prevention of COVID-19. Behind the scenes, physicians had been hearing of the favorable experiences encountered with these medications and how some centers were using them not just in the treatment of the disease, but in its prevention.

On March 16, Dr. Phillippe Gautret and Dr. Didier Raoult, infectious disease experts from Marseille, published their experience with hydroxychloroquine and azithromycin on MedRxIv.org, a website dedicated to the publication of non-peer-reviewed, scientific literature.[537] The study received wide publicity when Gregory Rigano, an adviser to the Stanford University School of Medicine's SPARK Translational Research Program announced on March 18 on Fox News's Tucker Carlson Tonight, the promising implications of the study's findings, including saying that this represented the second time where a cure had been found for a virus.[538]

The response from the press to Raoult's study was initially muted with only some small outlets giving it much attention. Medscape called the results "encouraging," and appropriately suggested the results should be viewed with caution.[539] *The Washington Examiner* neutrally reported the story, including Rigano's appearance of Fox.[540] And *Forbes* reported President Trump's announcement that "the FDA was fast-tracking the use of hydroxychloroquine and other anti-viral drugs for COVID-19 patients."[541]

Then, on March 19, President Trump touted the potential benefits of hydroxychloroquine in his daily CWHTF briefing, calling it a potential game-changer.[542] The President also tweeted about the combination of hydroxychloroquine and azithromycin on March 21, stating, "HYDROXYCHLOROQUINE & AZITHROMY-CIN, taken together, have a real chance to be one of the biggest game-changers in the history of medicine. The FDA has moved mountains—Thank You! Hopefully they will BOTH."[543]

Inexplicably, the narrative immediately changed. *Bloomberg* emphasized that the FDA had not approved hydroxychloroquine for the treatment of COVID-19.[544] *Business Insider* claimed that Trump was "creating a 'dangerous situation' by promoting an unproven coronavirus treatment."[545] And other outlets, like Politico, concentrated on the medication's potentially "dangerous side effects."[546] And by April 13, *The Hill* and *The Washington Post* were reporting that the CIA had warned its employees against their use because of their potential side effects.[547]

The press's staked position had become clear. It was going to zealously report against the potential role of a medication known to be safe and was demonstrating some promising results in a time-sensitive, but uncharted field. And the only thing that had changed from the time of Dr. Zaoult's enthusiastic report was the mere fact that President Trump was touting it. Indeed, the inquiries to the President during his nearly daily CWHTF Briefings reached such a level of raucous repetition that they could only be described as harassment.

"Mr. President, why do you tout a medication that has not been approved by the FDA?"

"Mr. President, don't you think you're endangering the public by recommending a medication that has been said to have serious side effects? "

"Mr. President, isn't it true that hydroxychloroquine can kill patients?"

"Mr. President, how do you respond to allegations that you have blood on your hands because of your recommendations for the use of hydroxychloroquine?"

And my personal favorite, "Mr. President, are you a doctor?"

And of course, the attacks upon the President became intensified after the misguided ingestion of fish tank cleaner by a couple in Arizona.

A related issue arose on April 21 when the National Institutes of Health (NIH) added more fuel to the press's attack upon the President by publishing its guidelines for the treatment of COVID-19 infections. In each case, from asymptomatic patients to those with severe disease, the NIH said, "There are insufficient data to recommend either for or against any antiviral or immunodilatory therapy in patients with COVID-19 [insert severity of illness]."[548] In the therapeutic options section of their guidelines, the NIH stated, "At present, no drug has been proved to be safe and effective for treating COVID-19."[549]

There are no Food and Drug Administration (FDA)-approved drugs specifically to treat patients with COVID-19. Regarding the use of chloroquine and hydroxychloroquine, the NIH panel again stated, "There are insufficient clinical data to recommend either for or against using **chloroquine** or **hydroxychloroquine** for the treatment of COVID-19 **(AIII)**,"[x, 550] and cautioned, "If chloroquine or hydroxychloroquine is used, clinicians should monitor the patient for adverse effects, especially prolonged QTC intervals **(AIII)**."[551] But amazingly, later on in its webpage, the panel went on to state,

---

[x] AIII is a rating assigned to the recommendation by the Panel. "A" means that there is a strong recommendation for the statement, and "III" means it is an "expert opinion." "Introduction COVID-19 Treatment Guidelines, "NIH, accessed Apr. 21, 2020, https://covid19treatmentguidelines.nih.gov/therapeutic-options-under-investigation/.

"Except in the context of a clinical trial, the COVID-19 Treatment Guidelines Panel (the Panel) **recommends against** the use of the following drugs for the treatment of COVID-19: The combination of **hydroxychloroquine plus azithromycin (AIII)** because of the potential for toxicities; **Lopinavir/ritonavir (AI)** or other **HIV protease inhibitors (AIII)** because of unfavorable pharmacodynamics and negative clinical trial data.[xi, 552]

Why the NIH would publish a statement in opposition to a treatment it has repeatedly stated it could neither endorse nor oppose is vexing. The statement, at best is confusing. At worst, it expresses an unsubstantiated opposition to the treatment. In fact, in covering the NIH's announcement the inconsistency of the panel's statement is the story, but instead, the medias' coverage focused on the confrontation. NPR's headline on the story is, "NIH Panel Recommends Against Drug Combination Promoted By Trump For COVID-19."[553] *Forbes* wrote, "NIH Panel Recommends Against Using Hydroxychloroquine and Azithromycin, Drug Combination Touted By Trump."[554] And The Hill reported, "NIH panel recommends against use of hydroxychloroquine and azithromycin to treat COVID-19."[555] Although each article quotes the President extensively and in a negative light, only the NPR article quoted any of the panel members: "'It's all based on the data,' said panel member Dr. Susan Swindells, a professor in the department of internal medicine at the University of Nebraska College of Medicine. 'We just plowed through everything that was, and apart from supportive care, there wasn't anything that was working terribly well.'"[556]

[xi] Lopinavir/ritonavir or other HIV protease inhibitors have not been covered extensively in this text because the author has not come across studies showing significant advantages of using these medications in the treatment of COVID-19.

The natural and more important question is, why, in the face of an admission of the cursory nature of the review of the data, with no evidence that anything is "working terribly well," and acknowledging there is insufficient evidence to make a determination one way or another would Dr. Swindell agree to a recommendation *against* a treatment?

But the press will never ask this question despite the fact that since publishing this statement the NIH has engaged in a massive study involving 2,000 adults to look at the applicability of hydroxychloroquine in the treatment of COVID-19.[557] Indeed, it seems that through its coverage of the medication and its potential benefits, the press lost its objectivity and instead concentrated its efforts on finding ways of discrediting the President.

Yet, the press's unfailing anti-Trump, and at times, anti-American bias, did not stop with its reporting on the risks of taking a tiny white pill. It extended to a concerted effort at minimizing the numerous misdeeds on the part of the Chinese government. Consider this story from CNN published on April 15, 2020:

> *The coronavirus outbreak, which began in the Chinese city of Wuhan in December last year, has spread to more than 180 countries and sickened close to 2 million people, including more than 80,000 in China. Yet according to the Chinese government, not a single serving member of the country's military has been infected.*
>
> *The reported absence of cases among China's armed forces comes despite the fact that thousands of military personnel were sent to Wuhan to assist in front line medical efforts. It also comes in sharp contrast to other military powers, notably the United States, which have seen an uptick in cases in recent weeks.*
>
> *As if to underscore this point, China's official military news agency has taken to proclaiming the navy's operational readiness in the face of the global pandemic. Earlier this week, a report detailing*

the deployment of a Chinese naval flotilla to the Pacific was offered
as evidence that the People's Liberation Army Navy has reportedly
done a better job controlling coronavirus than the US Navy.[xii]

CNN's face-value acceptance of a Chinese report and the willful repackaging of its contents served as a mouthpiece for Chinese propaganda. Not until eleven paragraphs of unchallenged pro-Chinese rhetoric does the author cast any doubt upon the veracity of the information by writing, "US observers have cast doubt on the PLA's claims that its naval operations have not been impacted by the virus."[558] As we have demonstrated repeatedly in this volume, there is incontrovertible evidence that China has repeatedly lied regarding the course of the Wuhan pandemic. From its indefensible claims of the absence of human-to-human transmission despite the lack of association between many of its patients with the Wuhan Wholesale Seafood Market to the explanation of a bat in the market as being the source of zoological transmission when no bats were sold at the Wuhan market at the time of the initial cases, to the concealment of its data from the rest of the world at a time when transparency could have saved lives, and its claim that no close contacts had contracted the disease while Dr. Li lay dying in a Chinese hospital, China's reporting of the developments regarding SARS-CoV-2 within its borders has been so brazenly disingenuous as to nullify any claims it may make about its navy's readiness or any success in the control of the virus's spread. To blindly accept its claims is to provide China with an authenticity it does not deserve. The liberal press's willingness to repeat this nefarious regime's claims stands as nothing less

---

[xii] Brad Lendon, "Chinese State Media Claims Country's Navy Is Not Affected by Coronavirus," CNN (blog), Apr. 15, 2020, accessed Apr. 17, 2020, https://www.cnn.com/2020/04/13/asia/china-coronavirus-aircraft-carrier-deployment-dp-hnk-intl/index.html.

than a zealous cooperation in the promotion of the Chinese global agenda.

And lest we forget, the press has been complicit with the Chinese in obfuscating any possibility of Chinese malfeasance in the development and spread of SARS-CoV-2. The mainstream media has repeatedly defended, not just reported, but defended, the position that the SARS-CoV-2 is the product of a naturally occurring mutation allowing it to be not only transmitted from a bat to humans, but also between humans. When questions were asked regarding the close association between the Wuhan market and two advanced biological laboratories, one of which was of the highest certifiable security levels in the world, the press did all it could to ridicule those who even cared to inquire.

Among the earliest skeptics was Senator Tom Cotton, a Republican from Arkansas, who on January 28, 2020, sent a letter to Secretary of Health and Human Services, Alex Azar, and Acting Secretary of Homeland Security Chad Wolf. The letter followed an earlier one sent to Azar on January 22. The January 28 letter called for an investigation into China's handling of the emerging Wuhan pandemic, stating, "Further, Chinese researchers have provided strong evidence in *The Lancet* that this coronavirus did not originate in the Wuhan seafood market, contrary to the official Chinese line. This evidence doesn't just cast doubt on Chinese reporting, but also suggests the risk of infectious pathways outside the seafood market."[559] Cotton also declared, "To the extent additional money or legal authorities are needed for a Manhattan Project-level effort to create a vaccine, I stand ready to assist in the Congress."[560]

His comments were reasonable and called for, but the castigatory reaction from the press was fierce and swift. On January 31, 2020, *The Huffington Post* released an article urging Americans not to listen to Cotton.[561] Stating that "health experts have rejected the suggestion that the virus is the result of some sort of bioweapon or manufactured cause," they dismissed his allegations as "fear mongering" and a "fringe theory."[562] They also suggested Cotton's "Manhattan-styled project" comment was part of "an absolute tear" on the Senator's part.[563] In short, the press's handling of the events regarding this pandemic has left all wondering whether they can even be trusted.

The answer, to America's great misfortune, is it cannot.

The Reopening

By April 30, the last day of the President's 30 Days to Flatten the Curve extension, the economy lay in ruins. The stock market was at 24,345.72. Over 30 million people were unemployed, and the GDP had gone from a consistent two to three percent increase to a drop of 4.8%. If there was one overarching conclusion, it was that the circumstance in which the United States found itself was unsustainable. Mental health concerns were increasing throughout the nation. Polling data was revealing that a larger share of Americans was reporting negative mental health impacts compared to pre-coronavirus times, [564] and many feared the compounding effects of the Wuhan pandemic on the ongoing opioid crisis in the United States.[565]

Another interesting negative consequence of the economic shutdown was to the health of the American public. In an effort to conserve resources and make sure that hospital beds would remain available, the CDC recommended that nonessential procedures not be performed in the nation's hospitals and surgery centers. Throughout the nation, governors and state health departments issued orders restricting them from performing anything other than emergent or urgent procedures. Some even prohibited doctors' offices from engaging in the nonessential care of patients. These orders coupled with images from New York and New Jersey showing hospitals overwhelmed with COVID-19 patients led people to stay away from hospitals and their doctors altogether.

But instead of being overrun with COVID-19 patients, hospitals throughout the nation lay barren. More importantly the incidence of events whose occurrence remained unchanged precipitously dropped. For example, the presentations for chest pain in the emergency rooms of my region's hospitals precipitously dropped. Cancer screenings were "way down."[566] Cancer treatments, particularly for slowly progressing ones like prostate cancer, were delayed. People were so scared of coming near the hospital due to potential exposures to SARS-CoV-2 they were having their heart attacks at home. For all these patients, whether they had been identified or not, a return to some state of normal operations was a matter of life or death.

But how should the nation reopen and when? There was a slew of opinions regarding the answer to these questions. Some advocated for a continued economic shutdown until the development of a vaccine.[567] Others argued that the United States needed to ramp up testing to the tune of 20 million tests per month before opening could be a consideration.[568] Still others felt the economy should be opened immediately. With such a diverging breadth of opinions, the only conclusion arrived at with certainty is that there was going to be no consensus as to how the "return to normalcy" was going to take place.

Predictably, the epidemiologists and public health experts wanted a structured approach to the reopening process. Politicians, on the other hand, were split mostly amongst political parties. Republicans were more apt to favor a rapid return to business. Democrats wanted

to return to business slowly, and although some on the Left articulated reasoned plans, others would get into trouble, as their hesitation
to reopen clashed with their constituents' desires. The President and
the CWHTF took a passive approach. President Trump's underlying
philosophy was that the economy needed to be reopened and was
opposed to the idea of extending the nation's shutdown. However,
he astutely recognized the varying situations afflicting the states and
thus understood that the solution for one state may not be viable for
another.

On April 16, the President unveiled his plan for reopening the
country. Although the CDC and he provided guidelines, the decisions regarding speed and aggressiveness were left up to the governors.[569] Essentially, the President laid out a three-step plan with
a series of criteria for each that would facilitate decision making
for the nation's governors.[570] In Phase One, vulnerable individuals would continue to shelter in place while all individuals were
requested to continue observing social distancing and avoiding
gatherings of more than ten people. Additionally, nonessential
travel should be minimized.[571] Employers in Phase One were encouraged to "telework," minimize travel, and close common areas
where personnel tend to congregate.[572] Under Phase One, schools
would remain closed, large venues restricted, gyms could open only
under certain criteria, bars would remain closed, and elective cases
could resume.[573] "States and regions,"[574] however, were asked not to
enter Phase One until they had a downward trend of flu-like and
COVID-like illnesses lasting a fortnight as well as an equally long
downward curve of new documented cases. They were also advised
to ascertain that their hospitals were able to "treat all patients without crisis care,"[575] and have a "robust testing program in place for
at-risk healthcare workers."[576]

Phase Two was recommended for "states and regions" that had entered Phase One and were demonstrating no evidence of a rebound. Here, gathering restrictions were increased to 50 and nonessential travel could resume. Schools could reopen, and bars may resume operating.[577]

Finally, Phase Three was reserved for states with no evidence of rebounding "and satisf[ied] the gating criteria a third time."[578] In Phase Three, vulnerable individuals could resume public interactions, but with caution, and low-risk populations should "consider minimizing time spent in crowded environments."[579]

Like everything else, the President's plan was met with great disparagement from the press. About the mildest critiques came from those claiming it was vague and lacked target dates.[580] Others criticized the plan for not implementing concrete testing requirements. Many were appalled that the President did not demand testing rates of 20 to 30 million per day before reopening.[581] A key component of the criticism against the President's reopening plan is the lack of a tracking and isolation strategy.[582] These proponents thought there was a roll for strong federal government oversight inclusive of implementing plans and granting permission for regions or states to move to the next stage. And of course, the chorus of those claiming that President Trump's plan would cost lives blared anew.

For their part, the people of the United States were eager to get back to some form of normalcy. Although polls like one by ABC News/Ipsos indicated that Americans were resistant to reopening by a margin of 30 points,[xiii, 583] the conduct about the country said otherwise.[584] Protests became more common and intense in areas perceived as hesitating in reopening. Regardless of what polls may

[xiii] Significantly, that poll of 532 general population adults did not disclose the ideological stance of its subjects or their party affiliations.

have been showing the growing message amongst political activists was that it was time to get back to work.

It was among the various governors that the divide regarding reopening became more palpable. Brian Kemp, from Georgia, was the first to lead his state on an aggressive campaign to reopen. Even though the state had not achieved the two weeks downslope on cases, Kemp ordered that businesses could reopen.[585] The move was viewed as too aggressive, even by President Trump, who publicly expressed his dissatisfaction with the Governor.[586] Nevertheless, in Georgia, businesses such as gymnasiums, restaurants, movie theaters, and hair salons reopened,[587] and in response, there was no rise in the number of daily cases,[588] nor was there an increase in the number of COVID-19 related deaths.[589] In fact, cases and deaths decreased.

Many states, Republican ones in particular, quickly followed. In Florida, a relaxation on business restrictions began on May 4.[590] Alaska reopened on April 24.[591] Arizona instituted a partial reopening on May 4.[592] And Colorado, a Democrat state, began its partial reopening on April 27.[593] In fact, by May 13, there were only 10 states that had not relaxed their restrictions, and except for Maryland and New Hampshire, all were Democrat states.[594]

In the meantime, the media continued to display their leftist bias and blared against these efforts. Jill Filipovic, in an article published by CNN, called the moves to reopen the country "utter idiocy,"[595] while claiming that these governors were "endangering American lives."[596] In another CNN piece, Yaneer Bar-Yam urged Americans to "save yourselves, your families and your communities by staying at home and ignoring your governor's 'ludicrous' policies."[597] Once again their one-sided, overtly biased reporting/opining ignored the complexities of the realities before them.

Some states ran into trouble over their reticence to reopen. In California, the opportunity for municipalities to extend stay-at-home orders was itself extended *indefinitely*![598] Of course, one questions whether the California executive branch even has the authority to issue a stay-at-home order without an endpoint. Although the governor's right to issue a stay-at-home order in the State of California was recently upheld, an order without an end date poses a totally different constitutional question.[599] Similarly, Los Angeles County's order has stumbled onto the same constitutional question when it extended its stay-at-home order until further notice.[600]

Michigan has also demonstrated hostility to reopening. There, Governor Gretchen Whitmer extended her Stay-At-Home Order until May 28.[601] Protesters responded by voicing their displeasure including openly carrying semi-automatic rifles inside the Capitol. During one rally held on May 14 outside the Capitol,[602] things got so intense that a scuffle ensued when a man holding an ax attempted to pry a flag with a nude female doll hanging from it from a protestor.[603]

Despite the intensity of the demonstrations, polls have indicated broad public support for Governor Whitmer regarding her handling of the pandemic,[604] but the Michigan State Legislature is having none of it. It took the Governor to court claiming that her extension was illegal since she lacks the authority to extend emergency orders beyond 28 days pursuant to a 1976 Michigan law.[605] Interestingly, the governor had sought the legislature's authorization on April 7 in order to extend the emergency executive orders till April 30. However, when the April 30 deadline arrived and the legislature had not yet acted, the Governor extended her emergency order on her own accord.[606] The matter is presently before the court.

A similar judicial confrontation is taking place in Wisconsin. On April 16, with the state having less than 3,555 confirmed cases and 170 deaths, the Department of Health Services extended Democratic Governor Tony Evers' Safer at-Home Order from its natural expiration of April 24 to May 26.[607] The Governor supported the action by stating, "Things won't get back to normal until there's a vaccine and treatment for this disease."[608] But Governor Evers' order was not made in accordance with the rulemaking procedures laid out under Wisconsin statutes and failed to comply with laws requiring the legislature's participation in orders invoking criminal sanctions.[609] Recall, this is the same governor who had issued an executive order suspending in-person voting the day prior to the election that was subsequently overturned by the judiciary.[610]

Governor Evers' extension was met with immediate public opposition. Initially, 700 protesters were expected to assemble in Madison. However, by the morning following the announcement, participation rose to 2400.[611]

And the outcry was met with governmental support. Sheriff Christopher Schmaling of Racine County refused to comply with the Governor's extended order, stating that he "could not in good faith participate in the destruction of Racine County businesses or interfere in the freedoms granted to all by our Constitution."[612] The Sheriff "would leave the enforcement of public health orders to health department officials."[613] The Republican legislature has also agreed with the protesters, arguing that the Governor had extended his statutorily prescribed authority and took him to court where the Supreme Court blocked the order.[614]

Other actions were a lot more personal. In Michigan, a barber had his license revoked because he refused to comply with the governor's order.[615] In defense of his actions, Karl Manke, the 77-year-old barber, said he needed to continue working. "The government is not my mother," he was quoted as saying. "I've been in business longer than they've been alive."[616]

In Hawaii, a New York tourist visiting the state was arrested for violating the mandatory 14-day quarantine requirement.[617] The evidence used against him? His Instagram photos depicting him at the beach holding a surfboard, sunbathing, and walking Waikiki at night.[618]

And in New York, in what is one of the most poignant displays of police overreach, a woman in the subway was forcibly arrested for not wearing a mask while her very young child is ripped away from her and helplessly looks on.[619]

In Ventura County, Dr. Robert Levin, the county's Health Director announced that the municipality was going to begin tracking individuals, who have tested positive for COVID-19, apparently regardless of their consent will get tracked, and the government will "make sure that they remain quarantined" making it "less and less possible for others in the county to run into someone with COVID-19 infection."[620] What's more, in those case where a one family member is infected with COVID-19, but the family shared the same bathroom, the authorities would removing the uninfected members into other kinds of housing that the municipality would have available.[621]

But among the most ominous cases was that of Shelley Luther, a salon owner who was imprisoned for the crime of opening her business. Luther had been forced to shut down her business on March 22 in response to an order from Texas Governor Greg Abbott. By April, Governor Abbott had allowed for the partial reopening of Texas businesses including restaurants and shopping malls, but hair salons were not yet allowed to reopen. Luther opened her salon anyway and on April 24 was presented with a cease and desist order from Dallas police.[622] Luther disobeyed and was arrested.

During her hearing, the judge called Luther "selfish," and told her she could avoid incarceration if she apologized for her "selfishness" and closed her salon. Luther's response was the retort heard around America. "I have to disagree with you, sir, when you say I'm selfish, because feeding my kids is not selfish. So, sir, if you think the law's more important than kids getting fed, then please, go ahead with your decision. But I am not going to shut the salon."[623]

And there it was, the conflict gripping America distilled down to its essence. The government and all the powers that be were trying to shut down the American people, but in so doing, they were paralyzing them and destroying everything for which they had worked. Instead of aiding Americans, the government was hurting them in a manner never before seen in this country. The question was whether this was a nation of liberty and free enterprise, or was it a country run by an autocracy free to demand everything from its citizens. The nation had given its all to control an emergency outbreak that was now becoming a protracted reality. But the government-certain governments-entrenched in the impossible effort to prevent even one tragedy was effectuating the ruin of all.

For a moment, it looked like the autocracy would prevail in the Luther case. The judge coldly sentenced her to seven days in jail and fined her $7,000,[624] and West Texan authorities charged eight others throughout the state with criminal charges for similar infractions.[625] As she was led to her cell, it appeared that Luther would be yet another victim of an overwhelming tide of power centralization and the belittling of American ideals.

But then the American people reacted. A GoFundMe page was set up by a group called Woke Patriots[626] raising over $500,000 in a matter of days.[627] The more conservative press reported on the seemingly absurd results. The Texas Attorney General called the sentence a political stunt, even though it was expressly allowed in the Governor's order, and "urged" the judge to release Luther.[628] A group of Texas judges retaliated in kind by calling the Attorney General "inappropriate" and his comment "unwelcomed."[629] Meanwhile, the Lieutenant Governor offered to serve a house arrest sentence in Luther's stead and pay her $7,000 fine.[xiv]

Despite the judges' disdain, the Governor recognized the absurdity of his own directive and modified it to prohibit confinement as punishment. On May 7, after serving two days in jail, Luther was ordered released by the Texas Supreme Court. Bitingly, hair salons were officially allowed to reopen, per executive order, at 12:01 in the morning, the very next day.[630]

[xiv] Texas Lieutenant Governor Dan Patrick ultimately contributed $7,000 to Luther's GoFundMe page.

Chapter 5

Trends and Correlations

From the data assembled, some early insights can be obtained regarding the proclivities of the Wuhan pandemic and the effectiveness of our responses. Of course, a proper, scientific evaluation requires much more data than we have time to acquire and much more sophisticated analysis that we are capable of performing here. Nevertheless, some interesting trends and correlations are developing allowing us to arrive at some preliminary conclusions.

Methods

The team at Healthcare Policy Solutions performed univariate analyses looking at the effects of a country's national healthcare ranking, per capita GDP, physician density, population density, number of tests per capita, and life expectancy on per capita COVID-19 cases and deaths. We selected the countries with the one hundred highest numbers of COVID-19 cases on May 2, 2020, according to Woldometer.com, and compared their numbers with the nation's healthcare ranking, per capita GDP, physician presence, population density, per capita testing numbers, and life expectancy. For the demographic data, we relied on data published by the World Bank. Specifically, for the per-capita GPD, we used the World Bank figures for 2018.[631] For physician presence, we used the most recently published numbers to a maximum of a decade number for physicians per 1000 citizens of each country.[632] For population density and life expectancy, we used the World Bank's 2018 figures.[633, 634] For the per capita testing, we relied on the data published by Worldometer.com as of May 2, 2020.[635] Although dated, we used the healthcare ranking published by the WHO in 2000, the last year it was done to determine each nation's standing with regard to its quality of healthcare.[636] All data visualizations and analyses were made using Tableau.[637] For scanograms, the appropriate trendline was applied to each visualization and determined its R^2 value or how well each set of data fit the various points on the graph. The p-value, or the probability value, which measures the possibility that the measured events occurred purely by chance, were also calculated. A p-value of less than 0.05 is usually considered to represent a non-random event and is given the designation of being "statistically significant." In other words, the correlation could not be readily explained as a purely random event.

Results

We found statistically significant correlations between a country's cases per capita and its deaths per capita and its life expectancy.

The correlation best fitting the cases per million and the life expectancy of citizens and cases per million was exponential with an R^2 and p-value of 0.458 with and p value of <0.0001 (Figure 5.1). Similarly, deaths per million had an exponential relationship with a nation's life expectancy with an R^2 of 0.422 and p-value of <0.0001 (Figure 5.2). Accordingly, as the nation's life expectancy increased, its per capita cases and per capita deaths increased exponentially.

Similarly, there was a statistically significant exponential correlation between the number of cases and deaths per million and the number of physicians per 1000 citizens, achieving an R^2 of 0.328 and p-value of <0.0001 for deaths (Figure 5.3) and an R^2 and p-value of 0.28 with a p value of <0.0001 for cases (Figure 5.4). Perhaps in contradiction to the intuitive expectation, the number of deaths and cases per capita actually exponentially increased for each country as the number of physicians increased. There was also a direct, linear relationship between a nation's GDP and its per capita cases. The R^2 was 0.484 with a p-value <0.0001 (Figure 5.5). For the correlation between per capita GDP and the deaths per million in the population, the relationship was exponential with an R^2 of 0.336 and a p-value of < 0.0001 (Figure 5.6). Again, the general pattern is the wealthier a nation is as measured by its per capita GDP, the more likely people in that nation were to contract COVID-19 and to die from it.

The healthcare rankings were also statistically correlated to the deaths and cases per capita, only inversely so. There was a power relationship between the nation's healthcare ranking and its deaths per million with an R^2 of 0.339 and a p-value of 0<.0001 (Figure 5.7). For the healthcare rankings and cases per million, the R^2 value was 0.373 with a p-value of <0.0001 (Figure 5.8). The higher the country's ranking, the worse its population faired with regard to deaths per capita and cases per capita.

We also looked at the relationship between a nation's per capita testing efforts and the number of cases and deaths per capita. Here there was an exponential correlation between the number of tests per capita and the number of cases (R^2 and p-value of 0.322 and a p value of <0.0001; Figure 5.9) and only a mild exponential correlation between tests per million and the number of deaths (R^2 and p-value of 0.097 and p-value =0.0022) as an exponential relationship (Figure 5.10). Again the relationship was direct for cases and deaths so that the greater the access to tests in a particular nation, the greater the number of cases per capita and the greater the number of deaths per capita.

There were no correlations between the number of cases or deaths per capita and population density.

Figure 5-1: Correlation Between Life Expectancy (2018) and Cases/1M Population

Life Expectancy (2018) vs Cases/ 1M Population

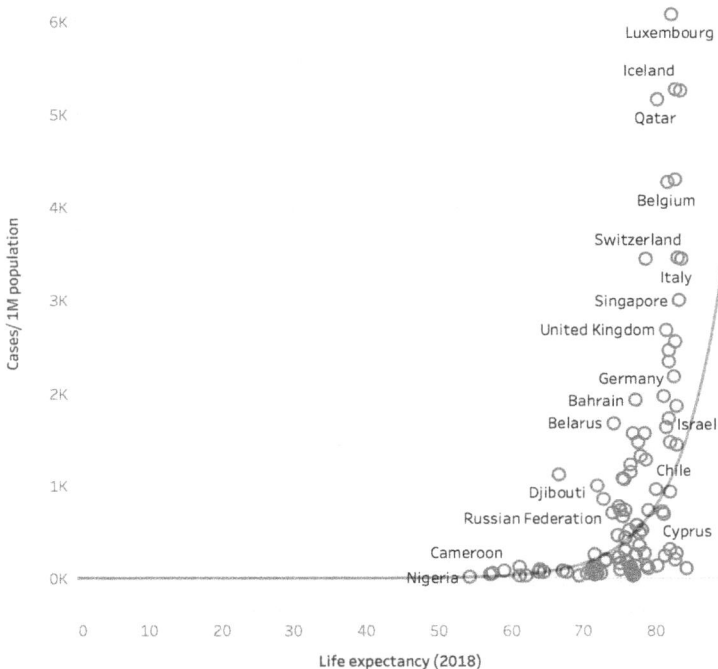

Figure 5-2: Correlation Between Life Expectancy (2018) and Deaths/1M Population

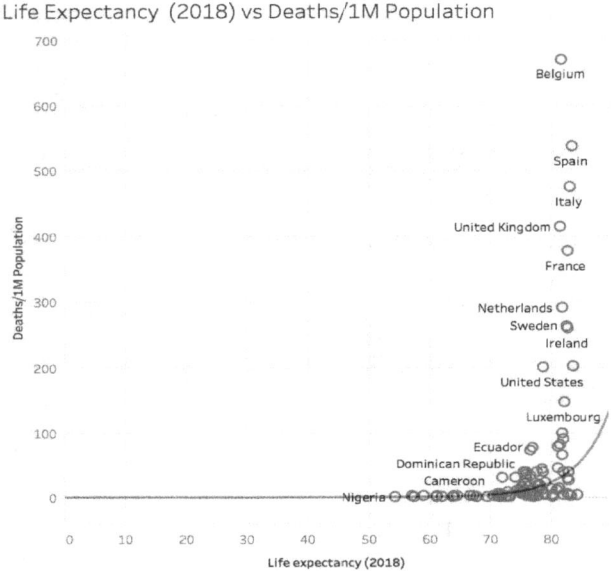

Life Expectancy (2018) vs Deaths/1M Population

Figure 5-3: Correlation Between Physicians/1,000 and Deaths/1M Population

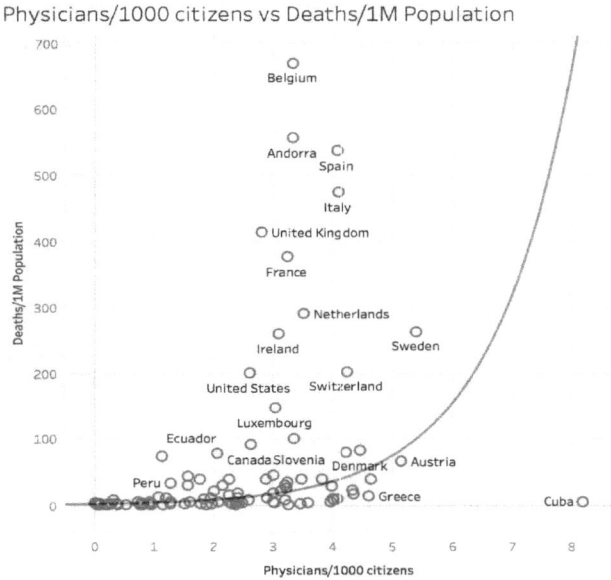

Physicians/1000 citizens vs Deaths/1M Population

Figure 5-4: Correlation Between Physicians/1,000 and Cases/1M Population

Physicians/1000 citizens vs Cases/1M Population

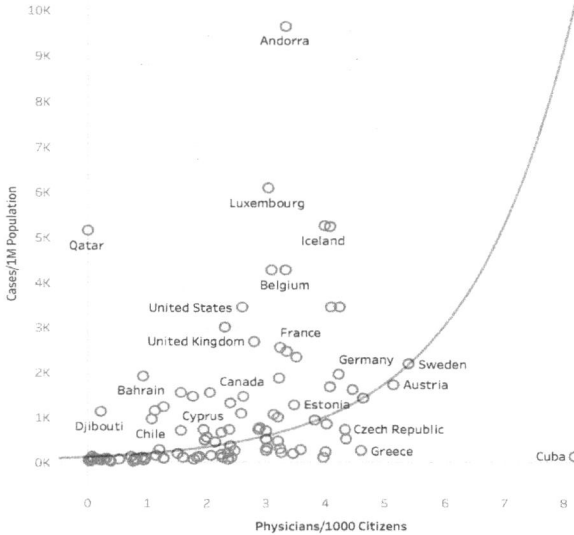

Figure 5-5: Correlation Between Per Capita GDP and Cases/1M Population

GDP Per Capita (2018) vs Cases/1M Population

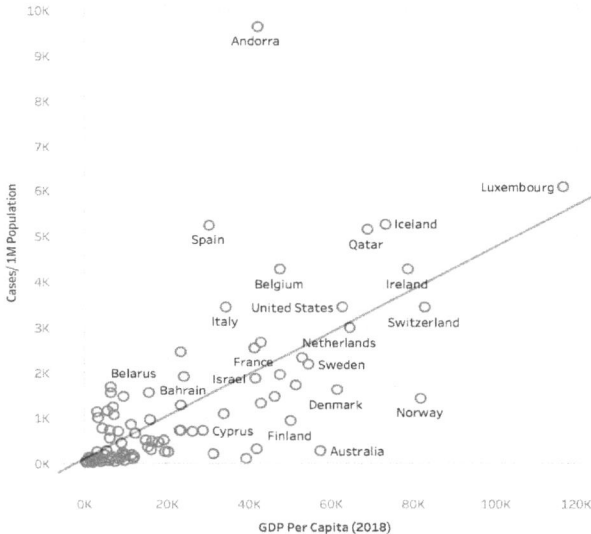

Figure 5-6: Correlation Between Per Capita GDP and Deaths/1M Population

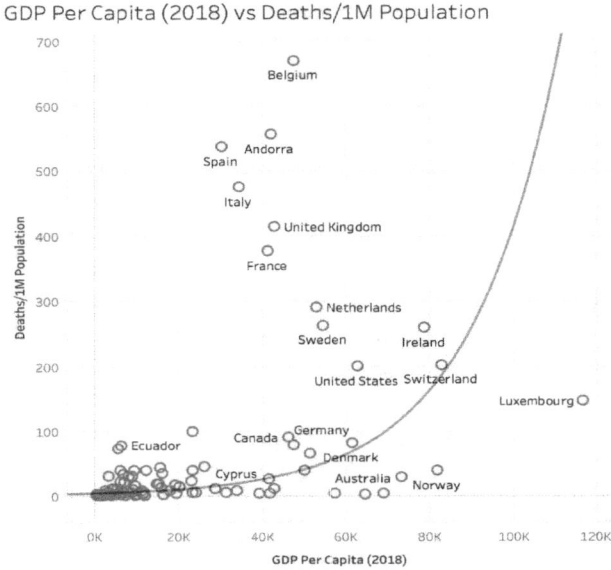

GDP Per Capita (2018) vs Deaths/1M Population

Figure 5-7: Correlation Between Healthcare Rankings and Deaths/1M Population

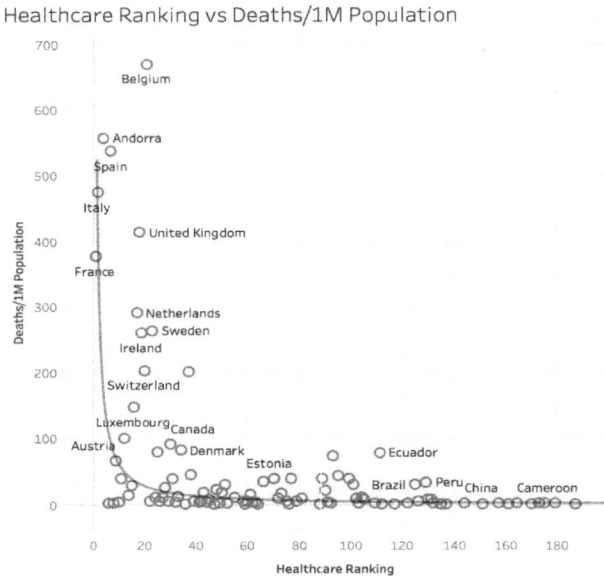

Healthcare Ranking vs Deaths/1M Population

180

Figure 5-8: Correlation Between Healthcare Rankings and Cases/1M Population

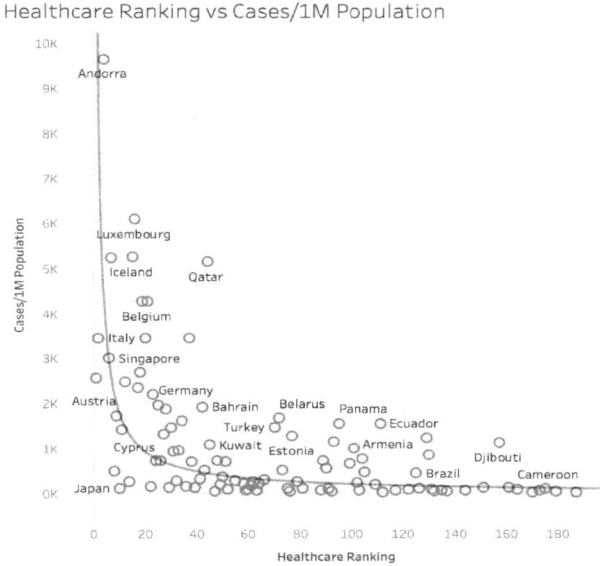

Healthcare Ranking vs Cases/1M Population

Figure 5-9: Correlation Between Per Capita Tests and Cases/1M Population

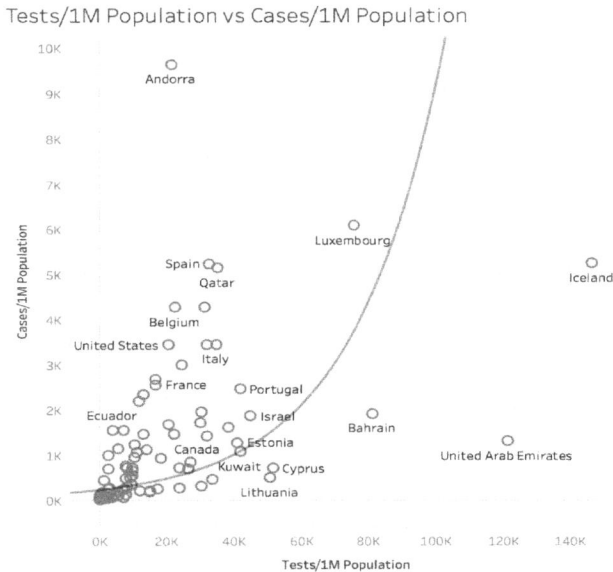

Tests/1M Population vs Cases/1M Population

181

Figure 5-10: Correlation Between Per Capita Tests and Deaths/1M Population

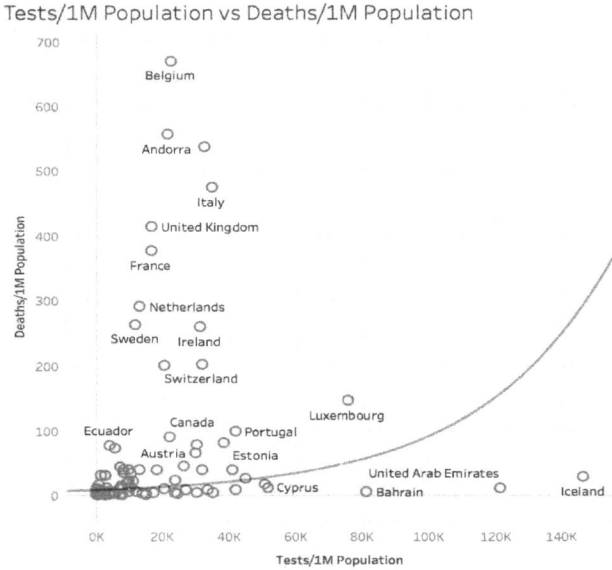

Tests/1M Population vs Deaths/1M Population

Conclusions

At the outset, it must be noted that our data is very preliminary. Advanced and more definitive conclusions based on SARS-CoV-2's behavior and spread awaits the accumulation of data maturation and further, much more sophisticated, multivariate analysis. Nevertheless, early on, certain preliminary conclusions can be made and directions in which to take further inquiries can be identified. For starters, it is remarkable that the nations with the higher number of physicians per capita, superiorly ranked healthcare systems and higher numbers of per capita testing faired worse. Specifically, in regard to per capita testing, one could expect a higher number of identified cases in countries where more tests were conducted because these countries ought to naturally capture a high percentage of actual cases compared to those that would be less aggressive about testing. However, this hypothesis would not apply to deaths, which are also higher in countries conducting more tests per capita. It would therefore seem that more aggressive national testing programs do not prevent COVID-19 deaths.

In fact, there are two interrelated factors that seem to be predictive of all other correlations, although the question of which is that the primary driver of cases and deaths cannot be definitively resolved purely with the numbers before us: the per capita GDP and the life expectancy for each nation. In each case, the numbers that we seek to improve, life expectancy and per capita GDP actually served as disadvantages with regards to preventing COVID-19 cases and deaths. One possible reason for this is that nations having higher per capita GDP engaged in greater degrees of international commerce requiring greater exposure to travel from abroad. It is apparent that this broad geographical intermingling is the primary factor that spreads the virus across the various global regions. From the experiences we described in Europe and Iran, we can see that such international travel that caused the virus to spread, not just across various segments of their respective continents, but to specific cities.

Similarly, nations with higher per capita GDPs generally tend to have greater life expectancies, and with greater life expectancies come higher mean population ages and higher percentages of elderly citizens. Once again, we saw the relentless affinity SARS-CoV-2 has for the elderly in Italy, France, Spain, and in the nursing homes in New York. It is possible that more sophisticated, multivariate analysis may demonstrate that per-capita GDP and life expectancy are each independent variables pushing a nation's per capita death and per capita case rates higher.

So is it a nation's wealth or its population's age that pushes the numbers up? In my view, although acting independently like the howling wind and the rising water in a ruthless tempest, they complement each other in delivering the ultimately devastating blows.

What then do we say of our responses? Are they immaterial? Likely not. Our responses have their purposes and their beneficial effects, but we must not believe that they are sufficient to overcome the overwhelming forces that the per capita GDP and a population's age has in promoting the devastation. In a *The Wall Street Journal* opinion piece, T.J. Rodgers presented a single-variate scanogram, much like the ones we have presented here, showing no correlation between the promptness of lockdown implementation and the cumulative number of deaths per million over a twenty-one-day period.[638] We should bear in mind that the things we think may help and do "in the name of science," may actually be futile, purposeless enterprises that end up hurting more than helping.

The conclusion that either a nation's per capita GDP, its expected lifespan, or both are the primary drivers of the numbers of cases and death a country experiences also explains the remaining identified correlations. Roughly speaking, nations with higher per capita GDP are associated with a higher number of physicians per capita, greater number of COVID-19 tests performed per capita, and better healthcare rankings. Consequently, the relationship between COVID-19 cases and deaths per capita and these other factors is not due to their independent deleterious effects on the spread of COVID-19. Such causative associations are clearly nonsensical. Rather, it is much more likely that factors such as physician prevalence, tests per capita, and better healthcare systems are associated with poorer outcomes because they are found in nations with greater wealth and older populations. We can also deduce that neither physicians, great healthcare systems, nor tests have been able to overcome the seemingly overwhelming challenges set up by a nation's greater wealth and older population.

Chapter 6

Coronalessons

The events stemming from the Wuhan pandemic are truly unprecedented. No segment of society has been left untouched. Whether one is in the healthcare fields, government, business, religious institutions, or simply trying to live out one's life in peace and tranquility, everyone has been affected by SARS-CoV-2 and restricted by the regulations that have been implemented in response. In our attempts to deal with the crisis, some of our actions were necessary and proper, others were undertaken in error, and still others were overt affronts into peoples' liberties driven by ideology, quests for personal power, and sheer opportunism. Deciphering which actions are which is fundamental, not only for the protection of our way of life but in preparation for our response to the next pandemic.

Admittedly, our experience with this virus is still unfinished, but sufficient data have materialized to allow for the incorporation of many lessons.

The initial intent of this work was to develop the criticisms and insights regarding the virus and our reactions to it as impartially as possible, and indeed this has been achieved. But a principal insight from this experience centers on the disturbing pattern of authoritarian overreach in which the Left and some jurisdictions subject to Democratic majorities have engaged compared to those on the Right. Indeed, we have already encountered this tendency throughout the events outlined in this text, and on many occasions have already called them out. Thus, any impartial review must acknowledge and oppose the partisan disparities in the handling of this virus.

Although not expressed as a freestanding coronalesson, one clear observation deals with the proclivity the Left has demonstrated for the repression of individual rights and freedoms. Its disdain for independent thought and decentralization of power has been denuded like never before and represents one of the principal questions each of us must answer moving forward. Do we wish to grant governing authority to those willing to restrict our most essential freedoms simply because they believe they are correct or do we entrust those who continuously strive to keep those tendencies in check? We have already entertained the results of the differences in attitude between the two camps. They will be developed even further in the sections that follow, but ultimately the answer to these overarching questions rests squarely on each one of us, our priorities, and the levels of trust we have upon our government.

Coronalesson No. 1: "Even though I walk through the valley of the shadow of death, I will fear no evil, for thou art with me, thy rod and thy staff comfort me." Pm. 23:4.

There is so much fear in our country. We fear speaking to others. We fear the future. We fear going to work. We fear not going to work. We fear getting sick. We fear making others sick. We fear dying.

How did we get to be so scared? We are the people who landed a man on the moon. We tamed the West. We conquered fascism. We defeated communism. We invaded Normandy. We landed on Iwo Jima. We invented the car, the plane, the telephone, and the light bulb. Fearful people cannot realize such accomplishments. They must be bold, tough as nails, and committed. That's always been America. But somehow, we have allowed ourselves to become intimidated by the future, by the unknown. We have cowered at the sight of any threat. Within days of engaging in a battle, whether it is a hostile enemy or a virus, we demand to get out. But why?

Certainly, one can point an accusatory finger at the media, which thrives on sensationalism and sows controversy merely to improve its ratings. We can blame technology since conversations that used to take months to sweep through America now blanket the continent in seconds. But there is a much more elemental reason, one to which neither social media nor a dysfunctional press can hold a candle.

We have lost faith in God.

Through the past fifty years, we have allowed prayer to be removed from schools. Moments of silence have been shunned, and our children have no longer been taught the Lord's Prayer. Such actions have consequences, and in our case, the consequences have been tragic.

Fear can only be conquered through a greater purpose. To achieve despite adversity, there must be a motivation so great that it overwhelms the threat faced by the actor. Ultimately, that source of motivation, that font of righteousness pushing one to achieve despite danger or threat can only be a god so good and so pure that He would create man in His image and continuously challenge us to be more like Him in His goodness and charity. Any other source of presumed righteousness can be molded, changed, and ultimately destroyed by man's hand. Any other source, even a nation as great as ours, can never serve as that unwavering guiding light motivating us to reach the stars.

The single, most important lesson gleaned from the COVID-19 experience is also the most elemental. We are all here to serve a great and loving God through whose service we will get through every tribulation we may encounter. It is the same lesson abandoned by every great society, whether it was the Israelites in the Old Testament, the Greeks, the Germans, the Chinese, the Egyptians, or the Romans. All of human history is encapsulated with the recurring tendency for mankind to learn and abandon this immutable lesson.

As the Wuhan pandemic made its way across the world, we stared into the face of adversity, and we feared death. We succumbed to the temptation of abandoning the very foundations we built to protect us from injustices much greater than the Wuhan pandemic. There is only one reason to explain our fear: our lack of faith. If you are a Christian, and you believe in a merciful God, in a God that gave His only son for our salvation, then you should know in your heart that we have already conquered death, and not only in a spiritual sense, but completely. "If for this life only we have hoped in Christ," wrote St. Paul in his First Letter to the Corinthians, "we are the most pitiable people of all."[639]

It is indeed interesting that a concept dealing with the core of our spirituality should be the first lesson learned from the purely worldly Wuhan pandemic, but it is indeed the most important. If we truly believed these truths, then no virus can conquer us. There is no death to mourn or fear. In fact, death is permanently extinguished.

When death fails to hold its mastery over us, we stop succumbing to its whims and threats. More importantly, we realize the existence of things immensely more important than our own individual lives; things like justice, love, charity, benevolence, fellowship, individual liberties, and the legacies we leave for our children. Understanding the overarching importance of the preservation of these virtues instills in us limitations in what we are willing to do and the institutions we are willing to sacrifice merely to lower an ephemeral viral mortality rate. A greater goal comes into view that drives to heights infinitely greater than fear. And it all starts with recalling the words in Psalms 23:4: "Even though I walk through the valley of the shadow of death, I will fear no evil, for thou art with me, thy rod and thy staff comfort me."

Guided by this correct mindset, on March 23, 2020, Texas Lieutenant Governor Dan Patrick appeared on Fox News and defended these selfless concepts. He asked, "Are you willing to take a chance on your survival in exchange for keeping the America that all Americans love for your children and grandchildren? And if that's the exchange, I'm all in."

Lieutenant Governor Patrick was correct. We should all be in because the alternative is giving up the greatness of our system of government, darkening the shining city on the hill, and threatening the freedoms and liberties we guarantee for our posterity. Governor Patrick's position was one of enlightenment, wisdom, and selflessness because it was one that acknowledges that Patrick himself was not the center of the universe.

The Left was quick to ridicule and scold Governor Patrick for his position. The likes of former presidential candidate Robert O'Rourke immediately exposed their short sidedness, buffoonery, and selfishness. "This kind of numbnuttery," tweeted O'Rourke, "will kill people in Texas. Young as well as old. We need a state-wide shelter in place order to stop the spread of coronavirus and save hundreds of thousands of lives."[640]

First, O'Rourke dismisses the intent and wisdom of Patrick's words, and then, in typical leftist fashion, uses the threat of death to cast fear upon the listener. O'Rourke knows that as long as death is feared, he can sell it as the ultimate threat. It becomes his most effective leverage.

According to O'Rourke's position, the government is the great savior. The solution, says he, lies with government action, in this case, a state-wide shelter-in-place order. To him, the consequences of governmental overreach, the infringement upon people's rights, or the destruction of the America we all love does not figure into the computation. The only thing that matters to O'Rourke and the Left is the statistical analysis of the number of American lives saved. He pays no attention to the number of lives ruined or the American institutions destroyed. It is only the government that saves, and it is the fear of death, a fear only possible in the absence of faith, that motivates.

These are the same precepts that have been employed by governors from the Left, and only from the Left, with the exception of Maryland Republican Governor Larry Hogan. For Whitmer in Michigan, Cuomo in New York, Newsom in California, and Pritzker in Illinois, to name a few, the same playbook is followed. Have the public concentrate on the number of deaths and cases while instilling fear in those who do not obey.

All these techniques, threats, and manipulations dissolve when we recognize that we are here for some purpose much greater than service to the government; that we are called to love God with all our might and to love our neighbors as we love ourselves.

"Even though I walk through the valley of the shadow of death, I will fear no evil, for thou art with me, thy rod and thy staff comfort me."

Coronalesson No. 2: Our Constitution is a wonderful, yet fragile thing.

The nineteenth-century British statesman and former Prime Minister, William Gladstone, once called the United States Constitution "the most wonderful work ever struck off at a given time by the brain and purpose of man." Of course, Gladstone was correct. But the Constitution is also amongst the frailest of documents.

Bruce Jacob, former Dean of the Stetson University College of Law, once remarked that the whole of the United States Constitution depended on the integrity of one clause. The clause is in Article VI, and it reads, "The Senators and Representatives before mentioned, and the Members of the several State Legislatures, and all executive and judicial Officers, both of the United States and of the several States, shall be bound by Oath or Affirmation, to support this Constitution . . . " He explained this one phrase could arguably be the most important because it required all serving in government, state, local, or federal, to be allegiant to the Constitution. And this oath demanded much more than merely a promise to pick up a musket and a pitchfork to protect one's fellow citizens from foreign invaders. The clause specifically requires anyone serving in public office to uphold the actual provisions within the Constitution of the United States. Because of this, Article VI, clause 3, no one in government could allow him or herself to propose any law or order offensive to the Constitution. Unless public officials restrained themselves from doing so, explained Dean Jacobs, the Constitution would quickly devolve into a meaningless piece of paper offering none of the guarantees it was supposed to offer.

Our experience with the Wuhan pandemic has certainly exposed the prophetic nature of Dean Jacobs's observations. Under the pretext of protection, practically every essential right has been infringed.

- The right to vote: The day before a primary election, Governor Evers issued an executive order that would have postponed it. If honored, the order would have substantially impacted the election's outcome.

- Freedom of speech: In Michigan, California, and other states, people were restrained from expressing their opinions and redressing their government. When people took to the streets, in cars or otherwise, to express their opposition to what they believed were draconian measures, they were called dangerous and reckless and were accused of endangering the lives of countless Americans. Some were arrested and their rallies prohibited in the name of public health.

- Freedom of the press: Any member of the press that dared come up with ideas contrary to the mainstream was bullied. Organizations billing themselves as social media platforms suppressed people from reporting events contrary to the platform's point of view.

- The right to peaceably assemble: People throughout the nation were kept from assembling in groups of greater than ten, and when they did, governors and other officials sought police actions against them.

- Equal protection under the law: At least forty-two states, but in particular, Michigan, California, Colorado, New Jersey, Pennsylvania, and even Texas shut down businesses, infringing on people's rights to contract, to engage in commerce, and to peaceably conduct their affairs. These people were arrested, fined, and delicensed.

In the name of protecting people from disease, some like Governor Evers overtly and repeatedly disregarded statutory limits on their emergency authorities so they could continue holding on to their newly found powers.

Similarly, in Michigan, Governor Whitmer stopped seeking the legislature's approval of her orders and went at it on her own, like a monarch, simply because the legislature refused to comply.

In California, Newsom indefinitely extended his state's emergency status, making his added powers and authorities the new norm. Clearly, in so doing Newsom ignored any semblance of restraint required by the Constitution.

- The judicially created right to privacy: The nation's experts, the members of the press, and many on the Left seriously proposed and defended having the federal government enact mandatory testing requirements, track citizens, and intercept them save they should come in contact with someone having COVID-19.

- Protections against search and seizure: The Ventura County Health Director initiated a program where people who had tested positive for COVID-19 would be tracked, their contacts identified, and quarantined. Most ominously, the plan included the removal of noninfected members of a family from a home if any member was infected and the family shared a common bathroom.

Scary as these infringements are perhaps even more violently attacked were the nation's religious rights. The little attention paid to honoring the freedom to worship, particularly in blue jurisdictions, was startling. As we saw in Greenville, governments actually prohibited church services from taking place even if worshipers attempted to comply with social distancing precautions.

Sometimes, as we previously noted, merely failing to mention such protections was enough to allow for the infringement upon religion to take place. Such was the case in California where the Governor's silence on the issue prompted a letter of concern from the DOJ. Even Florida, a state where Republicans dominate every chamber of state power, saw the display of the same disrespect for religious freedoms seen in some blue jurisdictions when a pastor in Tampa was arrested for holding church services. Although Governor Desantis's order did not prohibit stricter provisions from being implemented at the county or city level, no further actions against religious freedoms were observed following its implementation.

All this leads to one inescapable conclusion: in light of Congress's ineptitude and the gross disregard for religious freedoms displayed on the part of some of our leaders, the degree of infringements upon our religious liberties had Hillary Clinton been at the helm of the executive branch instead of President Trump would have been unparalleled in our Republic. By any measure, it appears no breaks would have been applied to cavalier public officials bent on suppressing religious rights or minimizing the importance of religious worship.

Even the Constitution's structural provisions were at risk. The previously noted "experts" argued for the implementation of robust contacting and tracking policies by the federal government when the Constitution specifically placed those provisions in the hands of the states. More palpably, CMS directed how physicians and hospitals undertook COVID-19 precautions by restricting their reimbursement, an intervention that stands well outside the agency's charter and a clear violation of the separation of powers doctrine.[i]

---

[i] I cover the limitations statutorily placed on CMS at length in *The Case for Free Market Healthcare.*

Why is this so important? Simple. Without the limitations placed upon our government and our public officials by the Constitution, the United States is just another Banana Republic. America remains a beacon of freedom because of the supremacy of the Constitution. Ignore it and any liberty can be infringed. Any property can be confiscated. Any person can be imprisoned. And any intrusion upon one's life can be made.

Yes, there are such things as emergency powers, but did you know they are not cited in the Constitution? The major reason for this is that, in the minds of the Framers, the major purveyor of emergency powers was not the federal government or even the President. They were the governors. Indeed, the only suggestion of emergency powers afforded to the federal government lies in the authority to suspend habeas corpus and that authority, "when in Cases of Rebellion or Invasion," lies with Congress.[641] The only other mentions of added powers during exigent circumstances relate to the federal government's mandate of protecting every state against invasion,[642] and its authority to call forth the militia.[643] Other than that, there really are no other provisions that would allow a president to take greater control of the nation and institute a state of emergency, quarantine, or a national lockdown. In fact, there isn't even an express power for the implementation of a mandatory, national vaccination campaign. The federal government has assumed each of those powers via interpretation, the judiciary's validations, and the states' passive consent.

What else can the federal government do without an expressed sanction from the Constitution? The truth is whatever it can get away with. And here, we come full circle with the issues brought up by the conduct of our national leaders and our experts concerning the proposed national responses to the Wuhan pandemic. Never mind that the actions they recommend are correct or incorrect from a public health standpoint, or whether they are based on sound or baseless assumptions, granting the federal government more power weakens the document that founded our country and lays waste to the protections it affords us.

In his Farewell Address, President George Washington addressed this very proclivity when he famously observed, "But let there be no change by usurpation; for though this, in one instance, may be the instrument of good, it is the customary weapon by which free governments are destroyed. The precedent must always greatly over-balance in permanent evil any partial or transient benefit, which the use can at any time yield." Scarcely in American history has Washington's words rung truer than when we reacted to the ravages of the Wuhan pandemic.

To President Trump's credit, despite comments he repeatedly made regarding his possession of plenary powers and despite the experts' preparations of the sweet apple of authority, he sagely re-sisted the temptation to centralize power. His approach of yielding to the states is completely consistent with the principles of federal-ism that have kept our nation strong. Amongst the many criticisms launched at the President, merited or not, was that his approach was disjointed since it allowed the states too much latitude. But in fact, his tactic protected the country from the opportunistic tendency to centralize power and stayed true to the constitutional precepts of constitutional federalism.

Coronalesson No. 3: When policymakers say they are using science to guide them in their decisions, they are not.

Curiously, when these governors are challenged, they seek ref-uge in something they call "science." How many times have you heard these men and women say that they rely on science to guide them in their decisions? In fact, they are not relying on science; they are relying on a statistic. There is a difference.

Science is a process by which humans learn about the world. It is a method through which we arrive at a physical truth. It relies on observation, inquiry, and experimentation. But it is a process that can take years, even decades, to play out. Arriving at some scientific truth about SARS-CoV-2 and COVID-19 will take decades, or years at the very least, not months or weeks.

Science is, by its nature, a retrospective process. By the time we definitively learn all we need to make sound policy decisions, the pandemic will have long since played itself out. The truth is that no one has yet arrived at a sound scientific understanding regarding SARS-CoV-2, thus making any decision in favor or against certain interventions based on faith. How ironic that faith is something leftist politicians adamantly deny using when in fact, it is exactly what they deploy!

Coronalesson No. 4: What press?

Perhaps the most appalling display throughout the Wuhan pandemic was that of the American press. In the United States, the press ranks amongst the most important of institutions. Its role is not to be taken lightly nor fooled with. Yet this is exactly what we witnessed in the pandemic's coverage.

A free society depends upon a certain minimum level of professionalism and ethics from the press. As the eyes and the ears of the people, journalists are the ultimate check on power. Without them, there can be nothing but tyranny. Thus, they serve an indispensable function. So integral to the proper workings of government is a free and unfettered press that President John F. Kennedy called it "a critical branch, the fourth estate."[644] But the press is not free if it has been sold. It is not unfettered if it is enslaved by its ideology.

Students of journalism are often told that their mission, their raison d'etre, is to "comfort the afflicted and afflict the comfortable." Although noble in its tone, the aspiration is negligent in its demand. The phrase was first delivered by a fictitious, nineteenth-century bartender named Mr. Dooley who lamented,

> *Th' newspaper does ivrything f'r us. It runs th' polis foorce an' th' banks, commands th' milishy, controls th' ligislachure, baptizes th' young, marries th' foolish, comforts th' afflicted, afflicts th' comfortable, buries th' dead an' roasts thim aftherward.*[ii]

It is indeed ironic that the actual quote called out the bias of journalists rather than extol their virtues. Dooley's expression, repackaged as a sort of rallying cry for journalists cannot escape its disgruntled origins. When the press afflicts any chosen class and comforts any other simply as a matter of right, it has failed by propagating the same dishonorable bias of which its original speaker complained. The role of the press must be to inform the people, free of favor or animus. Otherwise, democracy cannot exist. There will certainly be times for the press to comfort and to afflict as it delivers its opinions about the facts it is reporting. But the opinions, its scorn, and its praise must stand separately and independently from its political bias. Its accusations, as must its credits, necessarily follow the dignities and disgraces in their findings, not the other way around.

[ii] Mr. Dooley in David Shedden, "Today in Media History: Mr. Dooley: 'The job of the newspaper is to comfort the afflicted and afflict the comfortable,'" Poynter (blog), Oct. 7, 2014, accessed Apr. 21, 2020, https://www.poynter.org/reporting-editing/2014/today-in-media-history-mr-dooley-the-job-of-the-newspaper-is-to-comfort-the-afflicted-and-afflict-the-comfortable/.

Sadly, our nation has lost that free and unfettered press, for it has become the gun barrel of an agenda whose sight, once cast, becomes relentless. In our great nation, the coverage of the Wuhan pandemic has been anything but impartial. The events surrounding the spread of a virus, its treatment, and its prevention has been seen and reported through the lens of a sensationalistic press intent on punishing a president. A mere decade ago, the accusations regarding the deterioration of journalism had to do with money. Newspapers, it was felt, were all too eager to pursue the mighty dollar. In its quest to do so, the press changed its methods to enhance the sensationalism of the story and exalt the confrontation, all for the mighty buck.

Today, the zealous bastardization of a story for the sake of sales is no longer the prime motivation. Instead, the American press has picked a side in a political debate and has pushed it with the same ferocity as the candidates themselves. For the favored side, they hide, massage, and repackage the truth. For their enemies, they pillage, slander, and stain it. Yes, they still thirst for the almighty dollar, but now, the dollar is pursued through the rallying of the base and the serving of political red meat for consumption.

During the American coronavirus experience, the press has harangued a President merely because of its disdain for him. It has blindly berated a medication. It has ignored the lies and deceit of a communist dictatorship that harbors no regard for human life or decency. It spread fear and angst regarding the course of a pandemic while bullying and ridiculing those who stood up for their freedoms. And for those who disagreed with the press's prevailing narrative, there was only scorn and retribution. Tragically, there has been no impartiality in investigation, no truth in reporting.

For its performance at a time when there was no need for partisanship, the press earned an "F." And for that, our nation has suffered, as we all learned once again, that no democracy can long survive with such bleary and shaded eyes, and such clogged and muffled ears.

Coronalesson No. 5: "A house divided against itself cannot stand."

On June 16, 1858, Abraham Lincoln took to the podium at the Illinois State Republican Convention and famously said, "A house divided against itself cannot stand." At the time, the enemy was slavery, and Lincoln was making the point that the nation would someday come together on the issue, either as a slave nation or as a free one. It could not be both. His words were indeed prophetic, as they foretold the great schism that crystalized into a horrid Civil War pitting state against state, family against family.

Today, his words ring just as true, but in a different light. In this case, the enemy is not slavery but a virus, and our tense division has demonstrated how it is that under such conditions, we cannot stand. Our ideological division and the contempt each side harbors against the other have paralyzed us. For us, it is not that we will come together one way or another, as Lincoln was foreseeing. Rather, it is that if we continue on this track there will be nothing awaiting us but assured self-destruction.

In this particular fight, the bigger culprits have been the Never-Trumpers. They lost an incredibly important election, but their response has been anger, hatred, and animus to the point of losing all interest in addressing the problems that afflict us. Instead, they find it more productive to destroy the candidate who succeeded against them and denigrate those who supported him. Any idea President Trump proffers is immediately met with disdain, *even if they were the same ideas his opponents supported before his election*!

This time, their disdain burned us. We were so busy dealing with impeachment, so busy either promoting or opposing a Russia hoax, so busy denigrating border security for its own sake, that we took our eyes off the ball.

And what was that ball? The one that demands we improve our country and protect our fellow citizens. By the time the Wuhan pandemic hit, we were dug into our ideological trenches and aiming our political rifles at our brothers and sisters, all the time ignoring the approaching dragon that was about to breathe fire upon both sides of the battlefield.

Truly, this self-destructive condition can no longer exist. Either we learn to live with the results of an election where the winners listen to the defeated and the defeated work with the winners or the Union that President Lincoln saved will disappear, and the greatness of a nation will fade on a parched historical page.

America is the greatest nation in the world. Its strength comes from a foundation demanding that each citizen be in equal standing before the law and the presence of a diverse, strong, proud, and independent people. Together we form a rich mosaic depicting a blessed picture of freedom, opportunity, and accomplishment. Divided, we are nothing but a garbled mess.

Perhaps the saddest insight delivered to us by the Wuhan pandemic is a glimpse at the depth of our division. And perhaps the most life-saving coronalesson lies in the importance of our reunification under a common, unflickering light.

Coronalesson No. 6: Experts are to be heard, not obeyed, and models are predictions, not oracles.

"They're a tool, not an oracle."[645] Thus said *The Wall Street Journal* Editorial Board when speaking about predictive epidemiological models. The observation holds just as true for the experts who built them. But the events surrounding the Wuhan pandemic were so unique and rapid that they created a situation where the experts were essentially obeyed, serving as a laboratory experiment of sorts demonstrating what happens when a faction within society is followed without question.

A president with no healthcare or epidemiological experience was suddenly thrust into a situation replete with multiple, rapid, technical decisions. Naturally, he had to rely on those with knowledge and experience in the area. In this case, they were doctors, epidemiologists, and public health experts. Like all factions, this one was motivated by common interests, which may have included a desire to prevent disease, help others, and keep people safe. Admirable as these motivations are, they still represent only part of the picture. They gave little weight to the disruption their recommendations would cause to the lives of others. They did not account for the effects on macro and microeconomics. They did not consider the consequences to the prevention of other medical conditions. And they did not take into account the constitutionality of their recommendations.

So these advisors, who suddenly had the ear of the President, informed him of the virus and how lives may be saved through the policies they were recommending. They provided him with data, models, and all sorts of analytics in support of their contentions, and the President, who was forced to rely on them for information and guidance, acted on their suggestions.

In the meantime, the press, which had been particularly hateful to the President, continued the partisan assault on him by forcefully suggesting that he was either incompetent or unwilling to make the decisions that protect vulnerable Americans from death. The whole thing resulted in a perfect storm where the President was more aggressive in handling the situation while more reliant on the expert faction than he normally would. The experts' recommendations had even greater weight than usual, as they were essentially placed at the helm of a massive ship with priorities much greater than theirs.

And what did this faction of experts tell us? At first, it dismissed the virus as not a threat to the health and safety of the United States. Next, it said the virus was going to be the most colossal cause of destruction the United States had ever encountered. They actually told the President that 2.2 million people were going to die if he did not heed their warnings, which, as we have shown, was *impossible*. Then they told him that we should shut down the nation's economy for a fortnight. That doing so should be enough to "flatten the curve." Then they said it needed to be extended for another month, and that reopening should not occur until a vaccine was developed. Then they recommended we move forward with reopening only when we reached the capability of performing 20 million tests a month. And then they said that the federal government should undertake intrusive contact tracking programs so that it knows everyone who has the virus.

Nowhere in these expert analyses were the effects of these interventions on peoples' lives, their savings, and everything they had spent decades building articulated. And absolutely nowhere did they include any consideration to the rule of law and the foundational principles upon which the Constitution stood. Those things did not enter into their computation. They were the experts, and they were telling us what we had to do to save lives. Quite simply, if we didn't listen, people would die.

And thus we saw a basic tenet of the American Progressive Movement play out. Leave it the experts, the Progressives say. The experts will see us through.

But, did they? They had the nation engage in something called social distancing. People self-isolated. Groups of greater than ten were banished. Restaurants were closed. Public showings of movies were discontinued. And "non-essential" healthcare was no longer delivered.

What made the experts particularly effective was their use of the perfect backup with which to cover their errors. If 2.2 million people didn't die, it was not because they were wrong; it was because their recommendations were working! The President and the American people yielded to this elite class, and no one was allowed to challenge them or push back. Some questioned the appropriateness of the numbers these experts used to estimate the virus's contagiousness and lethality, but few suggested the very formula they used was inherently flawed, that the calculations they employed in arriving at their conclusions were inappropriate, and that as statisticians and epidemiologists, they should have been aware of it. In other words, what we got out of the COVID-19 experience was the perfect case study of what James Madison feared could take place when he wrote, "When a majority is included in a faction, the form of popular government, on the other hand, enables it to sacrifice to its ruling passion or interest both the public good and the rights of other citizens."[646]

But amazingly, drunk with the wine of power, the experts' recommendations did not stop at shutdowns. To them, the handshake was a thing of the past. Hugs were taboo. Masks should be worn in public. We should worship from our cars, if at all; unless we're worshipping science, of course. There should be no more theaters. And human interactions should be performed over the internet. Their recommendations would fundamentally transform human existence; all in the name of thwarting the evils the experts prioritized above all others.

But is this really the path we want to take? Now, that we have stabilized the spread of the virus to some extent, we should ask the questions we did not have the luxury of posing before. And we should deliver our inquiry with the knowledge that the Framers already had arrived at an answer, namely no faction, no matter how well-intentioned, should be given free rein over the nation's policy decisions.

Experts are to be heard, not obeyed. Their recommendations must be subjected to the same level of scrutiny as those posed by other factions, especially during a time of crisis where our society and our way of life is most at risk.

Coronalesson No. 7: On borders and walls.

SARS-CoV-2 taught us an important lesson about a nation's sovereignty and the importance of being able to secure one's borders: few things are as fundamental as a sovereign's ability to control its borders.

Prior to the appearance of COVID-19, one of the most important substantive conversations centered on American immigration and on the nation's inherent right to secure its borders. An increasingly loud call from the Left claimed that all nations' borders, particularly those of the United States, should be completely porous. Even Pope Francis staked his position on the issue when he said that Christians ought "to not raise walls but bridges, to not respond evil with evil, to overcome evil with good."[647] But in reality, as we have seen throughout the course of the Wuhan pandemic, walls, or at least the ability to secure a nation's border is a good, not an evil.

Throughout history, whole civilizations have been decimated because they were unable to control their borders. The Sea People destroyed the Miceans and the Hittites, among other cultures, in about 1200 B.C. because the latter were unable to ward off the former. Thousands were violently killed, the Bronze Age came to an end, and the world entered a dark age, not unlike the one following the fall of the Roman Empire. On the other hand, the Assyrians and the Egyptians survived the same pressures because they were able to ward off the invaders. In the middle ages, pagan tribes invaded the Roman Empire, as it weakened and was no longer able to secure its borders. Again western civilization was cast into an age of darkness and disarray when just a few centuries earlier, the world had seen the Pax Romana by a strong Rome that was able to control its borders.

The plague that began in the Middle East decimated populations as far west as Britannia because people carried the disease with them through porous borders. In modern times, the Germans marched through Europe because no continental country was strong enough to secure its borders.

In every one of these cases, people were saved and peace ensued because borders were observed and travel between nations was controlled. And when the borders became porous, particularly because the host nation was unable to control them, disease spread, wars erupted, and people died. When the invasion was widespread, mankind was sent backward, and darkness, hunger, and suffering prevailed, sometimes for centuries.

During the first three years of the Trump presidency, it seemed that whole segments of the American population had forgotten the necessity of borders for orderliness and the fostering of good-will amongst people. With increasing tenacity, the indisputable truth about the necessity of controlling America's borders was dismissed by the Left. For them, non-citizens had the ability to enter the country, as a matter of right. Any other approach was a grave injustice.

At times, it seemed there was no rhyme or reason to the argument being proffered other than to serve as an antagonist to President Trump. But when the Wuhan pandemic struck, all the claims from the Left about the injustices of borders and immigration control came to a screeching halt. The most successful first step in preventing death and disease for any country with the luxury of implementing it was the timely closure of its borders. Within weeks, New Zealand, Australia, South Korea, Singapore, the Caribbean nations all closed their borders, each with great success at containing the spread of the virus. Yet, when the United States tried it, the President was called a racist, and his actions were said to be part of a conspiratorial effort aimed at keeping "brown people" out. Subsequent events demonstrated the falsehood and baselessness of their claims.

The Wuhan pandemic forced us to relearn a lesson that had been inextricably sown into the fibers of history. A country cannot long subsist without maintaining control of its borders. Before COVID-19, the arguments were largely made from the standpoint of population control, economics, equal protection, government capabilities, and national defense. Yet our experience with SARS-CoV-2 has reminded us once again of the epidemiological and public health importance of securing a nation's borders. I believe it may not be the last time we have to relearn this lesson.

Coronalesson No. 8: Shutdowns don't work.

The insights gained from the relationships summarized in Chapter 5 and from our historical experience allow us to arrive at certain conclusions regarding the effectiveness of certain interventions aimed at combating the Wuhan pandemic and the futility of others. For starters, we can safely say that generally, shutdowns don't work. T.J. Rodgers' article in The Wall Street Journal demonstrating no correlation between a jurisdiction's promptness in implementing a shutdown and the total number of deaths experienced in the 21 days following it offers an early clue against the effectiveness of shutdowns. It certainly did not keep the United States from seeing the highest number of deaths and cases of any other country, nor did it help New York and New Rochelle in preventing the virus's overwhelming spread.

The reasons why shutdowns don't work are multifactorial. First, by the time the earliest cases were identified in the overwhelming majority of jurisdictions, SARS-CoV-2 had already silently embedded itself within the population and was already well on its way to extending its deathly tentacles. Second, very few countries have the tight command of their borders required to successfully keep a spreading virus out. Indeed, as we saw in our analysis, precious few countries had the opportunity to stop the influx of the virus. Such nations include New Zealand and Australia, two "island" countries blessed with the ultimate control of their borders. Australia shut down its borders, at least partially, by January 23 and required all entering the country to self-isolate by March 15. Similarly, New Zealand began restricting entry on February 3. In both cases, shutdown efforts were facilitated by the inescapable geographical separation with which they were blessed, and they enhanced their isolation with mandatory quarantines, social distancing requirements, and strict oversight methods. Nations like the Caribbean Islands were similarly as fortunate since the principal measure they employed in combating the Wuhan pandemic was closing.

Other nations benefited from prompt border control efforts followed by strict monitoring programs and isolation enforcement. These included jurisdictions like South Korea, Hong Kong, and Singapore. In each instance, the areas identified the threat early and sealed their borders to traffic from China, but they also implemented measures of testing and surveillance considered draconian by American standards. In South Korea, surveillance programs served as its primary method. In Hong Kong, an organic social distancing effort predated even the government's response. And in Singapore, a government-run surveillance program followed by selective stay-at-home orders allowed the virus to make its way through this relatively youthful nation with minimal loss of life.

But these measures could have never worked for the United States. First, America's borders are too large and too porous to allow for successful closure. Even without illegal immigration, travel to and from the United States from the far reaches of the world is too extensive to allow for the repulsion of the virus. Furthermore, the United States could not have acted with sufficient promptness to prevent those already silently carrying the virus from entering. By January 31, the day the United States restricted travel from China, thousands of potential carriers had already entered the country, making containment ineffective.

Moreover, sealing the border would have only been the first step. Regardless of the effectiveness of the closure, American efforts would have required extensive surveillance and tracking prohibited by the Constitution. For the United States, the only options were state-implemented isolation campaigns targeted at our hardest-hit areas and the protection of our senior citizens, particularly those residing within our nursing homes.

The effort at bending the curve was indeed valiant. Because the predictions were so flawed, we will never know how well they actually worked, if at all. We have already established the utter impossibility of the 2.2 million deaths the original estimates predicted. Short of that, it is impossible to say how many would have died had we not intervened in the manner we did. One thing stands as indisputable though; no effort could have spared 95% of predicted deaths.

Our more effective methods of resisting the effects of the virus dealt with mobilization. Indeed, America's deployment of the private sector was monumental. To have companies that had never produced a single ventilator, glove, medical gown, protective eyewear, or hand sanitizer change gears and crank them out as rapidly as they did is one of America's great achievements. Were it not for the private sector, our nation's suffering would have been overwhelming to the point of threatening the very structure of our society.

Imagine what would have happened had we not possessed the resources necessary to respond to this pandemic? If we did not have the number of ventilators we needed with no relief in sight. If we did not have the gloves, the gowns, the IVs, or the supportive equipment needed to care for each other. To what extent would some have gone to obtain those materials even when the law said they had no access to them? How long would Americans have stood for such a travesty? And what would they have done to save the lives of their loved ones in a world where insufficiency was the norm? What would *you* have done?

Indeed, America was extremely fortunate in having a private sector capable of responding to the challenges of a crisis and the leadership of a president who demanded such from it. It is imperative, moving forward, that it remains strong, robust, and minimally impeded.

Coronalesson No. 9: The importance of testing.

How important is testing? In reality, the importance of testing is defined by the manner in which we are planning to use the results.

Testing is supremely important for the individual wishing to know if he or she is infected and for the physician interested in knowing the best way of treating her patient. It is also important for the community, whether a municipality, or a smaller unit like a family that wishes to know if a particular person should be quarantined. But from a public health perspective, the importance of a robust testing program is determined by what the jurisdiction is capable and willing to do with the information.

For countries like Australia, New Zealand, South Korea, Singapore, and areas like Hong Kong, testing was paramount. For these jurisdictions, robust testing programs were the stalwarts of their efforts at averting a full breakdown of the social and medical systems. But these were jurisdictions that were able and willing to act on the results of their tests. Individuals who tested positive outside of the jurisdiction were not allowed entry. Those who tested positive domestically were quarantined. Their contacts were tracked. Depending on the jurisdiction if someone broke the isolation requirements, he or she may have been forcibly isolated. For them, there was a strong, public-health purpose for knowing a test result.

In the United States, the situation was decidedly different. We were not able to close our borders prior to the entry of the disease, so preventing entry was futile. Additionally, never in the history of the United States have people been detained and held against their will merely because of the result of a laboratory test. Would we have gone to that length? Were we prepared to chase down all the contacts of every individual, detain them, and even remove them from their homes to make sure the virus didn't spread (as Dr. Levin in Aventura County threatened to do)? Is it even constitutional for the government to engage in this kind of activity?

It is interesting that the questions regarding how we would act on a positive test in the name of preventing the spread of disease were rarely brought up on a national level. It is also of interest that the principal proponent of testing was the press, which rarely addressed the question of what they expected would be done with the results. Yes, they tossed the term "contact tracking," but they never cared to disclose what that would look like. Would it mean an arrest for the noncompliant? Would it mean separating parents from their children? The press never addressed it. They merely accused the administration of not performing sufficient tests. And when there were enough tests, so many that people were not subjecting themselves to them, as happened with ventilators, the press did not give the President credit. It merely stopped reporting on the issue.

In reality, while testing is important, the priority is the mobilization of resources and personnel to the places that need it, just like the President, FEMA, and most governors did. The role testing will play in future pandemics is dependent on the authorities we give government and the timing of such tests to a contagion's infiltration within our borders. Until we arrive at these answers, we cannot claim any specific importance to a massive testing campaign.

Coronalesson No. 10: China is not an ally.

It goes without saying. China is not our friend. China is not our ally. China cannot be trusted. But amongst many of our political and business leaders, these assertions seem to be foreign. To them, China is a valuable partner with whom ties need to be strengthened. In fact, the only national figure to have brazenly argued to the contrary was Donald J. Trump, and like with so many other things, the Wuhan pandemic confirmed the accuracy of his assertions.

During the twentieth century and into the twenty-first, China only harbored one overarching priority: to expand its sphere of influence throughout the world. And China is not engaged in this effort for the betterment of humanity. China's motivation for its quest for power is simply its quest for power. In a phrase, China wishes to manipulate the world into submission. No more. No less.

At every turn, China has aimed to bend international laws, steal intellectual property, manipulate currency, and increase the size of its military for one reason: to rob power and influence from the United States. Its quest to engage other countries in its BRI was undertaken only to benefit itself. Its efforts at cornering the market were only undertaken to improve its international position.

It is possible that SARS-CoV-2 spontaneously developed from its rat-infesting cousins and that China was running experiments at its Wuhan laboratory merely out of curiosity. But if so, I suspect China was not conducting experiments with the aim of finding the cure for cancer. China's interest in the coronavirus boils down to the same ones driving any other: the furtherance of its power and position in the world stage, and its conduct with regard to the SARS-CoV-2 sings of its motivations. If SARS-CoV-2 had spontaneously skipped into humans, then why suppress its presence?

China's early actions do not make any sense unless seen under the light of an entity engaged in nefarious conduct that got caught in doing so. When viewed in this manner, all of China's actions not only make complete sense, but they become predictable and foreseeable. China's actions towards those nations that entrusted it and entered financial relations with it are inexcusable. China knew of the virus's existence weeks prior to publicly admitting it. China also had all the evidence required to unmistakably conclude that SARS-CoV-2 demonstrated human-to-human transmission, but it kept this evidence from the rest of the world. Worse yet, it continued to allow Chinese citizens from high-risk areas to travel to places like Italy and Iran, which trusted China to foster goodwill and frankness with them. Those nations were instead rewarded with a continuous stream of infected individuals long after Chinese authorities knew the danger of their continued travel. Adding to the insult, when Italians began figuring out the undeniable, China actually sponsored a video decrying non-Chinese as racists for suspecting anything was up and encouraging Italians to hug Chinese people.

What does this malfeasance and persistent opacity on the part of the Chinese government tell us about our relationship with China? For starters, it says that President Trump was correct in harboring distrust for China and in using a heavy hand in dealing with the Chinese government.

China is not an upstanding member in the community of nations, and for the foreseeable future, ours is to counter China and its lackeys at every step. If China wishes to gain a stronger foothold in the United Nations, ours is to counteract that. If China wishes to compete in the international economic stage, ours is to defeat it. And if China wishes to push its military might about Asia and the Pacific, ours is to stare it down. We are a mightier country than China, and we stand for values the PRC has not even begun to appreciate. Until the day China recognizes the evil it is fomenting upon its citizens and upon the world, we cannot accept it as our partner. Will we have to conduct business with China? Most likely. But never as trusted friends, rather as a suspicious adversary.

Finally, China must pay. Whether the virus emanated purposely from a Chinese laboratory or spontaneously from a bat, the reckless disregard China demonstrated for human life is paralleled only by those harbored in other communist nations. China is directly responsible for the loss of hundreds of thousands of lives throughout the globe even if we exclude those deaths that could not have been prevented despite an earlier Chinese response. China has directly placed the trusting citizens of Italy and Iran at the mercy of its selfish whims, and a percentage of them have paid with their lives. China has also singlehandedly caused the disruption of the world's economies. For these actions and so many others, China must be held to account.

One final cautionary comment is in order: we cannot allow the people of China to be conflated with the actions of the Chinese government. We must be mindful that in China, the people are kept in the dark. We need no further evidence than the oppressive and intimidating actions of the Chinese government towards upstanding citizens like Drs. Li and Ai, and perhaps towards the batwoman herself. These are people who have been given no guarantees by their government and are most likely kept in the dark regarding the goings-on of their government's misdeeds. Indisputably, the Chinese people surely suffer and will continue to do so until the cold, evil grip of a communist dictatorship is wrestled away from their throats. Towards them, we must harbor nothing other than empathy and support.

Coronalesson No. 11: The World Health Organization is not.

How did the WHO lose its esteemed, selfless, and humanitarian role to become a mere lapdog for China? Clearly, the WHO is no longer a humanitarian, scientific organization looking purely at the interests of the health of the world's human population. Its loyalties, sadly, lie elsewhere. Its silence towards China is certainly telling, but its resistance towards Taiwan's participation and the brazenness with which it carries it out is appalling. If the WHO is truly entrusted with the health of everyone, then its rank favoritism in the manner in which it carries its alleged duties has disqualified it for such a responsibility.

One can offer a few explanations for the WHO's repeated failures with regards to China and its epidemics. One must suspect that both Chan's and Tedros's close ties to China impeded their abilities to demand more from the communist nation, or it may be, as Kathy Gilsinan observed, that the WHO's very structure keeps it from being effective.

Perhaps it is difficult for the agency to demand transparency from a country the size and might of China without jeopardizing its future resources. Or perhaps, less euphemistically, it is true that China has finally managed to nestle the WHO into its pocket. Regardless, it is obvious that the WHO is failing in its mission "to stimulate and advance work to eradicate epidemic, endemic and other diseases,"[648] and "to promote and protect the health of all peoples."[649]

If the WHO in its present state is unable to perform this function, then it must be reformed or replaced with another organization that can, perhaps one outside of the confines of the United Nations.

It is true that no organization can or ought to be in a position to impose its will upon an independent sovereign. The WHO cannot physically insert itself into a country and demand it be allowed to investigate. But when it comes across aberrancies or opaqueness in the handling of a disease, particularly when such a disease is due to the emergence of a new, poorly understood organism, it is incumbent, at the very least, for that organization to bring the matter to light and vociferously call for veracity in reporting the events surrounding the public health threat. For the past ten years, specifically, when it comes to events in China, the WHO has been unable or unwilling to do that.

The United States ought to proudly support an organization dedicated to the improvement of the human condition, particularly when its target is disease. The WHO is not that organization.

Coronalesson No. 12. The essential nature of capitalism to a free society.

Much has been said to minimize the value of capitalism. It has been called an evil system that reduces man to materialistic beings. It allows for the abuse of the poor at the expense of the rich. It supports a cutthroat mentality where all are seen as competition making the only manner of succeeding under such a system the willful destruction of another.

In reality, capitalism is the method by which the greatest degree of freedom may be achieved by the greatest number. It is the most versatile of all economic systems, allowing for society to quickly adapt to its changing demands and needs. If the measure of the greatness of an economic system is the facilitation of the advancement of man's quality of life, the diminution of poverty, the development of art and individual expression, and the elevation of opportunity for people to advance from the station into which they were born, then none can hold so much as a candle to the free market and free enterprise.

The events surrounding the Wuhan pandemic have once again demonstrated the irreplaceable value of the free market to our existence and survival. When the nation was forced to rapidly make up for a sudden shortage of supplies, it was the private sector that responded. Three million eight hundred twenty thousand N-95 masks, 3,260,000 surgical masks, 5,500,000 face shields, 4,700,000 surgical gowns, 30,300,000 gloves, 212,000 coveralls, 8,600 medical station beds, 11,000 ventilators, and 28,000,000 hydroxychloroquine tablets were committed within five weeks of initiating the effort. No government agency could ever achieve that.

In fact, to the extent that we were anemic in our response, it was specifically because we had previously regulated private enterprise into a weakened position. As we saw, the time following World War II was one of unparalleled productivity in the United States. But, through excessive governmental regulation, price caps, and production hurdles, our country naturally drove manufacturing into the hands of foreign powers. As a result, our nation tackled the Wuhan pandemic with 90% of its antibiotics being made in China, hydroxychloroquine manufacturing largely based out of India, N-95 masks being supplied by China, and only about a dozen companies capable of making ventilators in the United States. A country cannot independently survive when it depends on others for the production of so many of its essential products, particularly when those upon whom that country has become dependent are not its natural allies.

And the weaknesses in our supply chains were not confined merely to the medical manufacturing sector. A compounding factor to the destabilization of our markets was the price war between Saudi Arabia and Russia. When Saudi Arabia announced that it would be flooding the markets, oil prices crashed by 30%, or less than $30 barrel. Oil speculators scrambled, gasoline manufacturers shuttered, and the stock market careened down as it made its way to its eventual low of 18,591.93. If the United States loses an industry of this magnitude to an opportunistic foreign power it will not only see the loss of scores of thousands of jobs but the creation of a greater American dependence on foreign manufacturers, this time in the production of one of the most essential segments of our society, our energy sector.

The importance of domestic manufacturing is paramount to maintaining our nation's stability and malleability. At times it means paying a higher price for the product so we may keep it at home. At others, it requires deregulation. Regardless, the nation must maintain the production of essential products, the greatest extent possible, on American soil.

Coronalesson No. 13: Pay off your debt.

Public debt is a bad thing. It places a drag on the economy. If high enough, it can slow economic growth, make life more expensive for citizens, and make credit more difficult to obtain. Most agree that some amount of debt is necessary, as it would be difficult for a nation to contend with a spending limit that equaled its revenues. For example, America's present federal tax revenue is in the order of $3 trillion. Saying that the United States government is limited to spending $3 trillion per year is an unreasonable limitation when one considers that its military budget alone is over $600 billion, Medicare takes up $1.2 trillion and social security absorbs another trillion. If we imposed such strict budgeting constraints, then gone would be infrastructure maintenance and construction, border security, and agricultural support to name a few. More importantly, the country needs the latitude to accommodate sudden bursts of necessary spending such as in times of war and health crises.

So, how much is a healthy amount of debt? Economists disagree on the answer to this question. Many suggest that a nation's debt-to-GDP ratio ought not to exceed 60% in a country with a developed economy like the United States.[650] Others point out that so long as the yearly growth for a nation's GDP is greater than the amount it pays in interest each year, the debt does not really represent a threat to that nation's economy. History suggests anything greater than a debt-to-GDP ratio of 90% is destabilizing, particularly when it has been allowed to remain at such high levels for greater than five years, a situation called a public debt overhang.[651]

From other nations' experiences, however, we have been able to identify debt-to-GDP ratios that are clearly too high. Greece is the classic example of a country with an excessive debt-to-GDP ratio, which presently stands at 181%.[652] But even in 2011, when the Greek debt-to-GDP ratio stood at 165%, the nation had difficulty keeping its investors and eventually defaulted on its debt.[653] The result was massive inflation, social unrest, and economic instability. Spain and Italy, two other countries with economic challenges, have debt-to-GDP ratios of 95.5% and 134.8% respectively.[654] By comparison, economically healthier countries like Germany and Sweden carry deb-to-GDP ratios of 59.8% and 35.1% respectively.[655]

One notable exception is Japan, which has been able to tolerate a debt-to-GDP ratio of 234.99%.[656] The nation's ability to accommodate such high debt-to-GDP ratios could be due to the large amounts of personal savings the Japanese have and their willingness to buy government bonds. However, even though Japan has not been plagued by a financial crisis, it has suffered from weak economic growth.[657]

The United States has traditionally had a healthy debt-to-GDP ratio. In 1946, immediately following World War II, its debt-to-GDP ratio stood at a record 106%. In 1966, due to the boom in economic activity, the ratio decreased to 40.33%.[658] By 1980, the United States had successfully dropped its ratio to 30.60%[659] only to have it rise again to 105% by the end of President Obama's presidency in 2016.[660] His number, of course, is perilously close to what a nation's economy can withstand.

In 2020, the numbers will only worsen. With all the spending in response to the Wuhan pandemic, America's debt precipitously increased to over $25.6 trillion, placing our debt-to-GDP ratio at a staggering 121.88%.[661] And those numbers only deal with the numerator. A ratio is equally affected by its denominator, in this case, the GDP, which is estimated to fall by about 14% for the United States because of the shutdown.[662] Estimates are that the debt-to-GDP ratio will top 135% by September 30, 2020.[663]

Even when seen through the lens of the relationship between the debt interest and the GDP growth, America's numbers do not look good. As of 2018, U.S. interest paid on the nation's debt was $325 billion,[664] while the increase in GPD between Q4 2017 and Q4 of 2018 was $831 billion.[665] The result was a favorable difference at $506 billion. However, with the national economy predicted to contract, the interest rate on the debt will naturally exceed the GDP's growth, reversing a formerly favorable relationship.

It is clear that our country has not been responsible in handling its debt over the past thirty years. The rampant irresponsibility and drunken spending habits of the nation's leaders have left us with a massive debt even before accounting for the Wuhan pandemic. Our nation has never seen debt-to-GDP ratios anywhere near 135% over the past 100 years, and as opposed to the post-War period, there is no economic boom looming around the corner to bail us out. One thing is certain, however, that age-old mantra that all of us have heard since our childhood, "Pay off your debt," is definitely one we have not adhered to as a nation. As a result, one of the predictable consequences of our fiscal irresponsibility is now biting us. Because of our staggering debt going into this crisis, we simply do not have the flexibility to throw trillions of dollars into the economy to prevent its collapse. Ironically, doing so could cause its collapse. But we did it anyway. What the effects will be on our nation's stability and our continued ability to stave off foreign threats like China and Russia remain to be seen.

Dismal as our situation may be, however, we have two things going for us. First, we have a massive economy that other countries facing similar challenges do not. If there is an economy that can get through this, it is the United States, albeit with significant pain and suffering. The other advantage is that everyone else's economy is doing even worse.

Coronalesson No. 14: Our national stockpile needs to be actively maintained and its deployment procedures must be revamped.

It falls under many of the core responsibilities of the federal government, "To insure domestic tranquility, provide for the common defense, promote the general Welfare, and secure the Blessings of Liberty, to ourselves and our Posterity."[666] The SNS is one of those essential safeguards we keep to ascertain our ability to respond to national crises affecting the health of the American people, whether from military attack or massive disease outbreak. In the task of maintaining and resupplying it, Congress cannot ever let down its guard.

According to President Trump, there were issues with the size of the cache within the SNS. As mentioned previously, it is difficult to ascertain the size of our stockpile's shortcomings because the information, if not outright classified, is not readily available. If true, however, the withering away of the SNS represents a threat as great as not maintaining the nation's military.

President Clinton had an incredible idea when he conceived of the need for a national stockpile of medical relief supplies. His original conception dealt with antibiotics, but over time, advocates have recognized that such a reserve must include medical supplies as well. Until now, much of the public discussion regarding SNS preparation has been centered on regional or local demands for medical antibiotics or equipment. How do we respond to an anthrax attack on Chicago? What if there were an Ebola outbreak in San Francisco? Or what do we do in response to a full-fledged outbreak of Zika in Florida?

Much less has been said regarding handling a nation-wide contemporaneous assault on America's health and wellbeing. The lesson to be learned from SARS-CoV-2 is that we must now constantly entertain a response, not only to local events but to those spanning the whole nation. President Trump learned this lesson organically. He had to respond to the possibilities as they were materializing. Clearly, although forced upon him by necessity, this approach is suboptimal. The whole concept of being prepared lies in being prepared. It breads not a reactive posture, but a proactive one. As will be developed in the following chapter, we must now change our model for the SNS and its role in future crises.

Coronalesson No. 15: Protect our nursing homes.

It's a mistake that played itself out time and again throughout Europe and even within the United States: the failure to protect nursing homes. In Italy, 40% of deaths occurred in nursing homes, while in Sweden, they accounted for greater than 50% of the country's deaths. In France, COVID-19 took over 10,000 lives in nursing homes. In Spain, over 17,500 deaths are suspected to have taken place in nursing homes. And in the United States, 27% of all the state's deaths, or at least 5,215, are traceable to nursing homes.

On its face, it seems to be glaringly obvious. There is a highly contagious virus with a known predilection for people with serious medical conditions and advanced age heading to the United States. You protect your nursing homes. Why this would be such a great mystery defies credulity. The reality is that no one is going to be able to save all nursing home residents. If things go well with our lives, we live long ones and then pass away. Nursing home residents tend to be at the final stages of their lives, making it inevitable that many of them will pass away during their stay there. However, that does not, in any way, excuse their neglect, mistreatment, or lack of protection. It is precisely because these individuals are so frail and vulnerable that it is our duty to protect, shield, and comfort them.

This was exactly what Andrew Cuomo failed to do.

Cuomo's priority was preserving hospital beds. He took to television recurrently claiming that there were insufficient hospital beds, ICU beds, and ventilators, and pointed the accusatory finger squarely at the President. As it turns out, none of his predictions rang true, and even if they had, Governor Cuomo was provided a number of hospitals, including a hospital ship, to supplement his assets. Nevertheless and despite the vacant status of the supplemental, temporary hospitals provided to him, Cuomo chose to do everything possible to keep New York's permanent beds open, to the point of forcing COVID-19 patients, known or not, into the state's nursing homes. The decision was grossly ill founded and as explosive as tossing a lit match into a gasoline tank. The results were not only predictably catastrophic but they revealed the disregard Cuomo had for his state's senior citizens, particularly its weakest.

By contrast, Florida did it correctly. Governor DeSantis ordered his nursing homes to lock down. He made sure that only recently tested individuals were allowed admission to a nursing home, and visits were kept to a minimum. As a result, Florida, a slightly more populous state than New York, saw about one fifth the number of nursing home deaths (1,085) as of May 25, 2020.[667]

Relatedly, another issue arising from the actions taken during this pandemic deals with the preservation of the dignity of nursing home residents. All over the country, nursing home residents were dying alone. In our zeal to isolate them, we forced them to spend their last moments on earth away from the ones they loved. Companionship is a fundamental component of the dying process. As one prepares to leave the bounds of this life, fissures can be mended, appreciation and love can be expressed, and comfort can be provided, oftentimes without uttering a word. For those who survive, great contentment can be realized knowing that they were there for their loved ones as they slipped away. And alternatively, for those without the opportunity to console, the guilt regarding their failures can riddle them, often permanently. Under the effects of the pandemic, the government and certain facilities forcibly and inhumanely interfered with the manner in which that process played out. We must never let that circumstance be repeated.

Coronalesson No. 16: The relative lethality of COVID-19.

How lethal is SARS-CoV-2? The answer to this question is critical and not just for the obvious reason of providing information about our risk of dying from this contagion. Its contagiousness and lethality play central roles in the predictions of the virus's spread and the mortality associated with it. Recall that most criticisms regarding the prediction models used during the ramp-up of the coronavirus dealt with the appropriateness of the numbers selected. And although a major contention made in this volume regarding these models centers on the inappropriateness of assuming an equal chance of contact amongst all members of a population, it is equally important that an accurate number regarding the virus's infectiousness and its lethality be employed. The final answer regarding SARCoV-2's contagiousness and lethality is not out yet. In fact, they may be morphing. However, it is appropriate that we address it to some extent here.

The contagiousness, or the ease with which a contagion spreads, is best described by its basic reproduction number (Ro). This figure describes the number of people to which an infected person is apt to spread the contagion. In theory, one could determine the Ro by finding each person with a contagion and observing how many of his or her contacts develop the disease. Logistically, this exercise is nearly impossible. Instead, epidemiologists estimate the Ro using the shape of the curve of the contagion's spread. The higher the number, the more infectious the contagion is. Through these statistical calculations, the R_0 for Ebola was determined to be between 1.5 and 5. For MERS, it spanned between 0.8 and 6. Tuberculosis has an R0 between 0.3 and 4.25, and for SARS, the figure was somewhere between 2 and 4.[668]

On April 12, 2020, the CDC released a study based on the Chinese experience, estimating the SARS-CoV-2 Ro at 5.7.[669] It should be noted that factors external to the virus, such as population density, regional environment and containment efforts such as wearing masks and social distancing have effects on the virus's contagiousness. Additionally, many viruses morph over time so some viruses that were once highly contagious fizzle out and become more docile as the genome mutates. Consequently, the numbers and the statistical analyses based on these data are still developing. Towards this end, the CDC released data more recently estimating the SARS-CoV-2 Ro at 2.5.[670] The new numbers create a striking contrast with the prior data since under the original estimates COVID-19 appeared to be more contagious than the seasonal flu, Ebola, MERS, and SARS. It was even more contagious than the strain of influenza that caused the Spanish flu in 1918, which is estimated to have an Ro of 1.5 to 3. The newer numbers suggest SARS-CoV-2 is about as contagious as most other major contagions, but not more so.

Regardless of the Ro data, a major challenge to preventing the SARS-CoV-2's spread is its ability to be passed on while its host is still not showing any symptoms. If anything, this latter factor represents the biggest challenge in constraining the spread of this virus.

The virus's lethality is a different issue. The key figure regarding a virus's lethality is the ratio between the number of deaths due to the virus divided by the number of symptomatic cases. In other words, if you get sick from the SARS-CoV-2, what are the chances you will die from it? This is different from the deaths per case ratio as this latter number is much more difficult to quantify because of the unknown number of asymptomatic cases. As the virus made its way through China and Europe, symptomatic case fatality ratios as high as 6% were suggested. However, according to the CDC's latest data, the overall symptomatic case fatality rate (which is necessarily either equal to or higher than the overall case fatality rate) is 0.4%![671] This is dramatically lower than originally thought.

The CDC numbers also provide us with demographic insights. The highest death rates of 1.3% occurred in patients who were 65 years of age or older. For those who were sick with the virus and were 50-64 years of age, the death rate was 0.2% and for those who were 49-years-old or less, the rate was 0.05%,[672] reinforcing what Governor Cuomo should have known, that it was the elderly upon whom he should have been concentrating his protective efforts.

Finally, a few observations regarding racial and gender distributions of cases and deaths in the United States are necessary. There is data indicating that black Americans have a higher tendency to die from COVID-19 than would be predicted by their percentage of the population. In some reports, black Americans account for 42% of deaths while making up 21% of the population.[673] Although some have politicized this difference, the answer is much more complicated. Factors include relative poverty rates amongst black communities, population densities, the number of medical conditions per person, access to health care, and trust in the healthcare system.

A striking discrepancy also exists amongst the sexes. Even though men and women are equally likely to contract the virus, in China, 70% of those who died were men, 63% in Europe, and almost two thirds in New York.[674] Factors may include a higher tendency for men to hesitate in seeking medical treatment compared to women, men's propensity to engage in higher-risk activities like ignoring mitigation recommendations, and perhaps a

stronger female immune system.[675] Regardless of the posited causes for either demographic, the reality is more studies and much
more sophisticated statistical analyses are required before any scientifically valid conclusions can be formulated.

Coronalesson No. 17: Yes, it can happen in America.

This is perhaps the darkest, most frightening coronalesson. After
witnessing the events that have transpired since the beginning of
2020, we can never again say that the chaos, destruction, and instability afflicting other countries will never happen in America. If
there's one thing that has become evident from our common experience with Wuhan pandemic is the frailty of our American system
of governance and of our way of life. Up to this moment, many were
comfortable saying that our nation was too large, our people too
strong, our principles too deeply rooted, and our might too great to
ever allow the shenanigans we have witnessed in other countries to
take place here. But now, we have seen our economy, our stability,
our respect for government, and portions of our military brought to
its knees in just a few short weeks. *A few short weeks!*

On February 12, our stock market closed at 29,551,42. Our unemployment rate was at record lows. The country was prosperous.
Wages for working-class Americans were rising faster than the cost
of living, and we were flexing our muscles against opportunists like
the People's Republic of China.

But within a few short weeks, specifically by March 23, the stock
market lost nearly 40% of its value, businesses were shut down,
and over 20 million people became unemployed. Ominously, Time
Square lay empty. Except in a few decimated hotspots, hospitals
all over the country lay barren. Our nursing homes became death

grounds. Certain governors, nearly universally from the Left, took advantage of the chaos to overexert their power. Legislators attempted to fund a myriad of programs unrelated to healthcare or economic stabilization under the guise of helping the American people. And Americans were made to fear.

If all these horrible events destabilizing the nation can happen in six short weeks, imagine the depths to which we can sink if the fear is more sustained, the morals a little worse, or the attack more coordinated.

America can be brought to its knees, and easily. What we have learned from the Wuhan pandemic is that the fount of a nation's strength is not its economy, or its mighty warriors, or its enlightened legal corpus. The cornerstone of a nation's stability, and indeed its very strength, comes from its people, their ethics, resilience, and sense of purpose. In short, it rests on the character of its people.

President Trump astutely said that we must rebuild the nation, but the truth is that we cannot engage in this effort without fortifying our virtues, our beliefs, and our souls. If we build our economy on the backs of a weakened people, it is tantamount to building our homes, not on rock but on sand. As soon as the rains fall, the floods come, and the winds blow, our nation will collapse and lie in ruins.

Our exit strategy must be bolder and reach deeper than a mere economic reconstruction. It requires a fundamental reevaluation and reinvigoration of us as Americans.

But for that, we have the next chapter evaluating the path ahead.

Chapter 7

The Path Ahead

The trauma we have endured is truly unparalleled in our nation during a time of peace. None of us imagined a situation where our collective wealth would be so effectively slashed, our confidence so violently shaken, and our standing so greatly affected. But yet, it happened, and we survived. Now, as we stand before the rubble, we are challenged with charting a way forward, and it is here where the lessons we have learned help us most.

We need to reopen. We must get back to work. Our kids need to get back to school. Our athletes need to compete. Our entertainers must entertain. . . in person! Our youth need to continue to pursue their passions and to discover. Our healthcare providers need to get back to treating much more than COVID-19. There are lives to save. Dreams to fulfill. Rockets to be launched. And contributions to be made the likes of which we cannot even fathom. Everyone has a role to play in bettering our existence, but we cannot wait one more minute to resume realizing it.

SARS-CoV-2 is neither as lethal nor as contagious as we once thought. An Ro that was initially thought to be 5.7 appears to be 2.5, similar to that of the flu. And a symptomatic case death rate that we thought was as high a 6%, is in fact 0.04%, again, about as lethal as the flu. Yet we don't shut down for the flu. Additionally, whereby we feared the collapse of our healthcare system because of a rapid and tsunamic wave of patients, that is no longer a realistic possibility.

It is now time to go on with our lives. Yes, the furious search for a vaccine must continue. The research for treatments and preventive measures must endure. And case surveillance must still be undertaken, but they must continue while we move on in the fullest sense of the word.

There are at least 17 coronalessons we have learned from this experience. They tell us, loudly, that although we need to get back to work and we must continue with our lives, our newfound insights must also be applied. First, we must continue to track cases. Not as part of a massive contact tracking effort. As we saw, the time for massive and intrusive efforts is way past us. Rather, the various state health departments in coordination with the CDC must track the number of new COVID-19 cases. The public must continue to be reminded to frequently wash their hands, and those who are elderly and suffer from multiple medical conditions must be encouraged to use masks when entering crowded venues or publicly frequented indoor facilities like grocery stores or theaters. Local officials ought to communicate each community's daily caseloads and weekly trends using the local press and government websites. If an upward trend is spotted in a community, the public ought to be notified with instructions on what to do to counteract or prevent a potential outbreak.

At least as it relates to SASR-CoV-2, the priority must be the nursing homes as this is where the greatest harm is likely to take place. Nursing homes must be opened up to visitors, but policies calling for the routine and periodic COVID-19 PCR testing for those entering nursing homes should also be implemented. In between tests, those seeking entry should be screened for symptoms and undergo temperature checks. As implemented in Florida, all patients awaiting transfer from hospitals to extended care facilities, including assisted living facilities, must have a negative COVID-19 test within 48 hours of being discharged. If a resident in a nursing home tests positive for COVID-19, he or she must be isolated. Any caregivers and family members must use full PPE when attending to these residents. Provided the layout of the facility allows, it would be preferable if an infected resident or residents were placed in a separate area where friends and family may visit until they test negative. The tragedy of allowing the elderly to die alone by state decree can never be repeated.

The SNS must be restocked. There can never again be a time when Congress allows the SNS's medical supplies to be depleted. From now on, we must stand prepared for a strike from a novel virus. We must acknowledge that another attack will occur, either from nature or malfeasance, and it will threaten to overwhelm us. We must be prepared, not merely to respond to regional events like hurricanes, tornadoes, earthquakes, and localized outbreaks but for a pandemic that will grip the whole country. And the federal government cannot be expected to provide these resources by itself. The states need to build their own stockpiles as well, and Congress ought to consider withholding Medicaid and hospital support for those states not demonstrating sufficient progress towards that end.

Concurrently, FEMA, the White House, the U.S Public Health Service, the CDC Congress, and representatives from each state need to engage in a strategic initiative defining how medical supplies and support will be mobilized. The country can ill-afford to have a Cuomo claiming that he has no supplies when he is actually sufficiently stocked. Equally, the country cannot have a Cuomo begging for equipment as the primary method by which he or she applies for material and logistical support. These issues need to be hashed out ahead of time, and drilled, so that when the next pandemic hits, this country may execute the plan with military precision.

The President and the CWHTF have invented a new wheel made up of a broad network of manufacturers capable of supplying medical equipment in a very short time. This network must be formalized into a standing resource ready to respond. It must stand ready to provide ventilators, masks, face shields, protective medical gowns, gloves, alcohol swabs, collection tubes, study media, test kits, culture swabs, test reagents, and hand sanitizing solutions, to name a few. These companies must be identified and encouraged not only to network with the federal government but also with the states. The time to identify and engage these companies is now, well before we find ourselves staring at the harrowing face of another pandemic.

In the meantime, the experts (epidemiologists, statisticians, and public health experts) have some work to do. First, their post-mortem needs to acknowledge their recurring failures in handling this pandemic. Sadly, if there is one thing the experts demonstrated during this time, it is that they don't really know what they're talking about. Nevertheless, their substantiated input is desperately needed. A formula like SIR assuming that all members of a population in a geographical area as vast as the United States have an equal chance of coming into contact with any other is preposterously inappropriate for planning purposes. The experts can start by developing corrective coefficients that better estimate the chances that those in one area of the country will contact those in other area and spread disease. This correction should allow policymakers and emergency responders to better plan for outcomes and more effectively allocate resources, not to send them and the public into a spiraling tailspin.

From a messaging standpoint, experts must understand that theirs is to provide insight in support of decisions, not doubts for plans with which they may not agree. Whatever the optimal theoretical answer, the experts must also understand that theirs is not the only priority, or even the most important. Frankly, the days where a Dr. Fauci stands up before the podium and says that he is only speaking as a public health expert must be behind us. No one in the decision-making team can come out and speak on his behalf alone. He or she must understand the plan, hash out his or her differences, and deliver a message to the public that integrates all sides of the formula into one cohesive message.

We should remember that the private sector is the most versatile and responsive model to accommodate for rapid shifts in the market. The reason our nation was able to respond so quickly to the rapid and overwhelming onslaught of cases was because of the robust presence of the private sector. No government agency could have switched the production gears as rapidly and massively as the free market did. Yet, over the past five decades, we have done everything in our power to drive manufacturers out of our country and seek better environments elsewhere. We have been shown signs of how badly we can suffer for this grievous error. Fortunately, this time we have the privilege of saying that although there were some hardships in procurement and production, our collective experience was not as devastating as it could have been. Having recognized these weaknesses they must be corrected before we are in a situation where we have restricted ourselves so extensively we are unable to respond. Many of the recommendations made in *The Case for Free Market Healthcare* are applicable here. We should let the market compete in the healthcare arena as we do in any other sector. We must have government withdraw its restrictions on hospitals, manufacturers, and practices so that they may settle into the most efficient conditions possible. The FDA must be revamped as recommended in *The Case*, and all the regulatory encumbrances placed upon the healthcare sector must be removed. Ours is the greatest healthcare system in the world with the most qualified professionals. It can be even better if we let it.

Moving forward, we cannot place ourselves in a situation where we are dependent on China for anything. That China would be responsible for the production of 90% of our generic antibiotics is preposterous as is the thought that our nation has lost the ability to massively manufacture penicillin. There are many ways whereby we can lose our independence. One is to give foreign actors free rein over the production of our vital products. This situation can no longer exist.

China must pay for the reckless disregard of human life it demonstrated on a global scale. Plaintiffs must be allowed to sue China in U.S. courts and elsewhere for loss of life, pain and suffering, punitive damages, and economic harm. It must be made clear to China that actions endangering the lives of people around the world will not be tolerated. This is at least the second time when China responded to the appearance of a novel virus with secrecy and deceit. This time, the deadly consequences of China's actions were made worse by its continued interactions with countries like Italy and Iran who depended on its good faith and transparency, and on its commitment to avoid recklessly endangering the lives of foreign nationals, whether through shoddy workmanship or the irresponsible spread of disease.

Further, actions against China cannot be limited to legal recourses. China must suffer in its standing and the ease with which it continues to economically interact with other nations. The rectifications of Chinese behavior must go much further than merely their dealings in healthcare. Practically every inappropriate action China takes in the international arena must be countered, from its recurrent currency manipulation tactics to the manner in which it treats intellectual property rights. If China intends to build a world-class military, which it presently is attempting to do, it may not be allowed to do so off the backs of other countries.

Earlier, we noted that our country's debt-to-GDP ratio was likely going to increase to 135%. China's is now at 310%.[676] China cannot go toe-to-toe with the United States if we confront it; that is unless we sit on our laurels and watch as its rogue and inhumane government strengthens.

And then there's the WHO. As of this writing, President Trump has announced that he would be withdrawing the United States from the WHO.[677] With the recent conduct of the WHO, its protections of the Chinese government, and the dereliction of its duty to help the world combat disease, his move is appropriate. The real consideration is what's next. For starters, if the United States is to truly withdraw from the WHO, there must be a provision prohibiting Americans from contributing to the organization as individuals. The Gates Foundation is the second-largest funder of the WHO, second only to the United States. For the United States' position to be truly effective in its actions towards the WHO, money flowing from the Foundation must also be shut down. If Mr. Gates wishes to continue his humanitarian vaccine-promoting activities, he can certainly coordinate them with a novel organization headquartered in his country. The United States is certainly strong enough to create its own rival organization, and this time, one with some teeth and not bullied into submission.

Alternatively, the President could leverage his withdrawal from the WHO on negotiations providing a new direction for the organization. The WHO needs the United States a lot more than the United States needs the WHO. Most importantly, the world needs an organization that actually carries out its duties of disease surveillance and humanitarian aid free of political bias.

And let's not forget the United Nations. No matter how hostile to the United States the WHO may be, the UN is even worse. On the same day the President tweeted his position on withdrawing from the WHO, he asked Americans whether the United States should do the same with the UN. My answer to this question is a resounding no. The United States holds a seat at the UN's General Assembly with absolute veto power. The only check we have on the out-of-control, rogue tendencies of the UN is our ability to stop any adverse recommendation with a single vote. If we were not occupying that seat, I am confident this band of anti-Zionists, anti-American socialists will quickly organize against the United States and Israel. There's no telling how structured and broad that hostile alliance may become absent the restraining presence of the United States. Yes, the United States ought to discontinue all discretionary funding to the United Nations, but it must retain its membership, at least until the United Nations is dissolved.

In light of China's recurrent failures and deception in the arena of disease containment and the WHO's ineptness, a more robust attitude towards a distant outbreak is in order. But resolving to do this requires a more fundamental commitment, namely a large reduction in our partisanship. This recommendation goes out to both parties, but in this case, the greater culprit is Democratic leadership. Some have said that the President was distracted with all the impeachment proceedings. In reality, the House was distracted and was the major culprit in distracting others. The Senate was necessarily distracted because it was sucked into a trial it had no interest in holding. And the press, with its lust for President Trump's political blood, was most distracted of all. Each of them carried out a great disservice to our country.

The Wuhan pandemic demonstrates at least the second time in American history where our partisan division dearly cost us. All opponents to the President dropped the ball in their zeal to undo his rightfully won election, and they dragged the rest of us down with them. If there was one person who was not distracted, it was the person accused of being distracted: the President of the United States who, unlike the others, had the foresight to promptly restrict travel from China.

But a response to the Wuhan pandemic requires more fundamentally centered corrections. Indeed, these are vastly more important than any short-term recommendations we could make. Among the most threatening realization from our dealings with the Wuhan pandemic is the ignorance our citizens display regarding the structure and operation of the Constitution of the United States. The Constitution is designed to prevent the very events we witnessed with frustration. It is a document designed to decentralize power, deter the inappropriate assumption of power, and keep government from infringing upon the liberties of the people. From the recommendations made by many, including some public officials, poll responders, medical experts, and the members of the press, it is obvious that they know not how our government is supposed to function. The sad truth is, though, that they are merely repeating what they were taught in our schools. As evidenced by the unending stream of intrusions onto the Constitution undertaken by our nation's leaders, instruction on civics and American history has suffered greatly in this country. Much of it is due to an army of teachers from whose training any emphasis regarding American governmental design was removed. These men and women are now out in the field propagating their misrepresentations of American governance and imprinting them upon the next generation of leaders and voters. Absent a rapid correction on the education we receive, Americans will continue to lose sight of what they are defending and of what they stand for. Their rights will be eroded without knowing that they ever even had them.

If the deficit lies in our education, then the correction must reside there as well. Specifically, the manner in which we teach civics in this country and the emphases we place in teaching it must be changed. A proper rendition of our national structure must, at the very least, include a thorough understanding of the original incarnation of the Constitution and its intent. The focus must be on the importance of power decentralization, on checks and balances, and on teaching which department is responsible for what in our federalist design.

If our Republic is to survive, then every citizen must be aware of the limitations placed on the federal government, the roles of the states as the primary purveyors of the nation's police powers, and the differences between the two. Absent these fundamental understandings, the citizenry will not be in a position to check its own officials. And they must understand the salutatory purpose of the Second Amendment, which does not merely protect one's ability to hunt game or defend oneself against a physical attack. It really does allow the citizenry to provide yet another check on an overly zealous government.

Equally as important is the institution of a process by which the mismanagement of the people's treasury is stopped. We can never again find ourselves owing 135% of what we create each year in our country. It is unacceptable and a threat to our national security. More than at any other time in our nation's history the Wuhan pandemic has demonstrated the imminent need for a balanced budget amendment to the Constitution. Our Framers envisioned a government free to grow its expenditures during times of need, but also one sufficiently responsible to demand that expenditures drop once the crisis is past. Unfortunately, our leaders have been very effective at the former, but have failed miserably at the latter. It is time for the people to rectify the situation before it is too late. A balanced budget amendment must be passed.

Finally, we end with the rectification for the most important coronalesson of all: the restoration of our faith in God and in His primacy within the fabric of our nation. If, as a nation, we believe that Jesus Christ is God who humiliated himself in an act of mercy to undo the effects of the sin of Adam and that he demands that we spend every moment of our lives striving to live in a state of peace, not only with God but with our own neighbors, then we will be naturally compelled by our ethic to take on whatever evil may confront us. In that state, all fear and angst disappear and we become invincible soldiers in the defense of a better existence, a better healthcare system, and a greater system of government. The effects of our abandonment of these principles are clearly visible in our actions towards this virus and our attitudes towards each other. We must return, as a nation, to the loving arms of our Lord and Savior Jesus Christ and live out our lives as a unified body deeply respecting the rights, freedoms, and dignity of each individual. If we accomplish this, no virus will hurt us, no evil will threaten us, and no enemy can ever prevail over us.

Afterword

Take a look at what's happening around you. Take a good look. Objectively. Nonconspiratorially. All the events you are witnessing are interrelated. The Wuhan pandemic. The economic downturn. The quest for power. The unemployment rate. The run on our nation's debt. The absence of faith. And now, most recently, the rioting and looting. They are all part of a cascade. I am not saying that a great, worldly, nefarious weaver has strung together a series of preplanned events designed to elicit destruction and fear. Rather, I am acknowledging that there are opportunistic elements in our society that, for whatever reason, would like nothing more than to obliterate the system in which they find themselves in exchange for one they can better manipulate. They sit waiting, sometimes more patiently than others, for their opportunity to pounce.

Here, in the United States, we have created the greatest sociopolitical system in the world. It is admittedly flawed, but all of mankind is flawed, and it is clearly the greatest system ever devised. It is a system that rewards individual achievement and promotes movement between classes. It allows for individual expression and worship. And it divests power from the autocracy in an attempt to place it in the hands of the people. Although our system can be improved, there is no better one with which it can be replaced. May 2020 was marred by looting, rioting, and violence. The concerted destruction of stores and the burning of whole sections of American cities have sullied its warming trends and diminishing

COVID-19 numbers. And for what? Ostensibly, to protest the tragic and horrific murder of a black citizen by a white police officer in Minneapolis.

But clearly, racial disparities and overarching institutional injustices are not the motivations for these riots. One does not bring attention to injustice by causing even greater injustice. No. What we are witnessing are the actions of criminal opportunists who have been waiting for some fracture in America's social fabric to destroy the pinnacle of human sociopolitical design and replace it with something much more sinister.

In May 2020, America was in a weakened state. It had just come off the effects of an overreaction. Its economy was in tatters. Its people were suddenly unemployed. Its President, despite having accomplished much, was portrayed as caustic and divisive. Its debt-to-GDP ratio had just taken a precipitous leap. And its moral fiber, debilitated by decades of dismissing God, religion, and the family, was wanting. Each of these alone was sufficient to cause the political upheaval and instability we witnessed. Taken together, they made up a high-power explosive just waiting for a spark, and the spark came in the form of a murder.

It was gross, uncalled for, and cowardly, but it came at the hands of a white police officer in Minnesota who was arresting a black man named George Floyd. And it was filmed. Horrified, the country watched as George Floyd begged for mercy. He was on the ground. His hands restrained behind his back. He was surrounded by a number of police officers. Four? And he was clearly no longer a menace. Yet, one officer chose to pin his knee on Mr. Floyd's neck for nearly nine minutes. It is still unclear whether Floyd died of asphyxiation or a sudden shutdown of his physiology brought about by the physical stress the maneuver the police officer protractedly applied upon him caused. Either way, Floyd had the life snuffed out of him and died.

The outrage was immediate and unanimous. Everyone agreed! The events depicted were horrid. The police officer in question needed to be held to account. Justice needed to be served. Many were so appalled that they appropriately felt motivated to demonstrate and put a voice to their dismay. But there also arose an opportunity for those subversive elements to pounce on the vulnerabilities of a weakened nation. Thousands not from Minneapolis appeared at the protests. They threw bottles at the police, raided stores, and incinerated police cars. The looting spread to countless cities throughout the nation, and magically, mysteriously, pallets of bricks appeared on the sidewalks of major American cities where no construction was taking place but where more looting was about to occur.

The mayhem spread to all corners of the United States, including Washington, D.C, and continued for over a week. In the end, stores were destroyed, communities were decimated, and the looters retreated into the darkness, many within the shadows of homes hundreds of miles from where they inflicted their damage. These are not the actions of concerned citizens. These are the actions of subversives aiming to destroy society's foundational pillars to promote their own interests.

And what are those ends? We get an idea of what they desire from the "loose associations" of citizen groups whose views are voiced on social media. They include a call for justice. Although whose justice, they do not say. They call for equality, but theirs is not an equality of opportunity but an equality in outcomes administered according to the judgment of those they put in power. For them, property is not a right; it is at best a privilege bestowed by the state. At worst private property does not even exist. Personal desires are subservient to their justice. And the police, the major physical impediment to their agenda is to be disassembled, substituted by a utopian conglomerate of fellow humans empowered with amorphous authorities, again, all in the name of an undefined justice.

Looking at these events it is clear, objectively, that they are not spontaneous in origin. Rather, they represent an orchestrated response to a trigger set for a time of weakness. And America, in part due to the appearance of SARS-CoV-2, in part through the consequences of its response to the pandemic, and in great measure due to the moral apathy afflicting it, is weak. And so these elements, basted in the foul and rotted spices of socialism, communism, and a secular, one-world order pounced on the opportunity and gave form to each of the coronalessons we have previously explored. In physics, every action elicits an equal and opposite reaction. The same can be said in sociology. Our handling of the Wuhan pandemic has caused a reaction marked by economic debilitation, suffering, and death. That reaction has led to yet another pandemic, this one clearly manmade, and it too has resulted in economic debilitation, suffering, and death.

What will be our reaction to the reaction?

That is the piece we hold in our hands. I propose that instead of countering with more of the same, we counter with the calling given to us in both the Old Testament and the New. I say we choose to love God with all our strength; and that we love our neighbors, regardless of race, gender, religion, or ethnic origin with the same tenderness, charity, and protections that we do ourselves.

List of Illustrations

Citations

1. Taken from http://wjw.wuhan.gov.cn/front/web/showDetail/2020011109035, accessed Apr. 20, 2020. Translation obtained through Google.

2. "H1N1: The 2009 H1N1 Pandemic: Summary Highlights, April 2009-April 2010," CDC, Jun. 16, 2010, accessed Apr. 3, 2020, https://www.cdc.gov/h1n1flu/cdcresponse.htm

3. Mangia A, Piazzolla V, Giannelli A, et al. SVR12 rates higher than 99% after sofosbuvir/velpatasvir combination in HCV infected patients with F0-F1 fibrosis stage: A real world experience [published correction appears in PLoS One. 2019 Sep 25;14(9):e0223287]. *PLoS One*. 2019;14(5):e0215783. Published 2019 May 15. doi:10.1371/journal.pone.0215783.

4. Apoorva Mandavilli, "H.I.V. Is Reported Cured in a Second Patient, a Milestone in the Global AIDS Epidemic," *New York Times* (blog), Mar. 4, 2019, accessed Apr. 4, 2020, https://www.nytimes.com/2019/03/04/health/aids-cure-london-patient.html.

5. "H1N1: The 2009 H1N1 Pandemic: Summary Highlights, April 2009-April 2010," CDC, Jun. 16, 2010, accessed Apr. 3, 2020, https://www.cdc.gov/h1n1flu/cdcresponse.htm.

6. Ibid.

7. Owen Jarvis, "20 of the Worst Epidemics and Pandemics in History," Live Science (blog), Mar. 20, 2020, accessed Apr. 1, 2020, https://www.livescience.com/worst-epidemics-and-pandemics-in-history.html.

8. Ibid.

9. Ibid.

10. Julio Gonzalez, *The Case for Free Market Healthcare*, (Sarasota, FL: Bardolf & Co., 2020), 32.

11. Ibid.

12. Ibid.

13. Ibid. .

14. Owen Jarvis, "20 of the Worst Epidemics and Pandemics in History," Live Science (blog), Mar. 20, 2020, accessed Apr. 1, 2020, https://www.livescience.com/worst-epidemics-and-pandemics-in-history.html.

15. Ibid.

16. Ibid.

17. Ibid.

18. "Influenza (Flu): 1957-1958 Pandemic (H2N2 virus), CDC, accessed Apr. 4, 2020, https://www.cdc.gov/flu/pandemic-resources/1957-1958-pandemic.html.

19. "Influenza (Flu) Burden of Influenza," CDC, accessed Apr. 13, 2020, https://www.cdc.gov/flu/about/burden/index.html.

20. Jeffrey Kahn, Kenneth McIntosh, "History and Recent Advances in Coronavirus Discovery," *The Pediatric Infections Disease Journ.*, Vol. 24, No. 11, pS223-227, Nov. 2005, digital version accessed Apr. 6, 2020, https://journals.lww.com/pidj/fulltext/2005/11001/history_and_recent_advances_in_coronavirus.12.aspx.

21. Ewen Callaway, David Cyranoski, et al, "The Coronavirus Pandemic in Five powerful Charts," *Nature* (blog) 579, 482-483 (2020) Mar. 18, 2020, accessed Mar. 26, 2020, https://www.nature.com/articles/d41586-020-00758-2.

22. J.S. Peiris, "Coronavirus," Ch. 57, in *Medical Microbiology A Guide to Microbiological Infections: Pathogenesis, Immunity, Laboratory Diagnosis and Control.* (18th Ed) David Greenwood, Mike Barer, et al. ed. Elsevier, London, 2012, 590.

23. Ibid.

24. Ibid.

25. Owen Jarvis, "20 of the Worst Epidemics and Pandemics in History," Live Science (blog), Mar. 20, 2020, accessed Apr. 1, 2020, https://www.livescience.com/worst-epidemics-and-pandemics-in-history.html.

26. "H1N1: The 2009 H1N1 Pandemic: Summary Highlights, April 2009-April 2010," CDC, Jun. 16, 2010, accessed Apr. 3, 2020, https://www.cdc.gov/h1n1flu/cdcresponse.htm.

27. Ibid.

28. Ibid.

29. Ibid.

30. Ibid.

31. Ibid.

32. Ibid. .

33. Ibid.

34. "Influenza (Flu) 2009 H1N1 Pandemic," CDC (blog), accessed Apr. 2, 2020, https://www.cdc.gov/flu/pandemic-resources/2009-h1n1-pandemic.html.

35. "Influenza (Flu) 2009 H1N1 Pandemic," CDC (blog), accessed Apr. 2, 2020, https://www.cdc.gov/flu/pandemic-resources/2009-h1n1-pandemic.html.

36. Owen Jarvis, "20 of the Worst Epidemics and Pandemics in History," Live Science (blog), Mar, 20, 2020, accessed Apr. 1, 2020, https://www.livescience.com/worst-epidemics-and-pandemics-in-history.html.

37. "Influenza (Flu) 2009 H1N1 Pandemic," CDC (blog), accessed Apr. 2, 2020, https://www.cdc.gov/flu/pandemic-resources/2009-h1n1-pandemic.html."H1N1: The 2009 H1N1 Pandemic: Summary Highlights, April 2009-April 2010," CDC, Jun. 16, 2010, accessed Apr. 3, 2020, https://www.cdc.gov/h1n1flu/cdcresponse.htm.

38. "H1N1: The 2009 H1N1 Pandemic: Summary Highlights, April 2009-April 2010," CDC, Jun. 16, 2010, accessed Apr. 3, 2020, https://www.cdc.gov/h1n1flu/cdcresponse.htm.

39. "H1N1: The 2009 H1N1 Pandemic: Summary Highlights, April 2009-April 2010," CDC, Jun. 16, 2010, accessed Apr. 3, 2020, https://www.cdc.gov/h1n1flu/cdcresponse.htm; "Update on Influenza A (H1N1) 2009 Monovalent Vaccines," MMWR Weekly, CDC, Oct. 9, 2009, 58(39); 1100-1101, accessed Apr. 3, 2009, https://www.cdc.gov/mmwr/preview/mmwrhtml/mm5839a3.html.

40. Owen Jarvis, "20 of the Worst Epidemics and Pandemics in History," Live Science (blog), Mar. 20, 2020, accessed Apr. 1, 2020, https://www.livescience.com/worst-epidemics-and-pandemics-in-history.html.

41. Ibid.

42. "Ebola (Ebola Virus Disease): 2014-2016 Ebola Outbreak in West Africa," CDC, accessed Apr. 4, 2020, https://www.cdc.gov/vhf/ebola/history/2014-2016-outbreak/index.html.

43. Ibid.

44. Ibid.

45. Ibid.

46. Ibid.

47. Owen Jarvis, "20 of the Worst Epidemics and Pandemics in History," Live Science (blog), Mar. 20, 2020, accessed Apr. 1, 2020, https://www.livescience.com/worst-epidemics-and-pandemics-in-history.html

48. Jeffrey Kahn, Kenneth McIntosh, "History and Recent Advances in Coronavirus Discovery," *The Pediatric Infections Disease Journ.*, Vol. 24, No. 11, pS223-227, Nov. 2005, digital version accessed Apr. 6, 2020, https://journals.lww.com/pidj/fulltext/2005/11001/history_and_recent_advances_in_coronavirus.12.aspx.

49. Ibid.

50. J.S. Peiris, "Coronavirus," Ch. 57, in *Medical Microbiology A Guide to Microbiological Infections: Pathogenesis, Immunity, Laboratory Diagnosis and Control.* (18th Ed) David Greenwood, Mike Barer, et al. ed. Elsevier, London, 2012, 590.

51. Ibid.

52. Ibid.. p 587.

53. Ibid., p 590.

54. Michelle L. Holshue, Chas DeBolt, et al., "First Case of 2019 Novel Coronavirus in the United States, *NEJM*, 2020;382:929-36. DOI: 10.1056/NEJMoa2001191 , Jan 31, 2020, p 929, accessed March 25, 2020, https://www.nejm.org/doi/pdf/10.1056/NEJMoa2001191.

55. Jeremy Page, Wenxin Fan, and Natasha Khan, "How it All Started: China's Early Coronavirus Missteps," *The Wall Street Journal*, March 6, 2020, accessed March 19, 2020, https://www.wsj.com/articles/how-it-all-started-chinas-early-coronavirus-missteps-11583508932.

56. Madeleine Johnson, "Diagnostic Developers Leap Into Action on Novel Coronavirus Tests," Genoweb (blog), Jan. 23, 2020, accessed Apr. 29, 2020, https://www.genomeweb.com/pcr/diagnostics-developers-leap-action-novel-coronavirus-tests.

57. "WHO Makes Field Trip to Wuhan, China," in "Rolling Updates on Coronavirus Disease (COVID-19), WHO (blog), Jan. 21, 2020, accessed Apr. 29, 2020, https://www.who.int/emergencies/diseases/novel-coronavirus-2019/events-as-they-happen.

58. Madeleine Johnson, "Diagnostic Developers Leap Into Action on Novel Coronavirus Tests," Genoweb (blog), Jan. 23, 2020, accessed Apr. 29, 2020, https://www.genomeweb.com/pcr/diagnostics-developers-leap-action-novel-coronavirus-tests.

59. Taiesha Moss, "Sona Achieves Significant Milestone in Covid-19 Test Development," Sona Nanotech, Mar. 18, 2020, accessed Apr. 28, 2020, https://sonanano.com/sona-achieves-significant-milestone-in-covid-19-test-development/.

60. Alyssa Billingsley, "The Latest in Coronavirus (COVID-19) Testing Methods and Availability," GoodRx, Apr. 21, 2020, https://www.goodrx.com/blog/coronavirus-covid-19-testing-updates-methods-cost-availability/.

61. Jamie Ducharme, "Why Ventilators May Not Be Working as Well for COVID-19 Patients as Doctors Hoped," *Time* (blog), Apr. 16, 2020, accessed Jun. 6, 2020, https://time.com/5820556/ventilators-covid-19/.

62. Philippe Gautret, Jean-Christopher Lagier, "Clinical and Microbiological Effect of a Combination of Hydroxychloroquine and Azithromycin in 80 COVID-19 Patients with at Least a Six-Day Follow-Up: An Observational Study," *Mediterranée Infection* (blog) accessed Apr. 5, 2020, https://www.mediterranee-infection.com/wp-content/uploads/2020/03/COVID-IHU-2-1.pdf.

63. Zhaowenu Chen, Jija Hu, et al., "Efficacy of Hydroxychloroquine in Patients with COVID-19: Results of a Randomized Clinical Trail," MedRxiv (blog), Mar 22, 2020, accessed Apr. 4, 2020, https://www.medrxiv.org/content/10.1101/2020.03.22.20040758v2.

64. Jean Michel Molina, Constance Delaugerre, et al., "No Evidence of Rapid Antiviral Clearance or Clinical Benefit with the Combination of Hydroxychloroqinie and Azithromycin in Patients with Severe COVID-19 Infection," *Médecine et Maladies Infectieuses* (blog), Mar. 30, 2020, accessed Apr. 5, 2020, https://www.sciencedirect.com/science/article/pii/S0399077X20300858?via%3Dihub.

65. Manli Wang, Ruiyan Cao, et al., "Remdesivir and Chloroquine Effectively Inhibit the Recently Emerged Novel Coronavirus (2019-nCoV) in Vitro," *Cell Research, Nature (blog)*, vol. 30 269-271 (2020) elct published Feb. 4, 2020, accessed Apr. 4, 2020, https://www.nature.com/articles/s41422-020-0282-0#citeas.

66. "Advisort on the Use of Hydroxy-Chloroquine as Prophylaxis for SARS-CoV-2 Infection," National Task Force for COVID-19 in Balram Bhargava of the Indian Council for Medical Researh Open Letter, Mar. 22, 2020, accessed Apr. 22, 2020, https://www.mohfw.gov.in/pdf/AdvisoryontheuseofHydroxychloroquinasprophylaxis-forSARSCoV2infection.pdf.

67. Kai Kupferschmidt, "Trials of Drugs to Prevent Coronavirus Infection Begin in Health Care Workers," *Science* (blog), Apr. 7, 2020, accessed Apr. 22, 2020, https://www.sciencemag.org/news/2020/04/trials-drugs-prevent-coronavirus-infection-begin-health-care-workers.

68. Joseph Magagnoli, Siddharth Narendran, et al., "Outcomes of Hydroxychloroquine Usage in United States Veterans Hospitalized with Covid-19," MedRxIV.org, Apr. 16, 2020, accessed Apr. 21, 2020, https://www.medrxiv.org/content/10.1101/2020.04.16.20065920v1.full.pdf.

69. Mandeep R. Mehra, Sapan S. Desai, et al., "Hydroxychloroquine or Chloroquine With or Without a Macrolide for Treatment of COVID-19: A Multinational Registry Analysis," *The Lancet*, May 22, 2020, accessed May 25, 2020, https://www.thelancet.com/journals/lancet/article/PIIS0140-6736(20)31180-6/fulltext#sec1.

70. Gerhardt SG, McDyer JF, Girgis RE, Orens JB. "Maintenance of Azithromycin Therapy for Bronchiolitis Obliterans Syndrome," *Am. J. Respir. Crit. Care Med.*, 2003;168 :121–125, accessed Apr. 22, 2020, https://www.atsjournals.org/doi/pdf/10.1164/rccm.200212-1424BC.

71. Phillippe Gautret, Jean-Christophe Lagier, et al., "Hydroxychloroquine and Azithromycin as a Treatment of COVID-19: REsults of an Open-Label Non-Randomized Clinical Trial," Int. J. Anitmicrob. Agents," Mar. 20, 2020, accessed Apr. 22, 2020,

https://www.ncbi.nlm.nih.gov/pmc/articles/PMC7102549/.

72. Eve Bossebouf, Maite Aubry, et al., "Azithromycin Inhibits the Replication of Zika Virus," Antivirals Antiretrovirals. 2018;10(1):6–11, https://www.semanticscholar.org/paper/Azithromycin-Inhibits-the-Replication-of-Zika-Virus-Bosseboeuf-Aubry/52c1d80156463278c862cfea4152f5f819020bad.

73. Gerhardt SG, McDyer JF, Girgis RE, Orens JB. "Maintenance of Azithromycin Therapy for Bronchiolitis Obliterans Syndrome," *Am. J. Respir. Crit. Care Med.*, 2003;168 :121–125, accessed Apr. 22, 2020, https://www.atsjournals.org/doi/pdf/10.1164/rccm.200212-1424BC.

74. Amin Gasmi, Sadaf Noor, et al., "Individual Risk Management Strategy and Potential Therapeutic Options of the COVID-19 Pandemic," Clin. Immunol., Apr 7, 2020, Accessed Apr. 22, 2020, https://www.ncbi.nlm.nih.gov/pmc/articles/PMC7139252/

75. Ibid.

76. Letter from Denise M. Hinton to Ashley Rhoades, May 1, 2020, accessed May 11, 2020, https://www.fda.gov/media/137564/download.

77. Jonathan Grein, Norio Ohmagari, et al., "Compassionate Use of Remdesivir, for Patients with Severe Covid-19," *NEJM*, Apr. 10, 2020, 5, accessed Apr. 20, 2020, https://www.nejm.org/doi/pdf/10.1056/NEJMoa2007016.

78. Chenguang Shen, Zhaoqin Wang, et al., "Treatment of 5 Critically Ill Patients With COVID-19 With Convalescent Plasma," *JAMA* (blog), Mar. 27, 2020, accessed Apr. 5, 2020, https://jamanetwork.com/journals/jama/fullarticle/2763983.

79. Ibid.

80. Julio Gonzalez, *The Case for Free Market Healthcare*, (Sarasota, FL: Bardolf & Co., 2020), 86.

81. Bill Bostock, "Fauci Said It Will Take 12 to 18 Months to Get a Coronavirus Vaccine in the US. Experts Say a Quick Approval Could Be Risky," *Business Insider* (blog), Apr. 1, 2020, accessed Apr. 21 2020, https://www.businessinsider.com/coronavirus-vaccine-quest-18-months-fauci-experts-flag-dangers-testing-2020-4.

82. Ibid.

83. Ibid. .

84. Alana Wise, "Trump Promises 'Warp Speed' Coronavirus Vaccine Effort With New Program," NPR (blog), May 15, 2020, accessed May 16, 2020, https://www.npr.org/sections/coronavirus-live-updates/2020/05/15/857014274/trump-touts-operation-warp-speed-coronavirus-vaccine-effort.

85. W. Huisman, B.E.E. Martina, et al.,, "Vaccine-Induced Enhancement of Viral Infections," *Vaccine*, Vol. 27, Iss 4. Jan. 22, 2009, 505-512, accessed Apr. 21, 2020, https://www.sciencedirect.com/science/article/pii/S0264410X08015053#!.

86. WHO, *Programme Budget 2020-2021*, (Switzerland, WHO 2019), accessed May 5, 2020, https://www.who.int/about/finances-accountability/budget/WHOPB-PRP-19.pdf?ua=1.

87. Yanzhong Huang, "The SARS Epicemic and Its Aftermath in China: A Political Perspective," *Learning From SARS: Preparing for the Next Disease Outbreak: Workshop Summary* (Washington, D.C., Institute of Medicine National Academies Press 2004), accessed May 5, 2020, https://www.ncbi.nlm.nih.gov/books/NBK92479/.

88. Ibid.

89. "WHO Boss Has SARS Baggage," *Forbes* (blog), Apr. 29, 2009, accessed May 4, 2020, https://www.forbes.com/2009/04/29/wto-margaret-chan-face-epidemic.html#391ebb411d34.

90. Valerie Richardson, "WHO's China Ties Scrutinized After Botched Coronavirus Response," *The Washington Times* (blog), Apr. 9, 2020, accessed May 5, 2020, https://www.washingtontimes.com/news/2020/apr/9/who-china-ties-scrutinized-after-botched-coronavir/.

91. Tedros Adhanom Ghebreyesus in Andrew Joseph and Megan Thielking, "WHO Praises China's Response to Coronavirus, Will Reconvene Expert Committee to Assess Global Threat," STAT (blog), Jan. 29, 2020, accessed May 5, 2020, https://www.statnews.com/2020/01/29/who-reconvene-expert-committee-coronavirus/.

92. "Japan PM Abe Calls for Taiwan's Participation in WHO as Coronavirus Spreads," *Kyodo News* (blog), Jan. 30, 2020, accessed May 25, 2020, https://english.kyodonews.net/news/2020/01/cff2af87f289-abe-calls-for-taiwans-participation-in-who-as-coronavirus-spreads.html.

93. David Green, "WHO Bows to China Pressure, Contravenes Human Rights in Refusing Taiwan Media," *The News Lens* (blog), May 18, 2018, accessed May 25, 2020, https://international.thenewslens.com/article/95982.

94. Tom Grundy, "Video: Top WHO Doctor Bruce Aylward Ends Video Call After Journalist Asks About Taiwan's Status," *Hong Kong Free Press*, Mar. 29, 2020, accessed May 25, 2020, https://hongkongfp.com/2020/03/29/video-top-doctor-bruce-aylward-pretends-not-hear-journalists-taiwan-questions-ends-video-call/.

95. @StudioIncendo, Twitter, Mar. 28, 2020, 1034 AM, accessed May 25, 2020, https://twitter.com/studioincendo/status/1243909358133473285.

96. "Gross Domestic Product (GCP)," FRED, Apr. 29, 2020, accessed May 3, 2020, https://fred.stlouisfed.org/series/GDP.

97. Future Workers of Indiana: Projecting the Labor Force to 2040. INcontext Indiana University Kelly School of Business, vol 13, no 6 November-December 2012, http://www.incontext.indiana.edu/2012/nov-dec/article1.asp.

98. Thomas Franck, "Job Gains for the Manufacturing industry in the Last 12 Months Are the Most Since 1995," CNBC (blog), Aug, 3, 2019, accessed May 3, 2020, https://www.cnbc.com/2018/08/03/job-gains-for-the-manufacturing-industry-are-the-most-since-1995.html.

99. Table 2.1 Employment by Major Industry Sector," U.S. Bureau of Labor Statistics, last modified Sept. 4, 2019, accessed May 3, 2020, https://www.bls.gov/emp/tables/employment-by-major-industry-sector.htm.

100. Shannon K. O'Neil in "The Instability of Global Supply Chains in a Pandemic, With Shannon K. O'Neil," Council on Foreign Relations (podcast), Apr1, 2020, accessed May 4, 2020, https://www.cfr.org/podcasts/instability-global-supply-chains-pandemic-shannon-k-oneil.

101. Ana Swanson, "Coronavirus Spurs U.S. Efforts to End China's Chokehold on Drugs," *The New York Times* (blog), Mar. 11, 2020, accessed May 4, 2020, https://www.nytimes.com/2020/03/11/business/economy/coronavirus-china-trump-drugs.html.

102. Testimony of Mark Abdoo Before the US-China Economic & Security Review Commission, Jul. 31, 20219, accessed May 3, 2020, https://www.uscc.gov/sites/default/files/USCC%20Mark%20Abdoo%20FDA%20Hearing%20Statement%20073119.pdf.

103. "Chapter 3 Section 3-Growing U.S. Reliance on China's Biotech and Pharmaceutical Products," 2019 Report to Congress of the US-China Economic and Security Review Commission, November 2019, 250, accessed May 4, 2020, https://www.uscc.gov/sites/default/files/2019-11/Chapter%203%20Section%203%20-%20Growing%20U.S.%20Reliance%20on%20China%E2%80%99s%20Biotech%20and%20Pharmaceutical%20Products.pdf.

104. Testimony of Rosemary Gibson before the US-China Economic and Security Review Commission, Jul. 31, 2010, accessed May 3, 2020, https://www.uscc.gov/sites/default/files/RosemaryGibsonTestimonyUSCCJuly152019.pdf.

105. Austen Huffor and Mark Maremont, "Low Quality Masks Infiltrate U.S. Coronavirus Supply, *The Wall Street Journal* (blog), May 4, 2020, accessed May 4, 2020, https://www.wsj.com/articles/we-werent-protected-low-quality-masks-infiltrate-u-s-coronavirus-supply-11588528690?mod=searchresults&page=1&pos=1.

106. Julio Gonzalez, *The Case for Free Market Healthcare*, (Sarasota, FL: Bardolf & Co., 2020), 87.

107. Ibid., pp 88-90.

108. Olivia Waxman, "Coronavirus Is Putting the U.S. Strategic National Stockpile to the Test. Here's the Surprising Story Behind the Stash," Mar. 11, 2020, accessed May 1, 2020, https://time.com/5800393/coronavirus-national-stockpile-history/.

109. Anna Nicholson, Scott Wollek, et al., *The Nation's Medical Countermeasure Stockpile: Opportunities to Improve the Efficacy, Effectiveness, and Sustainability of the CDC Strategic National Stockpile*, (Washington, D.C.: The National Academies Press, doi: 10.17226/23532, 2016), 1.

110. Strategic National Stockpile 12-Hour Push Pacakge Product Catalog, CDC, accessed May 1, 2020, https://ftp.cdc.gov/pub/MCMTraining/Miscellaneous%20Resources%20and%20Documents/SNS_Push%20Package%20Catalogl_2-1-12.pdf.

111. Gregg Re, "Obama Administration Sought to Cut PPE Stockpile, but Biden Team Points to GOP-Led Budget Squeeze,'" Fox News (blog), Apr. 10, 2020, accessed May 16, 2020, https://www.foxnews.com/politics/obama-administration-sought-to-cut-ppe-stockpile-biden-gop.

112. Wolf Blitzer Staff, "Troops Put Rumsfeld in the Hot Seat," CNN (blog) Dec. 8, 2004, accessed May 11, 2020, https://www.cnn.com/2004/US/12/08/rumsfeld.kuwait/index.html.

113. Jeremy Page, Wenxin Fan, and Natasha Khan, "How it All Started: China's Early Coronavirus Missteps," *The Wall Street Journal*, March 6, 2020, accessed March 19, 2020, https://www.wsj.com/articles/how-it-all-started-chinas-early-coronavirus-missteps-11583508932.

114. Ibid.

115. Ibid.

116. Ibid.

117. Ibid.

118. Ibid.

119. Ibid.

120. Ibid.

121. Ibid.

122. Kathy Gilsinan, "How China Deceived the WHO," *The Atlantic* (blog), Apr. 12, 2020, accessed Apr. 19, 2020, https://www.theatlantic.com/politics/archive/2020/04/world-health-organization-blame-pandemic-coronavirus/609820/.

123. Michelle L. Holshue, Chas DeBolt, et al., "First Case of 2019 Novel Coronavirus in the United States, *NEJM*, 2020;382:929-36. DOI: 10.1056/NEJMoa2001191, Jan 31, 2020, p 929, accessed March 25, 2020, https://www.nejm.org/doi/pdf/10.1056/NEJMoa2001191.

124. Qun Li, Xuhua Guan, et al., "Early Transmission Dynamics in Wuhan, China, of Novel Coronavirus-Infected Pneumonia," *NEJM*, Jan. 29, 2020, pg. 4, accessed Mar. 25, 2020, DOI: 10.1056/NEJMoa2001316

125. Jeremy Page, Wenxin Fan, and Natasha Khan, "How it All Started: China's Early Coronavirus Missteps," *The Wall Street Journal*, March 6, 2020, accessed March 19, 2020, https://www.wsj.com/articles/how-it-all-started-chinas-early-coronavirus-missteps-11583508932.

126. Roujian Lu, Xiang Zhao, et al., "Genomic Characterization and Epidemiology of 2019 Novel Coronavirus: Implication for Virus Origins and Receptor Bonding," *The Lancet*, vol. 395 Iss 10224, 565-674, Feb 22, 2020, accessed Apr. 18, 2020, DOI: https://doi.org/10.1016/S0140-6736(20)30251-8.

127. Jane Qiu, "How China's 'Bat Woman' Hunted Down Viruses from SARS to the New Coronoavirus," *Scientific American* (blog), Mar. 11, 2020, accessed Apr. 18, 2020, https://www.scientificamerican.com/article/how-chinas-bat-woman-hunted-down-viruses-from-sars-to-the-new-coronavirus1/.

128. Ibid.

129. Ibid. .

130. Ibid.

131. Ibid.

132. Ian Birrell, "How China Muzzled Its Bat Woman: Beiking Authorities Hushed up the Findings of a Scientist who Unlocked the Genetic Mak-Up of the Coronavirus Within Days of the Outbreak-Which Is Vital for Tests and Vaccines," Apr. 12, 2020, accessed Apr. 18, 2020, https://www.dailymail.co.uk/news/article-8210951/Beijing-authorities-hushed-findings-Chinese-scientist.html.

133. Jeremy Page, Wenxin Fan, and Natasha Khan, "How it All Started: China's Early Coronavirus Missteps," *The Wall Street Journal*, March 6, 2020, accessed March 19, 2020, https://www.wsj.com/articles/how-it-all-started-chinas-early-coronavirus-missteps-115835089321158350508932.

134. Ibid.

135. Ibid.

136. Michelle L. Holshue, Chas DeBolt, et al., "First Case of 2019 Novel Coronavirus in the United States, *NEJM*, 2020;382:929-36. DOI: 10.1056/NEJMoa2001191, Jan 31, 2020, p 929, accessed March 25, 2020, https://www.nejm.org/doi/pdf/10.1056/NEJMoa2001191.

137. Jeremy Page, Wenxin Fan, and Natasha Khan, "How it All Started: China's Early Coronavirus Missteps," *The Wall Street Journal*, March 6, 2020, accessed March 19, 2020, https://www.wsj.com/articles/how-it-all-started-chinas-early-coronavirus-missteps-11583508932.

138. "Wuhan Neighborhood Sees Infections after 40,000 Families Gather for Potluck," The Star (blog), Feb. 6, 2020, accessed Mar. 26, 2020, https://www.thestar.com.my/news/regional/2020/02/06/wuhan-neighbourhood-sees-infections-after-40000-families-gather-for-potluck.

139. IHME COVID-19 Health Service Utilization Forecasting Team, "Forecasting COVID-19 impact on hospital bed-days, ICU-days, ventilator-days and deaths by US state in the next 4 months," 2, accessed Apr. 8, 2020, http://www.healthdata.org/sites/default/files/files/research_articles/2020/covid_paper_MEDRXIV-2020-043752v1-Murray.pdf.

140. Bret Baier and Gregg Re, "Sources Believe Coronavirus Outbreak Originated in Wuhan Lab as Part of China's Efforts to Compete with US," Fox News (blog), Apr. 16, 2020, accessed Apr. 18, 2020, https://www.foxnews.com/politics/coronavirus-wuhan-lab-china-compete-us-sources.

141. "Early and Combined Interventions Crucial in Tackling COVID-19 Spread in China," U. of Southampton News (blog), Mar. 11, 2020, accessed Apr. 19, 2020, https://www.southampton.ac.uk/news/2020/03/covid-19-china.page.

142. Jeremy Page, Wenxin Fan, and Natasha Khan, "How it All Started: China's Early Coronavirus Missteps," *The Wall Street Journal*, March 6, 2020, accessed March 19, 2020, https://www.wsj.com/articles/how-it-all-started-chinas-early-coronavirus-missteps-11583508932.

143. Kathy Gilsinan, "How China Deceived the WHO," *The Atlantic* (blog), Apr. 12, 2020, accessed Apr. 19, 2020, https://www.theatlantic.com/politics/archive/2020/04/world-health-organization-blame-pandemic-coronavirus/609820/

144. Ibid.

145. "Statement on the Meeting of the International Health Regulations (2005) Emergency Committee Regarding the Outbreak of Novel Coronavirus (2019-nCoV)," WHO (blog), Jan. 23, 2020, accessed May 4, 2020, https://www.who.int/news-room/detail/23-01-2020-statement-on-the-meeting-of-the-international-health-regulations-(2005)-emergency-committee-regarding-the-outbreak-of-novel-coronavirus-(2019-ncov).

146. Kathy Gilsinan, "How China Deceived the WHO," *The Atlantic* (blog), Apr. 12, 2020, accessed Apr. 19, 2020, https://www.theatlantic.com/politics/archive/2020/04/world-health-organization-blame-pandemic-coronavirus/609820/

147. Tedros Adhanom Ghebreyesus in Andrew Joseph and Megan Thielking, "WHO Praises China's Response to Coronavirus, Will Reconvene Expert Committee to Assess Global Threat," STAT (blog), Jan. 29, 2020, accessed May 5, 2020, https://www.statnews.com/2020/01/29/who-reconvene-expert-committee-coronavirus/.

148. Grace Panetta, "US Officials Were Reportedly Concerned that Safety Breaches at a Wuhan Lab Studying Coronaviruses in Bats Could Cause a Pandemic," *Business Insider* (blog), Apr. 14, 2020, accessed Apr. 18, 2020, https://www.businessinsider.com/us-officials-raised-alarms-about-safety-issues-in-wuhan-lab-report-2020-4.

149. In Bret Baier and Gregg Re, "Sources Believe Coronavirus Outbreak Originated in Wuhan Lab as Part of China's Efforts to Compete with US," Fox News (blog), Apr. 16, 2020, accessed Apr. 18, 2020, https://www.foxnews.com/politics/coronavirus-wuhan-lab-china-compete-us-sources.

150. IIbid.

151. Ibid.

152. Donald J. Trump during The Coronavirus White House Task Force briefing Apr. 19, 2020.

153. Eran Bendavid, Bianca Mulaney, et al., COVID-19 Antibody Seroprevalence in Santa Clara County, California, MedRxiv (blog), Apr. 11, 2020, accessed Apr. 18, 2020, https://www.medrxiv.org/content/10.1101/2020.04.14.20062463v1.full.pdf+html.

154. Peter Aitken, "One Third of Participants in Massachusetts Study Tested Positive for Coronavirus," Fox News (blog), Apr. 18, 2020, accessed Apr. 18, 2020, https://www.foxnews.com/science/third-blood-samples-massachusetts-study-coronavirus.

155. Ralph Baric in Jane Qiu, "How China's 'Bat Woman' Hunted Down Viruses from SARS to the New Coronoavirus," *Scientific American* (blog), Mar. 11, 2020, accessed Apr. 18, 2020, https://www.scientificamerican.com/article/how-chinas-bat-woman-hunted-down-viruses-from-sars-to-the-new-coronavirus1/.

156. Zhao lijian, @zlj517, Twitter, Mar. 12, 2020, 10:37 AM, accessed Apr. 25, 2020, https://twitter.com/zlj517/status/1238111898828066823.

157. "Coronavirus May Have Existed in Italy Since November: Local Researcher," CGTN, Mar. 22, 2020, accessed Apr. 19, 2020, https://news.cgtn.com/news/2020-03-22/Coronavirus-may-have-existed-in-Italy-since-November-local-researcher-P4i2As2OAg/index.html.

158. Ibid.

159. WHO, Feb. 28, 2020, accessed Apr. 19, 2020, https://www.who.int/docs/default-source/coronaviruse/transcripts/who-audio-emergencies-coronavirus-press-conference-full-28feb2020.pdf?sfvrsn=13eeb6a4_2.

160. Kathy Gilsinan, "How China Deceived the WHO," *The Atlantic* (blog), Apr. 12, 2020, accessed Apr. 19, 2020, https://www.theatlantic.com/politics/archive/2020/04/world-health-organization-blame-pandemic-coronavirus/609820/.

161. Tedros Adhanom Ghebreyesus in Jon Cohen, "'We Will Have Many Body Bags.' WHO Chief Responds to Trump's Criticisms," *Science* (blog), Apr. 12, 2020, accessed Apr. 19, 2020, https://www.sciencemag.org/news/2020/04/we-will-have-many-body-bags-who-chief-responds-trumps-criticisms.

162. Kathy Gilsinan, "How China Deceived the WHO," *The Atlantic* (blog), Apr. 12, 2020, accessed Apr. 19, 2020, https://www.theatlantic.com/politics/archive/2020/04/world-health-organization-blame-pandemic-coronavirus/609820/.

163. Alayna Treene and Jonathan Swift, "Trump Announces U.S. Will Halt Funding for WHO Over Coronavirus Response," Axios (blog), Apr. 15, 2020, accessed May 25, 2020, https://www.axios.com/trump-world-health-organization-funding-65de2595-2d5e-4a6c-b7c6-9c18aa4cb905.html.

164. Ibid.

165. Rob Picheta and Jessie Yeung, "Trump Is Threatening to pull the US Out of the WHO. What Does That Actually Mean? CNN (blog), May 19, 2020, accessed May 25, 2020, https://www.cnn.com/2020/05/19/us/trump-who-funding-threat-explainer-intl/index.html.

166. Ibid.

167. Hollie McKay, "Coronavirus: US Gives 10 Times the Amount of Money to WHO Than China," Fox News (blog), Apr. 10, 2020, accessed May 25, 2020, https://www.foxnews.com/world/coronavirus-us-china-who-world-health-organization-china.

168. Dario Cristiani, "Italy's Coronavirus Experience and the Challenge of Extreme Crises to Liberal Democracies," The German Marshall Fund of the United States, (blog) Mar. 20, 2020, accessed Apr. 25, 2020, http://www.gmfus.org/blog/2020/03/20/italys-coronavirus-experience-and-challenge-extreme-crises-liberal-democracies.

169. Helen Raleigh, "Iran and Italy Are Paying a Hefty Price for Close Ties with Communist China," The Federalist (blog), Mar. 17, 2020, accessed Apr. 26, 2020, https://thefederalist.com/2020/03/17/iran-and-italy-are-paying-a-hefty-price-for-close-ties-with-communist-china/.

170. Una Aleksander Berzina-Cerenkova, "BRI Instead of OBOR-China Edits the English Name of its Most Ambitious International Project," Latvian Institute of International Affairs (blog), Jul. 28, 2016, accessed Apr. 26, 2020, https://web.archive.org/web/20170206061842/http://liia.lv/en/analysis/bri-instead-of-obor-china-edits-the-english-name-of-its-most-ambitious-international-project-532.

171. Dario Cristani, "Italy Joins the Belt and Road Initiative: Context, Interests, and Drivers," China Brief, The Jamestown Foundation, (2020) vol. 19(8) Apr. 24, 2019, accessed Apr. 26, 2020, https://jamestown.org/program/italy-joins-the-belt-and-road-initiative-context-interests-and-drivers/

172. Independent Bureau, "Italy Becomes First G7 Nation to Join China's 'Belt & Road Initiative,'" The Indepedent (blog), Mar. 24, 2019, accessed Apr. 26, 2020, http://theindependent.in/italy-becomes-first-g7-nation-to-join-chinas-belt-road-initiative/.

173. IANS, "Corona-Hit Italy Suffers Due to Improved Ties With China?" Outlook (blog), Mar. 20, 2020, accessed May 4, 2020, https://www.outlookindia.com/newsscroll/coronahit-italy-suffering-due-to-improved-ties-with-china/1774564.

174. Naomi Xu Elegant, "China Locks Down 3 Cities and Suspends Flights: The Latest on the Deadly Wuhan Virus Outbreak," Fortune (blog), Jan. 23, 2020, accessed Apr. 26, 2020, https://fortune.com/2020/01/23/china-wuhan-lockdown-flights-suspended-virus-outbreak/.

175. Italy, Central Intelligence Agency Library, accessed Apr. 25, 2020, https://www.cia.gov/library/publications/the-world-factbook/geos/it.html.

176. Country Comparison: Median Age, Central Intelligence Agency Library, accessed Apr. 25, 2020, https://www.cia.gov/library/publications/the-world-factbook/fields/343rank.html#IT.

177. "Which Country Has the oldest Population? It Depends on How You Define 'Old,'" PRB (blog), accessed Apr. 26, 2020, https://www.prb.org/which-country-has-the-oldest-population/.

178. Dario Cristiani, "Italy's Coronavirus Experience and the Challenge of Extreme Crises to Liberal Democracies," The German Marshall Fund of the United States, (blog) Mar. 20, 2020, accessed Apr. 25, 2020, http://www.gmfus.org/blog/2020/03/20/italys-coronavirus-experience-and-challenge-extreme-crises-liberal-democracies.

179. "Italian Residents Hug Chinese People to Encourage Them in Coronavirus Fight," Feb. 4, 2020, accessed Apr. 26, 2020, https://www.youtube.com/watch?v=mN-Mdg4morQs.

180. Ibid.

181. Tales Azzoni and Andrew Dampf, "Game Zero: Spread of Virus Linked to Champions League Match," Associate Press (blog), Mar. 25, 2020, accessed Apr. 25, 2020, https://apnews.com/ae59cfc0641fc63afd09182bb832ebe2.

182. Ibid.

183. Ibid.

184. Ibid.

185. COVID-19 Coronavirus Pandemic, Worldometer, updated May 6, 2020, accessed May 6, 2020, https://www.worldometers.info/coronavirus/#countries.

186. Silvia Sciorilli Borrelli, "Rome Locks Down Northern Italy Amid Surge in Coronavirus Cases, Politico (blog), Mar. 8, 2020, accessed Apr. 25, 2020, https://www.politico.eu/article/rome-locks-down-northern-italy-as-coronavirus-cases-surge/.

187. Ibid.

188. Dario Cristiani, "Italy's Coronavirus Experience and the Challenge of Extreme Crises to Liberal Democracies," The German Marshall Fund of the United States, (blog) Mar. 20, 2020, accessed Apr. 25, 2020, http://www.gmfus.org/blog/2020/03/20/italys-coronavirus-experience-and-challenge-extreme-crises-liberal-democracies.

189. Margherita Stancati, "Italy's Coronavirus Lockdown Met With Confusion, Questions About Enforcement," The Wall Street Journal, Mar. 8, 2020, accessed Apr. 25, 2020, https://www.wsj.com/articles/italy-imposes-coronavirus-lockdown-on-large-parts-of-nations-north-11583668232?mod=article_inline.

190. Eric Sylvers and Giovanni Legorano, "As Virus Spreads, Italy Locks Down Country," The Wall Street Journal, Mar. 9, 2020, accessed Apr. 25, 2020, https://www.wsj.com/articles/italy-bolsters-quarantine-checks-after-initial-lockdown-confusion-11583756737?mod=article_inline.

191. The country brought thousands of ventilators, but it still faced personnel shortages. There simply weren't enough trained personnel to handle the onslaught of sick people.

192. Margherita Stancati, Italy, With Aging Population, Has World's Highest Daily Deaths From Virus," The Wall Street Journal, Mar. 9, 2020, accessed Apr. 25, 2020, https://www.wsj.com/articles/italy-with-elderly-population-has-worlds-highest-death-rate-from-virus-11583785086?mod=article_inline.

193. Maurizio Massari, "Italian Ambassador to the EU: Italy Needs Europe' Help," Politico (blog), Mar. 10, 2020, accessed Apr. 25, 2020, https://www.politico.eu/article/coronavirus-italy-needs-europe-help/.

194. Marcus Walker and Mark Maremont, "Lessons From Italy's Hospital Meltdown. 'Every Day You Lose, the Contagion Gets Worse,'" *The Wall Street Journal*, Mar. 17, 2020, accessed Apr. 25, 2020, https://www.wsj.com/articles/every-day-you-lose-the-contagion-gets-worse-lessons-from-italys-hospital-meltdown-11584455470?mod=article_inline.

195. Margherita Stancati, Italy, With Aging Population, Has World's Highest Daily Deaths From Virus," *The Wall Street Journal*, Mar. 9, 2020, accessed Apr. 25, 2020, https://www.wsj.com/articles/italy-with-elderly-population-has-worlds-highest-death-rate-from-virus-11583785086?mod=article_inline.

196. Marcus Walker and Mark Maremont, "Lessons From Italy's Hospital Meltdown. 'Every Day You Lose, the Contagion Gets Worse,'" *The Wall Street Journal*, Mar. 17, 2020, accessed Apr. 25, 2020, https://www.wsj.com/articles/every-day-you-lose-the-contagion-gets-worse-lessons-from-italys-hospital-meltdown-11584455470?mod=article_inline.

197. Ibid.

198. Ibid.

199. Margherita Stancati and Eric Sylvers, "Italy's Coronavirus Death Toll Is Far Higher Than Reported," *The Wall Street Journal*, Apr. 1, 2020, accessed Apr 25, 2020, https://www.wsj.com/articles/italys-coronavirus-death-toll-is-far-higher-than-reported-11585767179?mod=article_inline.

200. Noemie Bisserbe and Matthew Dalton, "How Coronavirus Outmaneuvered France's Health-Care System," *The Wall Street Journal* (blog), Apr. 26, 2020, accessed Apr. 26, 2020, https://www.wsj.com/articles/how-coronavirus-outmaneuvered-frances-health-care-system-11587906000?mod=searchresults&page=1&pos=6.

201. María Sosa Troya, "Data Shows Over 7,500 Confirmed or Probable COVID-19 Deaths at Spain's Care Homes," *El País* (blog) May 7, 2020, accessed May 28, 2020, https://english.elpais.com/society/2020-05-07/data-shows-over-17500-confirmed-or-probable-covid-19-deaths-at-spains-care-homes.html.

202. Jessie Yeung, Steve George and Ivan Kottaosvá, "First Case of Coronavirus Confirmed in Spain, CNN (blog), Jan. 31, 2020, accesses Apr. 26, 2020, https://www.cnn.com/asia/live-news/coronavirus-outbreak-02-01-20-intl-hnk/h_afcf3a4665521aab11c721c8cc80dd03

203. Ibid.

204. Giovanni Legorano, Xavier Fontdegloria, "Spain Seized by Fast-Growing Coronavirus Outbreak," *The Wall Street Journal* (blog), Mar. 24, 2020, accessed Apr. 26, 2020, https://www.wsj.com/articles/spain-seized-by-fast-growing-coronavirus-outbreak-11585074509?mod=searchresults&page=8&pos=1.

205. Ibid.

206. Elena Rodriguez, "Thousands March in Spain on Women's Day Despite Coronavirus Fears," Mar. 8, 2020, accessed Apr. 26, 2020, https://www.usnews.com/news/world/articles/2020-03-08/thousands-march-in-spain-on-womens-day-despite-coronavirus-fears.

207. Raphael Minder and Elian Peltier, "Spain Imposes Nationwide Lockdown to Fight Coronavirus," *The New York Times* (blog), Mar. 14, 2020, accessed Apr. 26, 2020, https://www.nytimes.com/2020/03/14/world/europe/spain-coronavirus.html.

208. Noemie Bisserbe and Matthew Dalton, "How Coronavirus Outmaneuvered France's Health-Care System," *The Wall Street Journal* (blog), Apr. 26, 2020, accessed Apr. 26, 2020, https://www.wsj.com/articles/how-coronavirus-out-maneuvered-frances-health-care-system-11587906000?mod=searchre-sults&page=1&pos=6.

209. Ibid.

210. Matthew Dalton and Nick Kostov, "ICUs on Rails: How France Coped With a Surge of Coronavirus Patients," *The Wall Street Journal* (blog), Apr. 25, 2020, accessed Apr, 26, 2020, https://www.wsj.com/articles/icus-on-rails-how-france-coped-with-a-surge-of-coronavirus-patients-11587807002?mod=article_inline.

211. Noemie Bisserbe and Matthew Dalton, "How Coronavirus Outmaneuvered France's Health-Care System," *The Wall Street Journal* (blog), Apr. 26, 2020, accessed Apr. 26, 2020, https://www.wsj.com/articles/how-coronavirus-out-maneuvered-frances-health-care-system-11587906000?mod=searchre-sults&page=1&pos=6.

212. Ibid.

213. Max Colchester, "Boris Johnson Set to Return to Work After Recovery From Covid-19," *The Wall Street Journal* (blog), Apr. 26, 2020, accessed Apr. 27, 2020, https://www.wsj.com/articles/boris-johnson-set-to-return-to-work-after-recov-ery-from-covid-19-11587907303?mod=searchresults&page=1&pos=5.

214. H.J. Mai, "Stockholm Expected to Reach Herd Immunity in May, Swedish Am-bassador Says," NPR (blog), Apr. 26, 2020, accessed Apr. 27, 2020, https://www.npr.org/2020/04/26/845211085/stockholm-expected-to-reach-herd-immuni-ty-in-may-swedish-ambassador-says.

215. Ibid.

216. COVID-19 Coronavirus Pandemic, Worldometer, updated May 6, 2020, accessed May 6, 2020, https://www.worldometers.info/coronavirus/#countries.

217. Ibid.

218. Ibid.

219. H.J. Mai, "Stockholm Expected to Reach Herd Immunity in May, Swedish Am-bassador Says," NPR (blog), Apr. 26, 2020, accessed Apr. 27, 2020, https://www.npr.org/2020/04/26/845211085/stockholm-expected-to-reach-herd-immuni-ty-in-may-swedish-ambassador-says.

220. Kate Baggaley, "Covid-19 Herd Immunity Isn't Happening Any Time Soon," *Popular Science* (blog), Apr. 22, 2020, accessed May 6, 2020, https://www.popsci.com/story/health/herd-immunity-covid-19-coronavirus/.

221. Benoir Faucon, Sune Engel Rasmussen, and Jeremy Page, "Strategic Partner-ship With China Lies at Root of Iran's Coronavirus Outbreak," *The Wall Street Journal* (blog), Mar. 11, 2020, accessed May 2, 2020, https://www.wsj.com/ar-ticles/irans-strategic-partnership-with-china-lies-at-root-of-its-coronavirus-out-break-11583940683/.

222. COVID-19 Coronavirus Pandemic, Worldometer, updated May 2, 2020, accessed May 2, 2020, https://www.worldometers.info/coronavirus/#countries.

223. Coronavirus Singapore, Worldometer, last updated May 2, 2020, accessed May 2, 2020, https://www.worldometers.info/coronavirus/country/singapore/.

224. Holly Secon, "Singapore's Coronavirus Response, Marked by Digital Surveillance and Quarantines in Hospitals Was Initially Successful. But It's Reaching a Tipping Point," *Business Insider* (blog), Apr. 8, 2020, accessed May 2, 2020, https://www.businessinsider.com/singapore-coronavirus-containment-new-challenges-2020-4.

225. Ibid.

226. Ibid.

227. Coronavirus Singapore, Worldometer, last updated May 2, 2020, accessed May 2, 2020, https://www.worldometers.info/coronavirus/country/singapore/.

228. Ibid.

229. Ibid.

230. Dewey Sim and Kok Xighui, "Coronavirus: Why So Few Deaths Among Singapore's 14,000 Covid-19 Infections?" *South China Morning Post* (blog), Apr. 27, 2020, https://www.scmp.com/week-asia/health-environment/article/3081772/coronavirus-why-so-few-deaths-among-singapores-14000.

231. Singapore, The World Factboook, CIA, May 3, 2020, accessed May 3, 2020, https://www.cia.gov/library/publications/the-world-factbook/geos/sn.html.

232. Dewey Sim and Kok Xighui, "Coronavirus: Why So Few Deaths Among Singapore's 14,000 Covid-19 Infections?" *South China Morning Post* (blog), Apr. 27, 2020, https://www.scmp.com/week-asia/health-environment/article/3081772/coronavirus-why-so-few-deaths-among-singapores-14000.

233. Coronavirus COVID-19 Coronavirus Pandemic, Worldometer, last updated May 6, 2020, accessed May 6, 2020, https://www.worldometers.info/coronavirus/#countries.

234. Coronavirus Hong Kong, Worldometer, last updated May 6, 2020, accessed May 6, 2020, https://www.worldometers.info/coronavirus/country/china-hong-kong-sar/.

235. Suzanne Staline, "Covid-19's Resurgence in Hong Kong Holds a Lesson: Defeating It Demands Presistnece," STAT (blog) Mar. 26, 2020, accessed May 6, 2020, https://www.statnews.com/2020/03/26/coronavirus-hong-kong-resurgenece-holds-lesson-defeating-it-demands-persistence/.

236. Ibid.

237. Ibid.

238. Jessie Yeung, "Two Weeks of Zero Local Infections: How Hong Kong Contained Its Second Wave of COVID-19," CNN (blog), May 5, 2020, accessed May 6, 2020, https://www.cnn.com/2020/05/05/asia/hong-kong-coronavirus-recovery-intl-hnk/index.html.

239. Coronavirus Hong Kong, Worldometer, last updated May 6, 2020, accessed May 6, 2020, https://www.worldometers.info/coronavirus/country/china-hong-kong-sar/.

240. Jessie Yeung, "Two Weeks of Zero Local Infections: How Hong Kong Contained Its Second Wave of COVID-19," CNN (blog), May 5, 2020, accessed May 6, 2020, https://www.cnn.com/2020/05/05/asia/hong-kong-coronavirus-recovery-intl-hnk/index.html.

241. Ibid.

242. Coronavirus COVID-19 Coronavirus Pandemic, Worldometer, last updated May 17, 2020, accessed May 17, 2020, https://www.worldometers.info/coronavirus/#countries.

243. Ibid.

244. Anup Malani, Arpit Gupta and Reuben Abraham, "Why Does India Have so Few Covid-19 Cases and Deaths?" Quartz India (blog), Apr. 16, 2020, accessed May 3, 2020, https://qz.com/india/1839018/why-does-india-have-so-few-coronavirus-covid-19-cases-and-deaths/.

245. Ibid.

246. Ibid.

247. Neetu Chandra Sharma, "Why India's COVID Count Remains High Despite Lockdown, LiveMint (blog), updated May 12, accessed May 17, https://www.livemint.com/news/india/why-india-s-covid-count-remains-high-despite-lockdown-11589300259404.html.

248. "Advisort on the Use of Hydroxy-Chloroquine as Prophylaxis for SARS-CoV-2 Infection," National Task Force for COVID-19 in Balram Bhargava of the Indian Council for Medical Researh Open Letter, Mar. 22, 2020, accessed Apr. 22, 2020, https://www.mohfw.gov.in/pdf/AdvisoryontheuseofHydroxychloroquinasprophylaxisforSARSCoV2infection.pdf.

249. Shaj Rahti, Pranav Ish, et al., "Hydroxychloroquine Prophylaxis for COVID-19 Contact in India," The Lancet, Apr. 17, 2020, accessed May 3, 2020, https://www.thelancet.com/journals/laninf/article/PIIS1473-3099(20)30313-3/fulltext.

250. IANS, "India Bans Exports of Wonder Drug Used to Treat Covid-19 Patients," Business Insider (blog), Mar 25, 2020, accessed May 3, 2020, https://www.businessinsider.in/india/news/india-bans-exports-of-wonder-drug-used-to-treat-covid-19-patients/articleshow/74802892.cms.

251. Lauren Frayer, "India Reverses Export Ban on Hydrozychloroquine, Other Drugs Following Trump Pressure," NPR (blog), Apr. 8, 2020, accessed May 3, 2020, https://www.npr.org/2020/04/08/830205883/india-reverses-export-ban-on-hydroxyclorquine-other-drugs-following-trump-press.

252. Aniruddha Ghosal, "India Scraps Plan to Test Hydorxyxhloroquine in Mumbai Slums," The Washington Times (blog), Apr. 29, 2020, accessed May 3, 2020, https://www.times.com/news/2020/apr/29/india-scraps-plan-test-hydroxychloroquine-mumbai-s/.

253. Anup Malani, Arpit Gupta and Reuben Abraham, "Why Does India Have so Few Covid-19 Cases and Deaths?" Quartz India (blog), Apr. 16, 2020, accessed May 3, 2020, https://qz.com/india/1839018/why-does-india-have-so-few-coronavirus-covid-19-cases-and-deaths/.

254. Tuberculosis, BCG Vaccine, CDC, last reviewed May 4, 2020, accessed May 3, 2020, https://www.cdc.gov/tb/publications/factsheets/prevention/bcg.htm.

255. Nigel Curtis, Annie Sparrow, et al., "Considering BCG Vaccination to Reduce the Impact of COVID-19," The Lancet, Apr. 30, 2020, accessed May 3, 2020, https://www.thelancet.com/journals/lancet/article/PIIS0140-6736(20)31025-4/fulltext.

Citations

256. Nicole L. Messina, Kaya Gardiner, et al., "Study Protocol for the Melbourne Infant Study: BCG for Allergy and Infection Reduction (MIS BAIR), A Randomized Controlled Trial to Determine the Non-Specific Effects of Neonatal BCG Vaccination in a Lw-Mortality Setting," BMJ Open, (2019) Vol. 9, Iss. 12, https://bmjopen.bmj.com/content/bmjopen/9/12/e032844.full.pdf.

257. Coronavirus COVID-19 Coronavirus Pandemic, Worldometer, last updated May 3, 2020, accessed May 3, 2020, https://www.worldometers.info/coronavirus/#countries.

258. South Korea, *The World Factboook*, CIA, May 3, 2020, accessed May 3, 2020, https://www.cia.gov/library/publications/the-world-factbook/geos/ks.html

259. Coronavirus South Korea, Worldometer, last updated May 3, 2020, accessed May 3, 2020, https://www.worldometers.info/coronavirus/country/south-korea/.

260. Charlie Campbell, "South Korea's Health Minister on How His Country Is Beating Coronavirus Without a Lockdown," *Time* (blog), Apr 30, 2020, accessed May 3, 2020, https://time.com/5830594/south-korea-covid19-coronavirus/

261. Park Neung-hoo in Charlie Campbell, "South Korea's Health Minister on How His Country Is Beating Coronavirus Without a Lockdown," *Time* (blog), Apr 30, 2020, accessed May 3, 2020, https://time.com/5830594/south-korea-covid19-coronavirus/

262. Ibid.

263. Alice Zwerling, Marcel A. Behr, et al., "The BCG World Atlas of Global BCG Vaccination Policies and Practicies," *PLoS Med*, (2011) 8(3): e 1001012, Mar. 22, 2011, accessed May 3, 2020, https://www.ncbi.nlm.nih.gov/pmc/articles/PMC3062527/.

264. Ibid.

265. COVID-19 Coronavirus Pandemic, Worldometer, last updated May 3, 2020, accessed May 3, 2020, https://www.worldometers.info/coronavirus/#countries.

266. Alice Klein, "Australia Seems to Be Keeping a Lid on COVID-19-How is It Doing It?" *New Scientist* (blog) Apr. 8, 2020, accessed May 3, 2020, https://www.newscientist.com/article/2240226-australia-seems-to-be-keeping-a-lid-on-covid-19-how-is-it-doing-it/.

267. Ibid.

268. Rosie Perper, "Australia and New Zealand Have Been Able to keep Their Number of Coronavirus Cases Low Thanks to Early Lockdown Efforts. Experts Say It's 'Probably Too Late' for Other Countries to Learn From Them," *Business insider* (blog), Apr. 17, 2020, accessed May 3, 2020, https://www.businessinsider.com/experts-australia-new-zealand-examples-how-to-slow-coronavirus-2020-4.

269. Ibid.

270. Alice Zwerling, Marcel A. Behr, et al., "The BCG World Atlas of Global BCG Vaccination Policies and Practicies," *PLoS Med*, (2011) 8(3): e 1001012, Mar. 22, 2011, accessed May 3, 2020, https://www.ncbi.nlm.nih.gov/pmc/articles/PMC3062527/.

271. Rosie Perper, "Australia and New Zealand Have Been Able to keep Their Number of Coronavirus Cases Low Thanks to Early Lockdown Efforts. Experts Say It's 'Probably Too Late' for Other Countries to Learn From Them," *Business insider* (blog), Apr. 17, 2020, accessed May 3, 2020, https://www.businessinsider.com/experts-australia-new-zealand-examples-how-to-slow-coronavirus-2020-4.

265

272. Coronavirus Brazil, Worldometer, last updated May 6, 2020, accessed May 6, 2020, https://www.worldometers.info/coronavirus/country/brazil/.

273. bid.

274. bid. .

275. Coronavirus COVID-19 Coronavirus Pandemic, Worldometer, last updated May 6, 2020, accessed May 6, 2020, https://www.worldometers.info/coronavirus/#countries.

276. Lucian Magalhaes and Christiana Sciaudone, "Coronavirus Sweeps Across Brazil, a Land Ill-Equipped to Fight It," *The Wall Street Journal* (blog), May 4, 2020, accessed May 6, 2020, https://www.wsj.com/articles/coronavirus-sweeps-across-brazil-a-land-ill-equipped-to-fight-it-11588603847.

277. Ibid.

278. Jair Bolsonaro in Lucian Magalhaes and Christiana Sciaudone, "Coronavirus Sweeps Across Brazil, a Land Ill-Equipped to Fight It," *The Wall Street Journal* (blog), May 4, 2020, accessed May 6, 2020, https://www.wsj.com/articles/coronavirus-sweeps-across-brazil-a-land-ill-equipped-to-fight-it-11588603847.

279. Lucian Magalhaes and Christiana Sciaudone, "Coronavirus Sweeps Across Brazil, a Land Ill-Equipped to Fight It," *The Wall Street Journal* (blog), May 4, 2020, accessed May 6, 2020, https://www.wsj.com/articles/coronavirus-sweeps-across-brazil-a-land-ill-equipped-to-fight-it-11588603847.

280. Lucian Magalhaes and Christiana Sciaudone, "Coronavirus Sweeps Across Brazl- bid.

281. Coronavirus COVID-19 Coronavirus Pandemic, Worldometer, last updated May 6, 2020, accessed May 6, 2020, https://www.worldometers.info/coronavirus/#countries.

282. Coronavirus Peru, Worldometer, last updated May 6, 2020, accessed May 6, 2020, https://www.worldometers.info/coronavirus/country/peru/.

283. Coronavirus Argentina, Worldometer, last updated May 6, 2020, accessed May 6, 2020, https://www.worldometers.info/coronavirus/country/argentina/.

284. Coronavirus COVID-19 Coronavirus Pandemic, Worldometer, last updated May 6, 2020, accessed May 6, 2020, https://www.worldometers.info/coronavirus/#countries.

285. Ibid.

286. Coronavirus Ecuador, Worldometer, last updated May 6, 2020, accessed May 6, 2020, https://www.worldometers.info/coronavirus/country/ecuador/.

287. Eisuke Nakasawa, Hiroyasu, Ino, and Akira Akabayashi, "Chronology of COVID-19 Cases on the Diamond Princess Cruise Ship and Ethical Considerations: A Report From Japan," *Disaster Med. Pub. Health Prep.*, Mar 24, 2020, accessed Apr. 22, 2020, https://www.ncbi.nlm.nih.gov/pmc/articles/PMC7156812/.

288. Smriti, Mallapaty, "What the Cruis-Ship Outbreaks Reveal About COVID-19, Nature (blog), Mar. 26, 2020, accessed Apr. 22, 2020, https://www.nature.com/articles/d41586-020-00885-w.

289. Eisuke Nakasawa, Hiroyasu, Ino, and Akira Akabayashi, "Chronology of COVID-19 Cases on the Diamond Princess Cruise Ship and Ethical Considerations: A Report From Japan," *Disaster Med. Pub. Health Prep.*, Mar 24, 2020, accessed Apr. 22, 2020, https://www.ncbi.nlm.nih.gov/pmc/articles/PMC7156812/.

290. Smriti, Mallapaty, "What the Cruis-Ship Outbreaks Reveal About COVID-19, *Nature* (blog), Mar. 26, 2020, accessed Apr. 22, 2020, https://www.nature.com/articles/d41586-020-00885-w.

291. Ibid.

292. Eisuke Nakasawa, Hiroyasu, Ino, and Akira Akabayashi, "Chronology of COVID-19 Cases on the Diamond Princess Cruise Ship and Ethical Considerations: A Report From Japan," *Disaster Med. Pub. Health Prep.*, Mar 24, 2020, accessed Apr. 22, 2020, https://www.ncbi.nlm.nih.gov/pmc/articles/PMC7156812/.

293. Ibid.

294. Timothy Russell, Joel Hellewell, et al., "Estimating the Infection and Case Fatality Ration for Coronavirus Disease (COVID-19) Using Age-Adjusted Date from the Outbreak on the Diamond Princess Cruise Shipe, February 2020," E*urosurveillance*, 2020;25(12), Mar. 26, 2020, accessed Apr. 22, 2020, https://www.eurosurveillance.org/content/10.2807/1560-7917.ES.2020.25.12.2000256#t2.

295. Smriti, Mallapaty, "What the Cruis-Ship Outbreaks Reveal About COVID-19, *Nature* (blog), Mar. 26, 2020, accessed Apr. 22, 2020, https://www.nature.com/articles/d41586-020-00885-w.

296. Timothy Russell, Joel Hellewell, et al., "Estimating the Infection and Case Fatality Ration for Coronavirus Disease (COVID-19) Using Age-Adjusted Date from the Outbreak on the Diamond Princess Cruise Shipe, February 2020," *Eurosurveillance*, 2020;25(12), Mar. 26, 2020, accessed Apr. 22, 2020, https://www.eurosurveillance.org/content/10.2807/1560-7917.ES.2020.25.12.2000256#t2.

297. Kenji Mizumoto, Katsushi Kagaya, et al., "Estimating the Asymptomatic Proportion of Coronavirus Disease 2019 (COVID-19) Cases on Board the Diamond Princess Cruise Ship, Yokohama, Japan, 2020," *Eurosurveillance*, 2020;25 (10), Mar. 12, 2020, accessed Apr. 22, 2020, https://www.eurosurveillance.org/content/10.2807/1560-7917.ES.2020.25.10.2000180.

298. Smriti, Mallapaty, "What the Cruis-Ship Outbreaks Reveal About COVID-19, *Nature* (blog), Mar. 26, 2020, accessed Apr. 22, 2020, https://www.nature.com/articles/d41586-020-00885-w.

299. Richard Paddock, Sui-Lee Wee, and Roni Caryn Rabin, "Coronavirus Infection Found After Cruise Ship Passengers Disperse," *The New York Times* (blog), Feb. 16, 2020, updated Feb. 20, 2020, accessed Apr. 22, 2020, https://www.nytimes.com/2020/02/16/world/asia/coronavirus-cruise-americans.html.

300. Ibid.

301. Ibid. .

302. Tomoya Onishi, "Cambodia's Hun Sen Welcomes Passengers from Shunned *Westerdam*," *Nikkei Asian Review* (blog), Feb. 15, 32020, accessed May 8, 2020, https://asia.nikkei.com/Spotlight/Coronavirus/Cambodia-s-Hun-Sen-welcomes-passengers-from-shunned-Westerdam.

303. "Coronavirus: How Did Cambodia's Cruise Ship Welcome Go Wrong?" BBC News (blog), Feb. 20, 2020, accessed Apr. 22, 2020, https://www.bbc.com/news/world-asia-51542241.

304. Richard Paddock, Sui-Lee Wee, and Roni Caryn Rabin, "Coronavirus Infection Found After Cruise Ship Passengers Disperse," *The New York Times* (blog), Feb. 16, 2020, updated Feb. 20, 2020, accessed Apr. 22, 2020, https://www.nytimes.com/2020/02/16/world/asia/coronavirus-cruise-americans.html.

305. Ibid.

306. Julie, "Updated Statement Regarding Westerdam," Holland America Cruise Line (blog) Mar. 4, 2020, accessed Apr. 22, 2020, https://www.hollandamerica.com/blog/ships/ms-westerdam/statement-regarding-westerdam-in-japan/.

307. "Public Health Responses to COVID-19 Outbreaks on Cruise Ships-Worldwide, February-March 2020, *MMWR* (blog), CDC, Mar. 27, 2020, accessed Apr. 23, 2020, https://www.cdc.gov/mmwr/volumes/69/wr/mm6912e3.htm.

308. Katie Canales, "Two-Thirds of Passengers from the Coronavirus-Stricken Grand Princess Cruise Ship Declined to be Tested While Quarantined at a California Miltary Base so They Could Go Home Sooner," *Business Insider* (blog), Mar. 19, 2020, accessed Apr. 23, 2020, https://www.businessinsider.com/coronavirus-grand-princess-cruise-ship-passengers-decline-testing-2020-3.

309. "Public Health Responses to COVID-19 Outbreaks on Cruise Ships-Worldwide, February-March 2020, *MMWR* (blog), CDC, Mar. 27, 2020, accessed Apr. 23, 2020, https://www.cdc.gov/mmwr/volumes/69/wr/mm6912e3.htm.

310. Katie Canales, "Two-Thirds of Passengers from the Coronavirus-Stricken Grand Princess Cruise Ship Declined to be Tested While Quarantined at a California Miltary Base so They Could Go Home Sooner," *Business Insider* (blog), Mar. 19, 2020, accessed Apr. 23, 2020, https://www.businessinsider.com/coronavirus-grand-princess-cruise-ship-passengers-decline-testing-2020-3.

311. "Public Health Responses to COVID-19 Outbreaks on Cruise Ships-Worldwide, February-March 2020, *MMWR* (blog), CDC, Mar. 27, 2020, accessed Apr. 23, 2020, https://www.cdc.gov/mmwr/volumes/69/wr/mm6912e3.htm.

312. Morgan Hines and Andrea Mandell, "Two Grand Princess Cruise Passengers with Coronavirus Die; 103 Have Tested Positive for COVID-19, *USA Today* (blog), Mar. 25, 2020, accessed Apr. 23, 2020, https://www.usatoday.com/story/travel/cruises/2020/03/25/coronavirus-cruise-grand-princess-two-passenger-deaths/5081851002/.

313. Alex Harris, Taylor, Dolven, and Michelle Kaufman, "Zaandam Was Cruising tot he 'End of the world.' Then COVID-19 Spread Across the Ship," *Miami Herald* (blog), Apr. 12, 2020, updated Apr. 15, 2020, accessed Apr. 23, 2020, https://www.miamiherald.com/news/business/tourism-cruises/article241740696.html.

314. ibid.

315. Ibid.

316. Ibid.

317. Ibid.

318. Ibid.

319. Ibid.

320. Ibid.

321. U.S. HHS and CDC, "Order Under Sections 361 & 365 of the Public Health Service Act (USC §§ 264,268) and 42 Code Federal Regulations Part 70 (Interstate) and Part 71 (Foreign): No Sail Order and Other Measures Related to Operations," 1, Mar. 14, 2020, accessed Apr. 22, 2020, https://www.cdc.gov/quarantine/pdf/signed-manifest-order_031520.pdf.

322. Brad Lendon, "Coronavirus May Be Giving Beijing an Opening in the South China Sea," CNN (blog), Apr. 7, 2020, accessed Apr. 25, 2020, https://www.cnn.com/2020/04/07/asia/coronavirus-china-us-military-south-china-sea-intl-hnk/index.html.

323. Matthias Gafni and Joe Garofoli, "Exclusive: Captain of Aircraft Carrier with Growing Coronavirus Outbreak Pleads for Help from Navy," *San Francisco Chronicle*, Mar. 30, 2020, accessed Apr. 24, 2020, https://www.sfchronicle.com/bayarea/article/Exclusive-Captain-of-aircraft-carrier-with-15167883.php.

324. Brett Crozier Memo: Request for Assistance in Response to COVID-19 Pandemic, Mar. 30, 2020, in Matthias Gafni and Joe Garofoli, "Exclusive: Captain of Aircraft Carrier with Growing Coronavirus Outbreak Pleads for Help from Navy," *San Francisco Chronicle*, Mar. 30, 2020, accessed Apr. 24, 2020, https://www.sfchronicle.com/bayarea/article/Exclusive-Captain-of-aircraft-carrier-with-15167883.php.

325. Matthias Gafni and Joe Garofoli, "Exclusive: Captain of Aircraft Carrier with Growing Coronavirus Outbreak Pleads for Help from Navy," *San Francisco Chronicle,* Mar. 30, 2020, accessed Apr. 24, 2020, https://www.sfchronicle.com/bayarea/article/Exclusive-Captain-of-aircraft-carrier-with-15167883.php.

326. Gina Harkins, "Modly Resigns as Acting SecNav Amid Backlash Over Carrier Captain's Firing," Military.com (blog), Apr. 7, 2020, accessed May 8, 2020, https://www.military.com/daily-news/2020/04/07/acting-navy-secretary-offers-resign-amid-growing-backlash-reports.html.

327. U.S. Pacific Fleet Public Affairs, "Navy Identifies USS Theodore Roosevelt Sailor Who Died of COVID-19," U.S. Navy, Apr. 16, 2020, accessed Apr. 24, 2020, https://www.navy.mil/submit/display.asp?story_id=112672.

328. Barbara Starr and Ryan Crowne, "Sailor from USS Teddy Roosevelt Found Unconscious, Transferred to Intensive Care," CNN Politics, Apr. 10, 2020, accessed Apr. 24, 2020, https://www.cnn.com/2020/04/09/politics/sailor-teddy-roosevelt-unconcious-covid-modly/index.html.

329. Ibid.

330. U.S. Pacific Fleet Public Affairs, "Navy Sailor Assigned to USS Theodore Roosevelt Dies of COVID-Related Complications," U.S. Navy, Apr. 13, 2020, accessed Apr. 24, 2020, https://www.navy.mil/submit/display.asp?story_id=112614.

331. "Daily Update: Apr. 23, 2020. Key Developments," Navy Line (blog), Apr. 23, 2020, accessed Apr. 24, 2020, https://navylive.dodlive.mil/2020/03/15/u-s-navy-covid-19-updates/.

332. Lolita C. Baldor, "Five USS Theodore Roosevelt Sailors Test Positive for Coronavirus a Second Time," *Time* (blog), May 15, 2020, accessed May 20, 2020, https://time.com/5837531/sailors-coronavirus-second-time/.

333. Brad Lendon, "Coronavirus May Be Giving Beijing an Opening in the South China Sea," CNN (blog), Apr. 7, 2020, accessed Apr. 25, 2020, https://www.cnn.com/2020/04/07/asia/coronavirus-china-us-military-south-china-sea-intl-hnk/index.html.

334. Cheng Chi-Wen, editor-in-chief Asia-Pacific Defense in John Xie, "China Claims Zero Infections in Its Military," VOA Cambodia (blog), Apr. 7, 2020, accessed Apr. 24, 2020. https://www.voacambodia.com/a/5362985.html

335. "China Confirms No Cases of Coronavirus Infection in Military," China Military (blog), Mar. 3, 2020, accessed Apr. 25, 2020, http://eng.chinamil.com.cn/view/2020-03/03/content_9758336.htm.

336. Brad Lendon, "Chinese State Media Claims Country's Navy Is Not Affected by Coronavirus," CNN (blog), Apr. 15, 2020, accessed Apr. 17, 2020, https://www.cnn.com/2020/04/13/asia/china-coronavirus-aircraft-carrier-deployment-dp-hnk-intl/index.html.

337. Paul Shinkman, "Military Warns of Coronavirus 'Breakouts' Aboard the USS Nimitz," *U.S. News & World Report* (blog), Apr. 9, 2020, accessed Apr. 24, 2020, https://www.usnews.com/news/national-news/articles/2020-04-09/military-warns-of-coronavirus-breakouts-aboard-uss-nimitz-aircraft-carrier.

338. Reuters, "EXCLUSIVE-US Navy Destroyer in Caribbean Sees Significant Coronavirus Outbreak-Officials," Thomson Reuters Foundation News (blog), Apr. 24, 2020, accessed Apr. 25, 2020, https://news.trust.org/item/20200424140331-zrivo.

339. Lolita C. Baldor, "Five USS Theodore Roosevelt Sailors Test Positive for Coronavirus a Second Time," *Time* (blog), May 15, 2020, accessed May 20, 2020, https://time.com/5837531/sailors-coronavirus-second-time/.

340. "COCVID-19 in China," *CDC Travelers' Health* (blog), CDC, Jan. 6, 2020, accessed Mar. 25, 2020, https://wwwnc.cdc.gov/travel/notices/warning/novel-coronavirus-china

341. Michelle L. Holshue, Chas DeBolt, et al., "First Case of 2019 Novel Coronavirus in the United States, *NEJM*, 2020;382:929-36. DOI: 10.1056/NEJMoa2001191 , Jan 31, 2020, p 929, accessed March 25, 2020, https://www.nejm.org/doi/pdf/10.1056/NEJMoa2001191.

342. Ibid.

343. Ibid.

344. Ibid.

345. "First Travel-Related Case of 2019 Novel Coronavirus detected in United States, CDC Newsroom (blog), CDC, Jan. 21, 2020, accessed Mar. 25, 2020, https://www.cdc.gov/media/releases/2020/p0121-novel-coronavirus-travel-case.html.

346. Michelle L. Holshue, Chas DeBolt, et al., "First Case of 2019 Novel Coronavirus in the United States, *NEJM*, 2020;382:929-36. DOI: 10.1056/NEJMoa2001191 , Jan 31, 2020, p 930, accessed March 25, 2020, https://www.nejm.org/doi/pdf/10.1056/NEJMoa2001191.

347. "Public Health Screening to Begin at 3 U.S. Airports for 2019 Novel Coronavirus ("2019-nCoV")," CDC Newsroom (blog), CDC, Jan. 17, 2020, accessed Mar. 25, 2020, https://www.cdc.gov/media/releases/2020/p0117-coronavirus-screening.html.

348. Michelle L. Holshue, Chas DeBolt, et al., "First Case of 2019 Novel Coronavirus in the United States, *NEJM*, 2020;382:929-36. DOI: 10.1056/NEJMoa2001191 , Jan 31, 2020, p 933, accessed March 25, 2020, https://www.nejm.org/doi/pdf/10.1056/NEJMoa2001191.

349. Ibid.

350. "First Travel-Related Case of 2019 Novel Coronavirus detected in United States, CDC Newsroom (blog), CDC, Jan. 21, 2020, accessed Mar. 25, 2020, https://www.cdc.gov/media/releases/2020/p0121-novel-coronavirus-travel-case.html.

351. Steve Eder, Henry Fountain, et al., "430,000 People Have Traveled From China to S.S. Since Coronavirus Surfaced," *New York Times* (blog), Apr. 4, 2020, accessed Apr. 4, 2020, https://www.nytimes.com/2020/04/04/us/coronavirus-china-travel-restrictions.html?referringSource=articleShare.

352. Ibid.

353. Elvia Malagón, Lauren Zumbach, and Dawn Rhodes, "Chicago Woman Who Traveled to China Diagnosed with Coronavirus, Health Officials Say," *Chicago Tribune* (blog), Jan. 25, 2020, accessed Mar. 26, 2020, https://www.chicagotribune.com/news/breaking/ct-coronavirus-china-epidemic-illinois-case-20200124-yx2x-d3yeovar3o25ei6bfvvbze-story.html.

354. Ibid.

355. David Jackson, "Trump Administration Declare Coronavirus Emergency, Orders First Quarantine in 50 Years," *USA Today* (blog) Jan. 31, 2020, accessed Apr. 14, 2020, https://www.usatoday.com/story/news/politics/2020/01/31/coronavirus-donald-trump-declares-public-health-emergency/4625299002/.

356. David Jackson, "Trump Administration Declare Coronavirus Emergency, Orders First Quarantine in 50 Years," *USA Today* (blog) Jan. 31, 2020, accessed Apr. 14, 2020, https://www.usatoday.com/story/news/politics/2020/01/31/coronavirus-donald-trump-declares-public-health-emergency/4625299002/.

357. "Could the Electoral College Elect Hillary Clinton Instead of Donald Trump?" *USA Today* (blog), updated Dec. 20, 2016, accessed Apr. 16, 2020, https://www.usatoday.com/story/news/politics/elections/2016/2016/11/16/fact-check-could-electoral-college-elect-hillary-clinton-instead-donald-trump/93951818/.

358. Kirstein Schmidt and Wilson Andrews, "A Historic Number of Electors Defected, and Most Were Supposed to Vote for Clinton," *The New York Times* (blog), Dec. 19, 2016, accessed Apr. 16, 2020, https://www.nytimes.com/interactive/2016/12/19/us/elections/electoral-college-results.html.

359. Matea Gold, "The Campaign to Impeach Trump Has Begun," *The Washington Post* (blog), Jan. 20, 2017, accessed Apr. 16, 2020, https://www.washingtonpost.com/news/post-politics/wp/2017/01/20/the-campaign-to-impeach-president-trump-has-begun/.

360. Melissa Chan, "There's Already a Campaign to Impeach President Donald Trump," *Time,* Jan. 20, 2017, accessed Apr. 16, 2020, https://time.com/4641233/donald-trump-inauguration-impeach/.

361. Kevin Breuninger, "Robert Mueller's Russia Probe Cost Nearly $32 Million in Total, Justice Department Says," CNBC (blog), Aug. 2, 2019, accessed Apr. 16, 2020, https://www.cnbc.com/2019/08/02/robert-muellers-russia-probe-cost-nearly-32-million-in-total-doj.html.

362. Susan Jones, "Mueller Probe: 22 Months, 19 Lawyers, 40 FBI, 2,800 Subpoenas, 500 Search Warrants, and 500 Witnesses, CNBC (blog), Mar. 29, 205, accessed Apr. 16, 2020, https://www.cnsnews.com/news/article/susan-jones/you-paid-22-months-19-lawyers-40-fbi-2800-subpoenas-500-search-warrants-500.

363. Rick Bright in interview with Norah O'Donnell, *60 Minutes*, May 17, 2020, accessed May 18, 2020, https://www.cbsnews.com/video/rick-bright-whistleblower-virologist-coroanvirus-pandemic-drug-research-60-minutes/.

364. Alex Azar in Stephanie Soucheray, "Officials Say Most Americans Not at Risk of Coronavirus," Center for Infectious Disease Research and Policy, Jan. 28, 2020, accessed Apr. 14, 2020, https://www.cidrap.umn.edu/news-perspective/2020/01/officials-say-most-americans-not-risk-coronavirus

365. Nancy Messonier in Stephanie Soucheray, "Officials Say Most Americans Not at Risk of Coronavirus," Center for Infectious Disease Research and Policy, Jan. 28, 2020, accessed Apr. 14, 2020, https://www.cidrap.umn.edu/news-perspective/2020/01/officials-say-most-americans-not-risk-coronavirus.

366. Logan Ratick, "Jan. Flashback: Dr. Fauci Said coronavirus 'Is Not a Threat to the People of the United States," SARA (blog), Apr. 3, 2020, accessed Apr. 14, 2020, https://saraacarter.com/jan-flashback-dr-fauci-said-coronavirus-is-not-a-major-threat-to-the-people-of-the-united-states.

367. Alex Azar in David Jackson, "Trump Administration Declare Coronavirus Emergency, Orders First Quarantine in 50 Years," *USA Today* (blog) Jan. 31, 2020, accessed Apr. 14, 2020, https://www.usatoday.com/story/news/politics/2020/01/31/coronavirus-donald-trump-declares-public-health-emergency/4625299002/.

368. "Pelosi Tours San Francisco's Chinatown To Quell Coronavirus Fears," KPX CBS SF BayArea (blog), Feb. 24, 2020, accessed Apr. 13, 2020, https://sanfrancisco.cbslocal.com/2020/02/24/coronavirus-speaker-house-nancy-pelosi-tours-san-franciscos-chinatown/.

369. Vox tweet in Gregg Re, "After Attacking Trump's Coronavirus-Related China Ban as Xenophobic, Dem and Media Have Changed Tune," Fox News (blog), Apr. 1, 2020, https://www.foxnews.com/politics/dems-media-change-tune-trump-attacks-coronavirus-china-travel-ban.

370. Nancy Pelosi in "Pelosi Statement on President Trump's Expanded Travel Ban," Nancy Pelosi Speaker of the House Newsroom (blog), Jan. 31, 2020, accessed Apr. 30, 2020, https://www.speaker.gov/newsroom/13120-2.

371. Joe Biden, @JoeBiden, Feb. 1, 2020, accessed Apr. 30, 2020, https://twitter.com/JoeBiden/status/1223727977361338370.

372. "About Us," STAT, accessed Apr. 30, 2020, https://www.statnews.com/about/.

373. Megan Thielking, "Health Experts Warn China Travel Ban Will Hinder Coronavirus Response," STAT (blog), Jan. 31, 2020, accessed Apr. 30, 2020, https://www.statnews.com/2020/01/31/as-far-right-calls-for-china-travel-ban-health-experts-warn-coronavirus-response-would-suffer/.

374. Michael Corkery and Annie Karni, "Trump Administration Restricts Entry Into U.S. From China," Jan. 31, 2020, *The New York Times* (blog) Jan. 31, 2020, accessed Apr. 30, 2020, https://www.nytimes.com/2020/01/31/business/china-travel-coronavirus.html.

375. Jessie Yeung, "As the Coronavirus Spreads, Fear is Fueling Racism and Xenophobia," CNN (blog), Jan. 31, 2020, accessed Apr. 30, 2020, https://www.cnn.com/2020/01/31/asia/wuhan-coronavirus-racism-fear-intl-hnk/index.html.

376. Eric Carter in Catherine E. Schoichet, The U Coronavirus Travel Ban Could Backfire. Here's How," CNN (blog), Feb. 7, 2020, accessed Apr. 30, 2020, https://www.cnn.com/2020/02/07/health/coronavirus-travel-ban/index.html.

377. Tom Howell, Jr., "Dems Ding Trump's $2.5 billion coronavirus request as 'too little, too late,'" *The Washington Times* (blog), Feb. 24, 2020, accessed May 1, 2020, https://www.washingtontimes.com/news/2020/feb/24/donald-trump-re-quests-25-billion-coronavirus-fight/.

378. Lauren Hirsch and Kevin Breuninger, "Trump Signs $8.3 billion Emergency Coronavirus Spending Package," CNCBC (blog), Mar. 6, 2020, accessed Apr. 30, 2020, https://www.cnbc.com/2020/03/06/trump-signs-8point3-billion-emergency-coronavirus-spending-package.html.

379. Donald J. Trump, "Oval Office Address to the Union," Mar. 11, 2020.

380. Ibid.

381. Ibid.

382. Olivia Niland, "Trump Is Extending the Europe Travel Ban to the UK and Ireland as the Coronavirus Pandemic Escalates," BuzzFeed News (blog), Mar. 14, 2020, accessed Apr. 15, 2020, https://www.buzzfeednews.com/article/olivianiland/trump-uk-ireland-travel-ban-europe-coronavirus.

383. Ibid.

384. Ibid.

385. Coronavirus Disease 2019: Social Distancing, CDC, Apr. 4, 2020, accessed Apr. 26, 2020, https://www.cdc.gov/coronavirus/2019-ncov/prevent-getting-sick/social-distancing.html.

386. Coronavirus Disease 2019: People Who Need Extra Precautions, CDC, Mar. 6, 2020, accessed May 1, 2020, https://www.cdc.gov/coronavirus/2019-ncov/need-extra-precautions/index.html.

387. Coronavirus Disease 2019: Social Distancing, CDC, Apr. 4, 2020, accessed May 2, 2020, https://www.cdc.gov/coronavirus/2019-ncov/prevent-getting-sick/social-distancing.html.

388. Sheri Fink, "Worst-Case Estimates for U.S. Coronavirus Deaths," *The New York Times* (blog), Mar. 13, 2020, accessed Apr. 9, 2020, https://www.nytimes.com/2020/03/13/us/coronavirus-deaths-estimate.html.

389. Ibid.

390. Meredith McGraw, " "Trump's New Coronavirus Argument: 2 Million People Are Being Saved," *Politico*, Apr. 1, 2020, accessed Apr. 13, 2020, https://www.politico.com/news/2020/04/01/trump-coronavirus-millions-saved-160814.

391. Doug Palmer, "U.S. Medical Stockpile Wasn't Built to Handle Current Crisis, Former Director Says," *Politico* (blog), Apr. 8, 2020, accessed May 1, 2020, https://www.politico.com/news/2020/04/08/national-stockpile-coronavirus-crisis-175619.

392. Ibid.

393. Sarah Kliff, Adam Stariano, et al., "There Aren't Enough Ventilators to Cope With the Coronavirus, *The New York Times* (blog), Mar. 18, 2020, accessed May 1, 2020, https://www.nytimes.com/2020/03/18/business/coronavirus-ventilator-shortage.html.

394. Anthony Fauci interview in State of the Union With Jake Tapper, CNN, Mar. 15, 2020, memorialized in @CNNSotu, Twitter, Mar. 15, 2020, 6:33 PM, accessed May 2, 2020, https://twitter.com/CNNSotu/status/1239318789856034817.

395. Peter Loftus, "Ventilator Makers Ramp Up Production Amid Coronavirus Crunch," *The Wall Street Journal* (blog), Mar. 19, 2020, accessed May 1, 2020, https://www.wsj.com/articles/ventilator-makers-ramp-up-production-amid-coronavirus-crunch-11584626858?mod=searchresults&page=4&pos=8.

396. Sarah Kliff, Adam Stariano, et al., "There Aren't Enough Ventilators to Cope With the Coronavirus, *The New York Times* (blog), Mar. 18, 2020, accessed May 1, 2020, https://www.nytimes.com/2020/03/18/business/coronavirus-ventilator-shortage.html.

397. Brett Samuels, "Trump Uses Defense Production Act to Require GM to Make Ventilators," *The Hill* (blog), Mar. 27, 2020, accessed May 2, 2020, https://thehill.com/homenews/administration/489909-trump-uses-defense-production-act-to-require-gm-to-make-ventilators.

398. Memorandum on Order Under the Defense Production Act Regarding 3M Company, Apr. 2, 2020, §2.

399. Rachel Sandler, "Trump Ends Feud With Mask Maker 3M, Announces Deal for 55 Million U.S. Masks per Month." *Forbes* (blog), Apr. 6, 2020, accessed May 2, 2020, https://www.forbes.com/sites/rachelsandler/2020/04/06/trump-ends-feud-with-mask-maker-3m-announces-deal-for-55-million-us-masks-per-month/#637691ce1209.

400. "President Donald J. Trump Has Led a Historic Mobilization to Combat the Coronavirus," The White House (blog), Apr. 14, 2020, accessed May 2, 2020, https://www.whitehouse.gov/briefings-statements/president-donald-j-trump-led-his-toric-mobilization-combat-coronavirus/.

401. "Coronavirus Disease 2019 Diagnostic Testing," CDC, last reviewed Apr. 14, 2020, accessed May 7, 2020, https://www.cdc.gov/coronavirus/2019-ncov/php/testing.html.

402. Ibid.

403. Adam Bernheim, Xueyan Mei, et al., "Chest CT Findings in Coronavirus Disease-19 (COVID-19): Relationship to Duration of Infection," *Radiology*, Feb. 20, 2020, accessed May 7, 2020, https://pubs.rsna.org/doi/10.1148/radiol.2020200463.

404. Maria Rachal, "Abbott Touts Speed, Scale of POC Coronavirus Test," Medtech Dive (bog), Mar. 30, 2020, accessed May 8, 2020, https://www.medtechdive.com/news/abbott-touts-speed-scale-of-poc-coronavirus-test/575092/

405. "Abbott Launches Molecular Point-of Care Test to Detect novel Coronavirus," Abbott Newsroom (blog), Mar. 27, 2020, accessed May 8, 2020, https://abbott.mediaroom.com/2020-03-27-Abbott-Launches-Molecular-Point-of-Care-Test-to-Detect-Novel-Coronavirus-in-as-Little-as-Five-Minutes.

406. Scott Gottlieb, @ScottGottliebMD, Twitter, Mar. 27, 2020, 8:26 PM, accessed May 8, 2020, https://twitter.com/ScottGottliebMD/status/1243696001958981632.

407. "Abbott Launches Molecular Point-of Care Test to Detect novel Coronavirus," Abbott Newsroom (blog), Mar. 27, 2020, accessed May 8, 2020, https://abbott.mediaroom.com/2020-03-27-Abbott-Launches-Molecular-Point-of-Care-Test-to-Detect-Novel-Coronavirus-in-as-Little-as-Five-Minutes.

408. Ibid.

409. Letter from Uwe Scherf to Christian Bixby, Re: EUA200090, Apr. 10 2020, accessed May 7, 2020, https://www.fda.gov/media/136876/download.

410. "Cleveland Company Approved to Make Swabs for Coronavirus Testing," Cleveland.com (blog), Apr. 24, 2020, accessed May 8, 2020, https://www.cleveland.com/open/2020/04/cleveland-company-approved-to-make-swabs-for-coronavirus-testing.html.

411. John Huotari, "ORNL Making Molds to Help Produce COVID-19 Test Tubes," *Oak Ridge Today* (blog), Apr. 21, 2020, accessed May 8, 2020, https://oakridgetoday.com/2020/04/21/ornl-making-molds-to-help-produce-covid-19-test-tubes/.

412. Brad Smith in "Remarks by President Trump, Vice President Pence, and Members of the Coronavirus Task Force in Press Briefing, Apr. 20, 2020, accessed May 8, 2020, https://www.whitehouse.gov/briefings-statements/remarks-president-trump-vice-president-pence-members-coronavirus-task-force-press-briefing-29/.

413. Coronavirus Disease 2019: Testing in US, CDC, updated May 7, 2020, accessed May 8, 2020, https://www.cdc.gov/coronavirus/2019-ncov/cases-updates/testing-in-us.html

414. COVID-19 Coronavirus Pandemic, Worldometer, updated May 8, 2020, accessed May 8, 2020, https://www.worldometers.info/coronavirus/#countries.

415. Ibid.

416. U.S. Constitution, Art. I, Sxn. 9, Cl 2.

417. U.S. Constitution, Art. V, Sxn. 4, Cl 1.

418. Taryn Luna, John Myers, "Large Gatherings Should Be Canceled Due to Coronavirus Outbreak, California Gov. Gavin Newsom Says," *Los Angeles Times* (blog), Mar. 11, 2020, accessed Apr. 15, 2020, https://www.latimes.com/california/story/2020-03-11/coronavirus-outbreak-large-gatherings-canceled-governor-gavin-newsom-california.

419. Order of the State Public Health Officer, Mar. 19, 2020.

420. Executive Department State of California, Executive Order N-33-20.

421. Sarah Mervosh, Denise Lu, and Venessa Seales, "See Which States and Cities Have Told Resident to Stay at Home," *The New York Times* (blog), Apr. 7, 2020, accessed Apr. 15, 2020, https://www.nytimes.com/interactive/2020/us/coronavirus-stay-at-home-order.html.

422. Justine Coleman, "All 50 States Under Disaster Declaration for First Time in US istory," *The Hill* (blog), Apr. 12, 2020, accessed Apr. 15, 2020, https://thehill.com/policy/healthcare/public-global-health/492433-all-50-states-under-disaster-declaration-for-first.

423. Michigan Executive Order 2020-42 (COVID-19)

424. Andrew O'Reilly, "Drivers Swarm Michigan Capital to Protest Coronavirus Lockdown Measures, Fox News (blog), Apr. 15, 2020, accessed Apr. 15, 2020, https://www.foxnews.com/politics/drivers-swarm-michigan-capital-to-protest-coronavirus-lockdown-measures.

425. Ibid.

426. State of Wisconsin Executive Order #74 Relating to Suspending In-Person Voting on April 7, 2020, due to the COVID-19 Pandemic," Apr. 6, 2020.

427. Natasha Korecki and Zack Montellaro, "Wisconsin Supreme Court Overturns Governor. Orders Tuesday Elections to Proceed," *Politico* (blog), Apr. 6, 2020, accessed Apr. 19, 2020, https://www.politico.com/news/2020/04/06/wisconsin-governor-orders-stop-to-in-person-voting-on-eve-of-election-168527.

428. State of New York Executive Order 202.10, Mar. 7, 2020.

429. Scott Neuman, "Man Dies, Woman Hospitalized After Taking Form of Chloroquine to Prevent COVID-19," NPR (blog), Mar. 24, 2020, accessed Apr. 15, 2020, https://www.npr.org/sections/coronavirus-live-updates/2020/03/24/820512107/man-dies-woman-hospitalized-after-taking-form-of-chloroquine-to-prevent-covid-19.

430. 2020-03-23 - COVID-19 Emergency Regulation Board of Pharmacy.

431. Letter from Deb Gagliardi and Forrest to Licensed Prescribers & Dispensers, Mar. 24, 2020.

432. Chuck Goudie, Bob Markoff, et al., "Coronavirus: New Questions About how Many Illinois State Prison Inmates Are Being Released Due to COVID-19," ABC7 (blog), Apr. 28, 2020, accessed May 18, 2020, https://abc7chicago.com/corona-virus-update-cases-illinois/6135977/; John Eligon, "'It's a Slap in the Face': Victims Are Angered as Jails Free Inmates," The New York Times (blog), Apr. 24, 2020, accessed May 18, 2020, https://www.nytimes.com/2020/04/24/us/coro-navirus-jail-inmates-released.html.

433. State of Florida Executive Order No. 20-91, Apr. 1, 2020.

434. State of Florida Executive Order No. 20-70, Mar. 20, 2020.

435. State of Florida Executive Order No. 20-71, Mar. 20, 2020.

436. State of Florida Executive Order No. 20-68, Mar. 17, 2020.

437. State of Florida Executive Order No. 20-89, Mar. 30, 2020.

438. State of Florida Executive Order No. 20-72, Mar. 20, 2020.

439. State of Florida Executive Order No. 20-91, Apr. 1, 2020.

440. Ibid.

441. Ellen Barry, "Days After a Funeral in a Georgia Town, Coronavirus 'Hit Like a Bomb," *The New York Times*, Mar. 30, 2020, accessed Mar. 30, 2020, https://www.nytimes.com/2020/03/30/us/coronavirus-funeral-albany-georgia.html?action=click&module=Top%20Stories&pgtype=Homepage.

442. Ibid.

443. Lee Brown, "New York City's First Coronavirus Patient Is a Healthcare Worker; Cuomo Says," *New York Post* (blog), Mar. 2, 2020, accessed May 8, 2020, https://nypost.com/2020/03/02/new-york-citys-first-coronavirus-patient-is-a-health-care-worker-cuomo-says/.

444. Tamer Lapin, "Coronavirus in NY: A Timeline of How the Disease Spread Through the Metro Area," *New York Post* (blog), Mar. 12, 2020, accessed May 8, 2020, https://nypost.com/2020/03/12/coronavirus-in-ny-a-timeline-of-how-the-dis-ease-spread-through-the-metro-area/.

445. "Coronavirus in NY: Cases, Maps, Charts, and Resources," Syracuse.com (blog), last updated May 7, 2020, accessed May 8, 2020, https://www.syracuse.com/coronavirus-ny/.

446. Lee Brown, "New York City's First Coronavirus Patient Is a Healthcare Worker; Cuomo Says," *New York Post* (blog), Mar. 2, 2020, accessed May 8, 2020, https://nypost.com/2020/03/02/new-york-citys-first-coronavirus-patient-is-a-healthcare-worker-cuomo-says/.

447. Ibid.

448. "Coronavirus in NY: Cases, Maps, Charts, and Resources," Syracuse.com (blog), last updated May 7, 2020, accessed May 8, 2020, https://www.syracuse.com/coronavirus-ny/.

449. Jimmy Vielkind, Leslie Brody, and Costas Paris, "Containment Area Planned for New York Suburb to Stem Coronavirus Spread," *The Wall Street Journal* (blog), Mar. 10, 2020, accessed May 8, 2020, https://www.wsj.com/articles/containment-area-planned-for-new-york-suburb-to-stem-coronavirus-spread-11583858117?mod=article_inline.

450. "Coronavirus in NY: Cases, Maps, Charts, and Resources," Syracuse.com (blog), last updated May 7, 2020, accessed May 8, 2020, https://www.syracuse.com/coronavirus-ny/.

451. Kyle Smith, "The Ventilator Shortage That Wasn't," *National Review* (blog), Apr. 17, 2020, accessed May 8, 2020, https://www.nationalreview.com/2020/04/coronavirus-crisis-ventilator-shortages-have-not-come-to-pass/.

452. Ibid.

453. Donald J. Trump in "Remarks by President Trump, Vice President Pence, and Members of the Coronavirus Task Force in Press Briefing, Apr. 20, 2020, accessed May 8, 2020, https://www.whitehouse.gov/briefings-statements/remarks-president-trump-vice-president-pence-members-coronavirus-task-force-press-briefing-29/

454. Michael R. Sisak, "Many Field Hospitals Went Largely Unused, Will Be Shut Down," *Military Times* (blog), Apr. 29, 2020, accessed May 8, 2020, https://www.militarytimes.com/news/coronavirus/2020/04/29/many-field-hospitals-went-largely-unused-will-be-shut-down/.

455. Ibid.

456. Elizabeth Koh, Jon Kamp, and Dan Froshc, "One Nursing Home, 35 Coronavirus Deaths: Inside the Kirkland Disaster," *The Wall Street Journal* (blog), Mar. 23, 2020, accessed Apr. 27, 2020, https://www.wsj.com/articles/one-nursing-home-35-coronavirus-deaths-inside-the-kirkland-disaster-11584982494.

457. Kate Feldman, "Life Care Center in Kirkland Epicenter of Washington's Coronavirus Outbreak, Sued for Wrongful Death," *New York Daily News* (blog), Apr. 12, 2020, accessed May 8, 2020, https://www.nydailynews.com/coronavirus/ny-coronavirus-kirkland-nursing-home-lawsuit-washington-20200412-ngbkjj7rffg2ld4f2s345lltii-story.html.

458. "State Data and Policy Actions to Address Coronavirus," The Henry J. Kaiser Foundation (blog) Apr. 23, 2020, Table: State Report of Long-Term Care Facility Cases and Deaths Related to COVID-19 (as of May 7, 2020), accessed May 8, 2020, https://www.kff.org/health-costs/issue-brief/state-data-and-policy-actions-to-address-coronavirus/.

459. Ibid.

460. Ibid.

461. Ibid.

462. Ibid.

463. Jim Mustian, Jennifer Peltz, and Bernard Condon, "NY's Cuomo Criticized Over Highest Nursing Home Death Toll," Spectrum News, Bay News 9 (blog), May 9, 2020, accessed May 9, 2020, https://abcnews.go.com/Health/wireStory/nys-cuomo-criticized-highest-nursing-home-death-toll-70596950.

464. "New Count Reveals 1,600 More Nursing Home Deaths in N.Y.," *The New York Times* (blog), May 5, 2020, accessed May 9, 2020, https://www.nytimes.com/2020/05/05/nyregion/covid-ny-update.html.

465. Ibid.

466. Jim Mustian, Jennifer Peltz, and Bernard Condon, "NY's Cuomo Criticized Over Highest Nursing Home Death Toll," Spectrum News, Bay News 9 (blog), May 9, 2020, accessed May 9, 2020, https://abcnews.go.com/Health/wireStory/nys-cuomo-criticized-highest-nursing-home-death-toll-70596950.

467. Ibid.

468. Carolyn J. Berdzik, Jonathan Berkowitz, Lisa M. Robinson., "New York State Department Releases Advisory Prohibiting Nursing Homes From Denying Admissions Due to Coronavrius," Goldberg Segalla Knowledge (blog), Mar. 27, 2020, accessed May 8, 2020, https://www.goldbergsegalla.com/news-and-knowledge/knowledge/nys-health-dept-releases-coronavirus-advisory.

469. Ibid.

470. Jim Mustian, Jennifer Peltz, and Bernard Condon, "NY's Cuomo Criticized Over Highest Nursing Home Death Toll," Spectrum News, Bay News 9 (blog), May 9, 2020, accessed May 9, 2020, https://abcnews.go.com/Health/wireStory/nys-cuomo-criticized-highest-nursing-home-death-toll-70596950.

471. Ibid.

472. Jared Moskowitz, State of Florida Division of Emergency Management DEM ORDER NO. 20-006, Mar. 15, 2020, accessed May 8, 2020, https://s33330.pcdn.co/wp-content/uploads/2020/03/DEM-ORDER-NO.-20-006-In-re-COVID-19-Public-Health-Emergency-Issued-March-15-2020.pdf.

473. Ibid.

474. "Nursing Homes," Florida COVID-19 Response, accessed May 8, 2020, https://floridahealthcovid19.gov/nursing-homes/.

475. "State Data and Policy Actions to Address Coronavirus," The Henry J. Kaiser Foundation (blog) Apr. 23, 2020, Table: State Report of Long-Term Care Facility Cases and Deaths Related to COVID-19 (as of May 7, 2020), accessed May 8, 2020, https://www.kff.org/health-costs/issue-brief/state-data-and-policy-actions-to-address-coronavirus/.

476. Ibid. .

477. Anjeanette Damon, "COVID-19 cases and Death in Nevada Nursing Homes Continue to Climb," *Reno Gazette Journal* (blog), Apr. 30, 2020, accessed May 8, 2020, https://www.rgj.com/story/news/2020/05/01/nevada-coronavirus-covid-19-cases-nursing-homes-deaths/3061863001/.

478. Memo from Nevada Department of Health and Human Services to Health Care Providers-Read Receipt Requested, "Coronavirus Disease 2019 (COVID-19)-REVISED, Mar. 25, 2020, accessed May 8, 2020, https://nvhealthresponse.nv.gov/wp-content/uploads/2020/03/COVID-19-TB-3.23.20-1.pdf.

479. Christopher Helman, "Bloodbath for America's Oil Frackers as Saudis Declare Price War on Russia," *Forbes* (blog), Mar. 9, 2020, accessed May 10, 2020, https://www.forbes.com/sites/christopherhelman/2020/03/09/bloodbath-for-oil-frackers-as-saudis-declare-price-war-on-russia/#22ceb5892198.

480. Rosie Perper, Sarah Al-Arshani, and Holly Secon, "More Than Half of the US Population Is Now Under Orders to Stay Home-Here's a List of Xoronavirus Lockdowns in US States and Cities," *Business Insider* (blog), Mar. 15, 2020, last updated Apr. 1, 2020, accessed May 8, 2020, https://www.businessinsider.com/states-cities-shutting-down-bars-restaurants-concerts-curfew-2020-3.

481. Jack Kelly, "A Record-Setting 3.3 Million People Filed for Unemployment," *Forbes* (blog), Mar. 26, 2020, accessed May 8, 2020, https://www.forbes.com/sites/jackkelly/2020/03/26/a-record-setting-33-million-people-filed-for-unemployment/#54e2f3597ccf.

482. Ibid.

483. Matt Krantz, "These 13 Stock Completely Erase Their Massive Coronavirus Losses," *Investors Business Daily* (blog), Apr. 9, 2020, accessed May 11, https://www.investors.com/etfs-and-funds/sectors/sp500-stocks-completely-erase-massive-coronavirus-losses-bounce/.

484. Jack Brewster, "Trump Signs $2 Trillion Coronavirus Relief Bill Into Law, Largest Aid Package in U.S. History," *Forbes* (blog), Mar. 27, 2020, accessed May 9, 2020, https://www.forbes.com/sites/jackbrewster/2020/03/27/trump-signs-2-trillion-stimulus-bill-into-law-largest-aid-package-in-us-history/#6e3d83ab4ea5.

485. Ibid.

486. Joseph Zeballos-Roig, "Trump Signs the $2 Trillion Coronavirus Economic Relief Bill Into Law, Which Includes Checks for Americans and Business Loans," *Business Insider* (blog), Mar. 27 2020, accessed May 8, 2020, https://www.businessinsider.com/trump-signs-coronavirus-economic-relief-aid-bill-checks-for-americans-2020-3.

487. Ebony Bowden and Steven Nelson, "President Trump Sign Into Law $2 Trillion Coronavirus Bailout," *New York Post* (blog), Mar. 27, 2020, accessed May 8, 2020, https://nypost.com/2020/03/27/president-trump-signs-into-law-2-trillion-coronavirus-bailout/.

488. "The CARES Act Provides Assistance to Small Businesses," U.S. Department of the Treasury, accessed May 8, 2020, https://home.treasury.gov/policy-issues/cares/assistance-for-small-businesses.

489. Andrew Duehren, "Funding Exhausted for $350 Billion Small-Business Paycheck Protection Program, *The Wall Street Journal* (blog), Apr. 16, 2020, accessed May 10, 2020, https://www.wsj.com/articles/funding-exhausted-for-350-billion-small-business-paycheck-protection-program-11587048384.

490. Jeffrey Bartash, "U.S. Unemployment Rate Has Likely Reached 15% Economists Say," MarketWatch (blog), Apr. 16, 2020, accessed May 8, 2020, https://www.marketwatch.com/story/jobless-claims-soar-again-by-525-million-as-coronavirus-pushes-unemployment-to-15-2020-04-16.

491. Natalie Andrews, "Trump Signs Coronavirus Stimulus Bill as Focus Shifts to State Funding," *The Wall Street Journal* (blog), Apr. 24, 2020, May 10, 2020, https://www.wsj.com/articles/trump-signs-coronavirus-stimulus-bill-as-focus-shifts-to-state-funding-11587749963.

492. Jeff Cox, "Here Is Everything the Fed Has Done to Save the Economy," CNCBC (blog), Apr. 13, 2020, accessed May 13, 2020, https://www.cnbc.com/2020/04/13/coronavirus-update-here-is-everything-the-fed-has-done-to-save-the-economy.html.

493. Kimberly Amadeo, "Reserve Requirement and How It Affects Interest Rates," The Balance (blog), Mar. 16, 2020, accessed May 13, 2020, https://www.thebalance.com/reserve-requirement-3305883.

494. Jeff Cox, "Here Is Everything the Fed Has Done to Save the Economy," CNCBC (blog), Apr. 13, 2020, accessed May 13, 2020, https://www.cnbc.com/2020/04/13/coronavirus-update-here-is-everything-the-fed-has-done-to-save-the-economy.html.

495. Sarah Chaney and Eric Morath, "April Unemployment Rate Rose to a Record 14%, *The Wall Street Journal* (blog), May 8, 2020, accessed May 11, 2020, https://www.wsj.com/articles/april-jobs-report-coronavirus-2020-11588888089.

496. Patricia Cohen and Tiffany Hsu, "For Workers, No Sign of 'What Normal Is Going to Look Like,'" *The New York Times* (blog), May 7, 2020, accessed May 11, 2020, https://www.nytimes.com/2020/05/07/business/economy/coronavirus-unemployment-claims.html.

497. Patricia Mazzei, "Florida Pastor Arrested AFter Defying Virus Orders," *The New York Times* (blog), Mar. 30, 2020, accessed Apr. 14, 2020, https://www.nytimes.com/2020/03/30/us/coronavirus-pastor-arrested-tampa-florida.html.

498. Ibid.

499. Ibid.

500. Executive Order of the Hillsborough County Emergency Policy Group Safer-At-Home Order in Response to a County Wide Threat from the COVID-19 Virus, § 3.ii, Mar. 27, 2020, accessed May 12, 2020, https://www.hillsboroughcounty.org/library/hillsborough/media-center/documents/administrator/epg/saferathomeorder.pdf.

501. Michael Ruiz, "Mississippi City's Coronavirus Shutdown Bans Drive-In Church Services Ahead of Easter," Fox News (blog), Apr. 11, 2020, accessed May 11, 2020, https://www.foxnews.com/us/mississippi-coronavirus-shutdown-city-bans-drive-in-church-services-easter.

502. Sophie O'Hara, "Report: Judge Overrules Democrat Mayor Who Banned Easter Drive-In Church Services," Wayne Dupree (blog), Apr. 11, 2020, accessed May 8, 2020, https://www.waynedupree.com/louisville-mayor-church/.

503. William Barr, "Attorney General William P. Barr Issues Statement on Religious Practice and Social Distancing; Department of Justice Files Statement of Interest in Mississippi Church Case," Department of Justice Office of Public Affairs, Fn. 1., Apr. 14, 2020, accessed May 21, 2020, https://www.justice.gov/opa/pr/attorney-general-william-p-barr-issues-statement-religious-practice-and-social-distancing-0.

504. Ibid.

505. "Governor Northam Announces New Measures to Combat COVID-19 and Support Impacted Virginians," Virginia Governor Ralph S. Northam, Mar. 17, 2020, accessed Apr. 14, 2020, https://www.governor.virginia.gov/newsroom/all-releases/2020/march/headline-854487-en.html.

506. Executive Order 2020-11 (COVID-19).

507. "Coronavirus, Executive Order 2020-11 FAQs," Michigan.gov, accessed Apr. 15, 2020, https://www.michigan.gov/coronavirus/0,9753,7-406-98178_98455-522357--,00.html.

508. Letter Eric S. Dreiband to Gavin Newsom, May 19, 2020, in @KerriKupecDOJ, Twitter, May 19, 2020, 7:57 PM, accessed May 21, 2020, https://twitter.com/KerriKupecDOJ/status/1262895160318480384.

509. Ibid.

510. State of Florida Office of the Governor Executive Order 20-91, (Essential Services and Activities During Covid-19, §3.A.i.

511. Lee Brown, "Virginia Pastor Who Defiantly Held Church Service Dies of Coronavirus," *New York Post* (blog), Apr. 13, 2020, accessed Apr, 14, 2020, https://nypost.com/2020/04/13/virginia-pastor-who-held-packed-church-service-dies-of-coronavirus/.

512. Deliverance Evangelistic Church, Facebook Post of April 12, 0744, accessed Apr. 14, 2020, https://www.facebook.com/OfficialNDEC/videos/233789087982971/?__tn__=-R.

513. Neil Ferguson, Daniel Laydon, et al., "COVID-19 Impact of Non-Pharmaceutical Intervention (NPIs) to Reduce COVID-19 Mortality and Healthcare Demand," Imperial College COVID-19 Response Team, Mar. 16, 2020, accessed May 13, 2020, https://www.imperial.ac.uk/media/imperial-college/medicine/sph/ide/gida-fellowships/Imperial-College-COVID19-NPI-modelling-16-03-2020.pdf.

514. Lydia Ramsey, "A Leaked Presentation Reveals the document US Hospitals Are Using to Prepare for a Major Coronavirus Outbreak. It Estimates 96 Million US Coronavirus Cases and 480,000 Deaths, *Business Insider* (blog), Mar. 6, 2020, accessed Apr. 13, 2020, https://www.businessinsider.com/presentation-how-hospitals-are-preparing-for-us-coronavirus-outbreak-2020-3.

515. "IHME COVID-19 model FAQs," healthdata.org (blog), accessed Apr. 8, 2020, http://www.healthdata.org/covid/faqs#differences%20in%20modeling.

516. Ibid.

517. IHME COVID-19 Health Service Utilization Forecasting Team, "Forecasting COVID-19 impact on hospital bed-days, ICU-days, ventilator-days and deaths by US state in the next 4 months," accessed Apr. 8, 2020, http://www.healthdata.org/sites/default/files/files/research_articles/2020/covid_paper_MEDRXIV-2020-043752v1-Murray.pdf.

518. Ibid.

519. Ibid.

520. Video in Ian Schwartz, CNN's Acosta: Trump 'Propaganda' Video 'Looked Straight Out of Beijing or Pyongyang," Real Clear Politics (blog), Apr. 13, accessed May 13, 2020, https://www.realclearpolitics.com/video/2020/04/13/cnns_acosta_trump_propaganda_video_looked_straight_out_of_beijing_or_pyongyang.html.

521. Jim Acosta in transcript of *Anderson Cooper 360 Degrees*, Apr. 13, 2020, accessed May 13, 2020, http://transcripts.cnn.com/TRANSCRIPTS/2004/13/acd.01.html.

522. Sean Collins, "Fauci Acknowledged a Delay in the US Coronavirus Response. Trump Then Retweeted a Call to Fire Him," Vox (blog), Apr. 13, 2020, accessed Apr. 16, 2020, https://www.vox.com/covid-19-coronavirus-us-response-trump/2020/4/13/21218922/corona-virus-fauci-trump-fire-tweet.

523. Eric Lipton, David E. Sanger, et al., "He Could Have Seen What Was Coming: Behind Trump's Failure on the Virus," *The New York Times* (blog) Apr. 11, 2020, updated, Apr. 14, 2020, accessed Apr. 16, 2020, https://www.nytimes.com/2020/04/11/us/politics/coronavirus-trump-response.html.

524. Grace Panetta, "Trump Reportedly Squandered 3 Crucial Weeks to Mitigate the Coronavirus Outbreak after a CDC Official's Blunt Warnings Spooked the Stock Market," *Business Insider* (blog) Apr. 12, 2020, accessed Apr. 16, 2020, https://www.businessinsider.com/trump-wasted-3-weeks-coronavirus-mitiga-tion-time-february-march-nyt-2020-4.

525. Ed Pilkington, Victoria Bekiempis, and Oliver Laughland, "Pelosi Accuses Trump of Costing US Lives with Coronavirus Denials and Delays," *The Guardian* (blog), Mar. 29, 2020, accessed Apr. 14, 2020, https://www.theguardian.com/us-news/2020/mar/29/pelosi-trump-coronavirus-response-inaction-delays

526. Mark von Rennenkampff, "Trump's Hubris and Ideological Rigidity Will Cost American Lives," *The Hill* (blog), Mar. 30, 2020, accessed Apr. 14, 2020, https://thehill.com/opinion/white-house/490045-trumps-hubris-and-ideological-rigidi-ty-will-cost-american-lives.

527. David Remnick in "Remnick: Cost of Trump's Delays Will Be 'Paid in Human Lives,'" CNN Business (blog), accessed Apr. 13, 2020, https://www.cnn.com/videos/business/2020/03/29/remnick-cost-of-trumps-delays-will-be-paid-in-hu-man-lives.cnn.

528. David Frum, "This Is Trump's Fault; The President Is Failing, and Americans Are Paying for His Failures," *The Atlantic* (blog), Apr. 7, 2020; accessed Apr. 14, 2020, https://www.theatlantic.com/ideas/archive/2020/04/americans-are-paying-the-price-for-trumps-failures/609532/.

529. Mary Petrone and Nathan Grubaugh, "Coronavirus Mutations: Much Ado About Nothing," CNN Health (blog), Mar. 7, 2020, accessed, Apr. 16, 2020, https://www.cnn.com/2020/03/07/health/coronavirus-mutations-analysis/index.html.

530. Michael Crowley, "Some Experts Worry as a Germ-Phobic Trump Confronts Growing Epidemic," *The New York Times* (blog), Feb. 10, 2020, accessed Apr. 16, 2020, https://www.nytimes.com/2020/02/10/us/politics/trump-coronavi-rus-epidemic.html.

531. Vox in Timothy P. Carney, "Coronavirus Revisionism: When the Media Pretends Their Narrative is 'Reality'," *Washington Examiner* (blog), March 31, 2020, accessed Apr. 16, 2020, https://www.washingtonexaminer.com/opinion/coronavi-rus-revisionism-when-the-media-pretends-their-narrative-is-reality.

532. Nick Robins-Early, "Don't Listen to Sen. Tom Cotton About Coronavirus," Huffpost (blog) Jan. 31, 2020, accessed Apr. 16, 2020, https://www.huffpost.com/entry/tom-cotton-coronavirus-china_n_5e34a3b7c5b6f26233294378.

533. Alex Azar in Stephanie Soucheray, "Officials Say Most Americans Not at Risk of Coronavirus," Center for Infectious Disease Research and Policy, Jan. 28, 2020, accessed Apr. 14, 2020, https://www.cidrap.umn.edu/news-perspective/2020/01/officials-say-most-americans-not-risk-coronavirus

534. Nancy Messonier in Stephanie Soucheray, "Officials Say Most Americans Not at Risk of Coronavirus," Center for Infectious Disease Research and Policy, Jan. 28, 2020, accessed Apr. 14, 2020, https://www.cidrap.umn.edu/news-perspective/2020/01/officials-say-most-americans-not-risk-coronavirus.

535. Logan Ratick, "Jan. Flashback: Dr. Fauci Said coronavirus 'Is Not a Threat to the People of the United States," SARA (blog), Apr. 3, 2020, accessed Apr. 14, 2020, https://saraacarter.com/jan-flashback-dr-fauci-said-coronavirus-is-not-a-major-threat-to-the-people-of-the-united-states

536. Philippe Gautret, Jean-Christopher Lagier, " Hydroxychloroquine and Azithromycin as a Treatment of COVID-19: Results of an Open-Label Non-Randomized Clinical Trial," medrxiv.org (blog) Mar. 16, 2020, accessed Apr. 21, 2020, https://www.medrxiv.org/content/10.1101/2020.03.16.20037135v1.full.pdf.

537. Author, personal observation of Gregory Rigano in Tucker Carlson Tonight, Fox News, Mar. 18, 2020; Tim Pierce, "Malaria Drug See Promising Signs as Future Coronavirus Treatment," *Washington Examiner*, (blog), March 18, 2020, accessed Apr. 20, 2020, https://www.washingtonexaminer.com/news/malaria-drug-sees-promising-signs-as-future-coronavirus-treatment.

538. Aude Lecruvier, "COVID-19: Could Hydroxychloroquine Really Be an Answer? Medscape (blog), Mar. 18, 2020, accessed Apr. 21, 2020, https://www.medscape.com/viewarticle/927033.

539. Author, personal observation of Gregory Rigano in Tucker Carlson Tonight, Fox News, Mar. 18, 2020; Tim Pierce, "Malaria Drug See Promising Signs as Future Coronavirus Treatment," *Washington Examiner*, (blog), March 18, 2020, accessed Apr. 20, 2020, https://www.washingtonexaminer.com/news/malaria-drug-sees-promising-signs-as-future-coronavirus-treatment.

540. Mary Beth Pfeiffer, "Researchers Look to Old Drug for a Possible Coronavirus Treatment-It Might Just Work," *Forbes* (blog), Mar. 18, 2020, accessed Apr. 21, 2020, https://www.forbes.com/sites/marybethpfeiffer/2020/03/18/science-works-to-use-old-cheap-drugs-to-attack-coronavirus--it-might-just-work/#41b380655c49.

541. Tal Axelrod, "Trump Steps up Effort to Tout Malaria Drug as Coronavirus 'game changer' Despite Doubts from FDA," *The Hill* Mar. 21 2020, accessed Apr. 21, 2020, https://thehill.com/homenews/administration/488796-trump-steps-up-effort-to-tout-malaria-drug-as-coronavirus-game.

542. Donald J. Trump, @realDonaldTrump, Twitter, Mar. 21, 2020, in Joe Palca, "NIH Panel Recommends Against Drug Combination Promoted By Trump For COVID-19," NPR (blog), Apr. 21, 2020, accessed Apr. 21, 2020, https://www.npr.org/sections/coronavirus-live-updates/2020/04/21/840341224/nih-panel-recommends-against-drug-combination-trump-has-promoted-for-covid-19.

543. Anna Edney, "Trump Touts Drug That FDA Says Isn't Yet Approved for Virus," *Bloomberg* (blog) Mar. 19, 2020, accessed Apr. 17, 2020, https://www.bloomberg.com/news/articles/2020-03-19/trump-touts-malaria-drug-as-potential-coronavirus-treatment.

544. *Business Insider* (blog) Apr. 9, 2020, accessed Apr. 17, 2020, https://www.businessinsider.com/trump-unproven-coronavirus-treatment-chloroquine-dangerous-expert-2020-4.

545. Sarah Owermohle, "What You Need to Know About the Malaria Drugs Trump Keeps Touting," *Politico*, Apr. 6, 2020, accessed Apr. 17, 2020, https://www.politico.com/news/2020/04/06/malaria-drug-coronavirus-trump-hydroxychloroquine-169103.

546. David Barrett, "Anti-Malarial rug Touted by Trump Was Subject of CIA Warning to Employees," *The Washington Post* (blog), Apr. 13, 2020, accessed Apr. 17, 2020, https://www.washingtonpost.com/; Marina Pitofsky, "CIA Warned Employees Against Using Hydroxychloroquine for Coronavirus: Report," The Hill (blog), Apr. 14, 2020, accessed Apr. 17, 2020, https://thehill.com/homenews/administration/492649-internal-cia-document-warns-against-using-hydroxychloroquine-for.

547. "Management of Persons with COVID-19," NIH, accessed Apr. 21, 2020, https://covid19treatmentguidelines.nih.gov/overview/management-of-covid-19/.

548. "Therapeutic Options for COVID-19 Currently Under Investigation," NIH, accessed Apr. 21, 2020, https://covid19treatmentguidelines.nih.gov/therapeutic-options-under-investigation/.

549. Ibid.

550. Ibid.

551. Ibid.

552. Joe Palca, "NIH Panel Recommends Against Drug Combination Promoted By Trump For COVID-19," NPR (blog), Apr. 21, 2020, accessed Apr. 21, 2020, https://www.npr.org/sections/coronavirus-live-updates/2020/04/21/840341224/nih-panel-recommends-against-drug-combination-trump-has-promoted-for-covid-19.

553. Rachel Sandler, "NIH Panel Recommends Against Using Hydroxychloroquine and Azithromycin, Drug Combination Touted By Trump." *Forbes* (blog), Apr. 21, 2020, accessed Apr. 21, 2020, https://www.forbes.com/sites/rachelsandler/2020/04/21/nih-panel-recommends-against-using-drug-combination-touted-by-trump-outside-clinical-trials/#506477d4b405.

554. Joseph Guzman, "NIH Panel Recommends Against Use of Hydroxychloroquine and Azithromycin to Treat COVID-19." *The Hill* (blog), Apr. 21, 2020, accessed Apr. 21, 2020, https://thehill.com/changing-america/well-being/prevention-cures/493995-nih-panel-recommends-against-use-of.

555. Susan Swindells in Joe Palca, "NIH Panel Recommends Against Drug Combination Promoted By Trump For COVID-19," NPR (blog), Apr. 21, 2020, accessed Apr. 21, 2020, https://www.npr.org/sections/coronavirus-live-updates/2020/04/21/840341224/nih-panel-recommends-against-drug-combination-trump-has-promoted-for-covid-19.

556. "NIH Begins Clinical Trial of Hydroxychloroquine and Azithromycin to Treat COVID-19," NIH (blog), May 14, 2020, accessed May 19, 2020, https://www.nih.gov/news-events/news-releases/nih-begins-clinical-trial-hydroxychloroquine-azithromycin-treat-covid-19.

557. Brad Lendon, "Chinese State Media Claims Country's Navy Is Not Affected by Coronavirus," CNN (blog), Apr. 15, 2020, accessed Apr. 17, 2020, https://www.cnn.com/2020/04/13/asia/china-coronavirus-aircraft-carrier-deployment-dp-hnk-intl/index.html.

558. Tom Cotton Letter to Mike Pompeo, Alex Azar, and Chad Wolf, Jan 28, 2020.

559. Ibid.

560. Nick Robins-Early, "Don't Listen to Sen. Tom Cotton About Coronavirus," Huffpost (blog) Jan. 31, 2020, accessed Apr. 16, 2020, https://www.huffpost.com/entry/tom-cotton-coronavirus-china_n_5e34a3b7c5b6f26233294378.

561. Ibid.

562. Ibid.

563. Ashley Kirzinger, Audrey Kearney, et al., "KFF Tracking Poll-Early April 2020: The Impact of Coronavirus on Life in America," KFF (blog), Apr. 2, 2020, accessed May 14, 2020, https://www.kff.org/coronavirus-covid-19/report/kff-health-tracking-poll-early-april-2020/.

564. Peter Grinspoon, "A Tale of Two Epidemics: When COVID-19 and Opioid Addiction Collide," *Harvard Health Publishing* (blog), Apr. 20, 2020, accessed May 14, 2020, https://www.health.harvard.edu/blog/a-tale-of-two-epidemics-when-covid-19-and-opioid-addiction-collide-2020042019569.

565. Olivia Goldhill, "Cancer Screenings Are Way Down During the Coronavirus," Quartz (blog), May 8, 2020, accessed May 14, 2020, https://qz.com/1853670/cancer-screenings-are-way-down-during-coronavirus/.

566. Emma Reynolds, "Lockdowns Shouldn't Be Fully Lifted Until Coronavirus Vaccine Found, New Study Warns," CNN (blog), Apr. 9, 2020, accessed May 8, 2020, https://www.cnn.com/2020/04/09/world/lockdown-lift-vaccine-coronavirus-lancet-intl/index.html.

567. Terri Whitcraft, Bill Hutchinson, and Nadine Shubailat, "'Road Map' to Recovery Report: 20 Million Coronavirus Tests per Day Needed to Fully Open Economy," ABC News (blog), Apr. 20, 2020, accessed May 14, 2020, https://abcnews.go.com/US/road-map-recovery-report-20-million-coronavirus-tests/story?id=70230097.

568. Ed O'Keefe and Kathryn Watson, "'You're Gonna Call Your Own Shots,'" Trump Tell Governors About Guidelines to Reopen States," CBS News (blog), Apr. 16, 2020, accessed May 14, 2020, https://www.cbsnews.com/news/trump-guidelines-on-opening-up-america-leave-much-up-to-governors/.

569. White House and CDC, "Guidelines Opening Up America Again," whitehouse.gov, accessed May 14. 2020, https://www.whitehouse.gov/openingamerica/.

570. Ibid.

571. Ibid.

572. Ibid.

573. Ibid.

574. Ibid.

575. Ibid.

576. Ibid.

577. Ibid.

578. Ibid.

579. David Smith, "Trump's 'Science Based' Reopening Strategy Is Still Full of Unanswered Questions," The (blog), Apr. 16, 2002, accessed May 14, 2020, https://www.theguardian.com/world/2020/apr/16/trumps-science-based-reopening-strategy-is-still-full-of-unanswered-questions.

580. Teri Whitcraft, Bill Hutchinson, and Nadine Shubailat, "'Road Map' to Recovery Report: 20 Million Coronavirus Tests per Day Needed to Fully Open Economy," ABC News (blog) Apr. 20, 2020, accessed May 7, 2020, https://abcnews.go.com/US/road-map-recovery-report-20-million-coronavirus-tests/story?id=70230097.

581. James C. Capretta, "Opinion: This Conservative Economist Says President Trump's Plan to Reopen the Economy Fails in Crucial Ways," MarketWatch (blog), Apr. 26, 2020, accessed May 14, 2020, https://www.marketwatch.com/story/this-conservative-economist-says-president-trumps-plan-to-reopen-the-economy-fails-in-crucial-ways-2020-04-24.

582. ABC News/Ipsos Poll, May 6-7, 2020, accessed May 14, 2020, https://www.ipsos.com/sites/default/files/ct/news/documents/2020-05/topline-abc-coronavirus-wave-8.pdf.

583. Kendall Karson, "Reopening the Country Seen as Greater Risk Among Most Americans: POLL," ABC News (blog), May 8, 2020, accessed May 14, 2020, https://abcnews.go.com/Politics/reopening-country-greater-risk-americans-poll/story?id=70555060.

584. Brian Kempf, The State of Georgia Executive Order Providing Flexibility for Healthcare Practices, Moving Certain Businesses to Minimum Operation and Providing for Emergency Response, Apr. 20, 2020, accessed May 14, 2020, https://gov.georgia.gov/executive-action/executive-orders/2020-executive-orders.

585. Russ Bynum, "Georgia Lets Clos-Contact Businesses Reopening Despite Rise in Coronavirus Cases," Time (blog), Apr. 24, 2020, accessed May 14, 2020,

586. Brian Kempf, The State of Georgia Executive Order Providing Flexibility for Healthcare Practices, Moving Certain Businesses to Minimum Operation and Providing for Emergency Response, Apr. 20, 2020, accessed May 14, 2020, https://time.com/5826943/georgia-reopen-coronavirus/.https://gov.georgia.gov/executive-action/executive-orders/2020-executive-orders.

587. Fig. COVID-19 Cases Over Time, Georgia Department of Public Health Daily Status Report, Georgia Department of Public Health, accessed May 14, 2020, https://dph.georgia.gov/covid-19-daily-status-report.

588. Ibid.

589. Jiachuan Wu, Robin Muccari, et al., "Reopening America Some States Are Staring to Reopen and Lift Lockdowns, Even as the Battle Against the Coronavirus Rages on," NBC News (blog), updated May 11, 2020, accessed May 14, 2020, https://www.nbcnews.com/news/us-news/reopening-america-see-what-states-across-u-s-are-starting-n1195676.

590. Ibid.

591. Ibid.

592. Ibid.

593. Sarah Mervosh, Kasmine C. Lee, et al., "See Which States Are Reopening and Which Are Still Shut Down," *The New York Times* (blog), updated May 13, 2020, accessed May 14, 2020, https://www.nytimes.com/interactive/2020/us/states-re-open-map-coronavirus.html.

594. Jill Filipovic, "Governors Reopening Their States Are Endangering American Lives," CNN (blog), Apr. 21, 2020, accessed May 14, 2020.

595. Ibid.

596. Yaneer Bar-Yam, "Don't Let Governors Fool You About Reopening," CNN (blog), May 12, 2020, accessed May 14, 2020, https://www.cnn.com/2020/05/12/opinions/governors-reopen-states-opinion-bar-yam/index.html.

597. Sonia Y Angell, Order of the State Public Health Officer, May 7, 2020, accessed May 15, 2020, https://www.cdph.ca.gov/Programs/CID/DCDC/CDPH%20Document%20Library/COVID-19/SHO%20Order%205-7-2020.pdf.

598. Ibid.

599. Kellie Hwang, "Los Angeles to Extend Stay-At-Home Order, While Some California Counties Are Cleared to Reopen," *San Franciso Chronicle* (blog), May 14, 2020, accessed May 15, 2020, https://www.sfchronicle.com/bayarea/article/LA-to-extend-stay-home-through-July-while-two-15265751.php.

600. Gretchen Whitmer, Executive Order 2020-68 (COVID-19), "Declaration of States of Emergency and Disaster Under the Emergency Management Act, 176 PA 390, Apr. 30, 2020, accessed May 15, 2020, https://www.michigan.gov/whitmer/0,9309,7-387-90499_90705-527716--,00.html.

601. David Eggert, "Hundred Protest Stay-At-Home Order Outside Michigan Capitol, *The News Tribune* (blog), May 14, 2020, accessed May 15, 2020, https://www.thenewstribune.com/news/nation-world/national/article242737811.html.

602. Ivan Pereira, "Protester With Ax Involved in Clash at Michigan Rally Against Stay-At-Home Orders, May 14, 2020, accessed May 15, 2020, https://abc7.com/protester-with-ax-involved-in-clash-at-michigan-rally-against-stay-at-home-orders/6183213/.

603. David Eggert, "Hundred Protest Stay-At-Home Order Outside Michigan Capitol, *The News Tribune* (blog), May 14, 2020, accessed May 15, 2020, https://www.thenewstribune.com/news/nation-world/national/article242737811.html.

604. Gus Burns, "Judge to Determine if Michigan's Extended Coronavirus State of Emergency Is Legal," MLive (blog), updated May 15, 2020, accessed May 15, 2020, https://www.mlive.com/public-interest/2020/05/judge-to-determine-if-michigans-extended-coronavirus-state-of-emergency-is-legal.html.

605. Ibid.

606. State of Wisconsin Department of Health Emergency Order #28 Safer at Home Order, Apr. 16, 2020, accessed Apr. 19, 2020, https://content.govdelivery.com/attachments/WIGOV/2020/04/16/file_attachments/1428995/EMO28-SaferAtHome.pdf.

607. Tony Evers in Scott Bauer, "Wisconsin Gov. Tony Evers Extends Stay-at Home Orders for Another Month, Closes Schools for Remainder of Academic Year," *Hartford Courant*, Apr. 16, 2020, accessed Apr. 19, 2020, https://www.courant.com/coronavirus/ct-nw-wisconsin-stay-at-home-order-extended-20200416-eajw46fjqvegpf4x43yenweqfm-story.html.

608. *Wisconsin Legislature v. Secretary-Designee Andre Palm, et al.*, Wisc. No. 2020AP765-OA, May 13, 2020, accessed May 15, 2020, https://www.wicourts. gov/sc/opinion/DisplayDocument.pdf?content=pdf&seqNo=260868&mod=article_inline.

609. State of Wisconsin Executive Order #74 Relating to Suspending In-Person Voting on April 7, 2020, due to the COVID-19 Pandemic," Apr. 6, 2020.

610. Jason Calvi and AP Wire Service, "Wisconsin Republicans to Challenge Extension of 'Safer at Home' Order; Interest in Rally Explodes, Fox6Now.com (blog), Apr. 17, 2020, accessed Apr. 19, 2020, https://fox6now.com/2020/04/17/interest-in-rally-explodes-after-gov-evers-extension-of-safer-at-home-order/.

611. Christopher Schmaling Media Release, Apr. 17, 2020, accessed Apr. 19, 2020, https://www.racinecounty.com/government/sheriff-s-office

612. Ibid.

613. *Wisconsin Legislature v. Secretary-Designee Andre Palm, et al.*, Wisc. No. 2020AP765-OA, May 13, 2020, accessed May 15, 2020, https://www.wicourts. gov/sc/opinion/DisplayDocument.pdf?content=pdf&seqNo=260868&mod=article_inline.

614. Ed White, "Michigan Barber Who Pledged to Stay Open 'Until Jesus Comes' Has License Suspended for Defying Coronavirus Orders," *Time* (blog), May 13, 2020, accessed May 16, 2020, https://time.com/5836393/michigan-barber-license-suspended/.

615. Karl Manke in Ed White, "Michigan Barber Who Pledged to Stay Open 'Until Jesus Comes' Has License Suspended for Defying Coronavirus Orders," *Time* (blog), May 13, 2020, accessed May 16, 2020, https://time.com/5836393/michigan-barber-license-suspended/.

616. Madeline Holcombe, "New York Tourist Is Arrested in Hawaii After Posting Beach Pictures on Instagram," CNN (blog), May 16, 2020, accessed May 16, 2020, https://www.cnn.com/2020/05/16/us/hawaii-arrest-coronavirus-trnd/index. html.

617. Ibid.

618. @theCJPearson, Twitter, May 14, 1227 PM, accessed May 17, 2020, https://twitter.com/thecjpearson/status/1260969917345603586?s=12.

619. Robert Levin in Ventura County presentation, KTLA 5, YouTube, May 4, 2020, at 3:20-5:20, accessed May 22, 2020, https://www.youtube.com/watch?v=0Kf_gWrBio4.

620. Ibid.

621. Neil Vigdor, "Dallas Salon Owner Is Jailed for Defying Order of Stay Closed," *The New York Times* (blog), Apr. 24, accessed May 15, 2020, https://www.nytimes. com/2020/05/05/us/dallas-salon-opens-coronavirus.html.

622. Shelley Luther in Neil Vigdor, "Dallas Salon Owner Is Jailed for Defying Order of Stay Closed," The New York Times (blog), Apr. 24, accessed May 15, 2020, https:// www.nytimes.com/2020/05/05/us/dallas-salon-opens-coronavirus.html.

623. Manny Fernandez and David Montgomery, "Dallas Salon Owner Who Was Jailed for Reopening Is Released," *The New York Times* (blog), May 7, 2020, accessed May 15, 2020, https://www.nytimes.com/2020/05/07/us/dallas-salon-owner-shelley-luther.html.

624. Neil Vigdor, "Dallas Salon Owner Is Jailed for Defying Order of Stay Closed," *The New York Times* (blog), Apr. 24, accessed May 15, 2020, https://www.nytimes.com/2020/05/05/us/dallas-salon-opens-coronavirus.html.

625. Emily Czachor, "GoFundMe Raises More Than $500,000 for Dallas Hair Salon Owner Arrested fro Opening Business Despite Coronavirus Restrictions," *Newsweek* (blog), May 12, 2020, accessed May 15, 2020, https://www.newsweek.com/gofundme-raises-more-500000-dallas-hair-salon-owner-arrested-opening-business-despite-1503496.

626. Manny Fernandez and David Montgomery, "Dallas Salon Owner Who Was Jailed for Reopening Is Released," *The New York Times* (blog), May 7, 2020, accessed May 15, 2020, https://www.nytimes.com/2020/05/07/us/dallas-salon-owner-shelley-luther.html.

627. Ibid.

628. Letter from various Dallas Circuit Court Judges to Ken Paxton, undated, in @HowertonNews, Twitter, May 6, 2020, 710 PM, accessed May 15, 2020, https://twitter.com/HowertonNews/status/1258172318414770181.

629. Greg Abbott, Executive Order GA 21 Relating to the Expanded Reopening of Services as Part of the Sage, Strategic Plan to Open Texas in Response to the COVID-19 Disaster, May 5, 2020, accessed May 16, 2020, https://www.cityofazle.org/DocumentCenter/View/6692/EO-GA-21-expanding-Open-Texas-COVID-19-salons-barber-shops-05-05-2020?bidId=.

630. GDP per Capita, The World Bank, May 2020, https://data.worldbank.org/indicator/NY.GDP.PCAP.CD.

631. Physicians per 1,000 People, The World Bank, May 2020, https://data.worldbank.org/indicator/SH.MED.PHYS.ZS.

632. Population density (people per sq. km of land area), The World Bank, May 2020, https://data.worldbank.org/indicator/EN.POP.DNST?end=2018&start=1961.

633. Life expectancy at birth, total (years), The World Bank, May 2020, https://data.worldbank.org/indicator/SP.DYN.LE00.IN.

634. COVID-19 Coronavirus Pandemic, Worldometer, updated May 2, 2020, accessed May 3, 2020, https://www.worldometers.info/coronavirus/#countries.

635. Tandon, Ajay & Murray, Christopher & Lauer, Jeremy & Evans, David. (2000). Measuring Overall Health System Performance for 191 Countries. Global Programme on Evidence for Health Policy Discussion Paper No. 30, accessed May 23, 2020, https://www.who.int/healthinfo/paper30.pdf.

636. Tableau.com, accessed Amy 23, 2020, https://www.tableau.com/trial/tableau-software?utm_campaign_id=2017049&utm_campaign=Prospecting-CORE-ALL-ALL-ALL-ALL&utm_medium=Paid+Search&utm_source=-Google+Search&utm_language=EN&utm_country=USCA&kw=tableau&adgroup=CTX-Brand-Priority-Core-E&adused=RESP&matchtype=e&-placement=&gclid=CjwKCAjwk6P2BRAIEiwAfVJ0rEgswhgXWmCm2qDVwTwn3J-jDE-Sl65deGiqtc2IDX18-RTwd-GGacRoCf7wQAvD_BwE&gclsrc=aw.ds.

637. T. J. Rodgers. "Do Lockdowns Save Many Lives? In Most Places, the Data Say No," *The Wall Street Journal*, Apr. 26, 2020, accessed May 24, 2020, https://www.wsj.com/articles/do-lockdowns-save-many-lives-is-most-places-the-data-say-no-11587930911.

638. 1 Cor. 19

639. Robert O'Rourke, @BetoO'Rourke, Twitter, Mar 23, 2020, 8:55 PM, accessed May 21, 2020, https://twitter.com/BetoORourke/status/1242253546625683458.

640. United States Constitution Art. I, §9, cl.2.

641. United States Constitution Art. IV, §4.

642. United States Constitution Art. I, §8, cl.15.

643. John F. Kennedy, Press Conference of May 9, 1962, *Public Papers of the Presidents of the United States: John F. Kennedy,* 1962, p. 376 (1963) quoted in Library of Congress, Respectfully Quoted: A Dictionary of Quotations, (New York: Dover Publications, Inc., 2010) q. 1520.

644. *The Wall Street Journal* Editorial Board, "The Art of Coronavirus Modeling," WSJ (blog), Apr. 7, 2020, accessed Apr. 8, 2020, https://www.wsj.com/articles/the-art-of-coronavirus-modeling-11586301975.

645. James Madison "The Federalist No. 10," Nov. 23, 1787

646. Pope Francis in "Don't Build Walls, Pope Francis Says," Reuters (blog), Feb. 8, 2017, accessed Apr. 15, 2020, https://www.reuters.com/article/us-pope-wall-idUSKBN15N1ZW.

647. Constitution of the World Health Organization Ch.II, Art. 2(g), Apr. 7, 1948, amended Sept. 15, 2005, accessed May 4, 2020, https://apps.who.int/gb/bd/PDF/bd47/EN/constitution-en.pdf?ua=1.

648. Ibid.

649. Anis Chowdhury and Iyanatul Islam, "Is There an Optimal Debt-to-GDP Ratio?" VOX Centre for Economic Research Policy Portal (blog), Nov. 9, 2010, accessed May 27, 2020, https://voxeu.org/debates/commentaries/there-optimal-debt-gdp-ratio.

650. Carmen Reinhart, Vincent Reinhart, and Kenneth Rogoff, "Public Debt Overhangs: Advanced Economy Episodes Since 1800," *Journ. Eco Perspective*, (Summer 2012) Vol. 26, No. 3, pp. 69-86, accessed May 27, 2020, https://pubs.aeaweb.org/doi/pdfplus/10.1257/jep.26.3.69.

651. Government Debt as Percent of GDP, accessed May 27, 2020, https://www.google.com/publicdata/explore?ds=ds22a34krhq5p_&ctype=l&strail=false&bcs=d&nselm=h&met_y=gd_pc_gdp&scale_y=lin&ind_y=false&rdim=country_group&idim=country:el:it:de&ifdim=country_group&hl=en&dl=en&ind=false.

652. Romina Boccia, "How the United States' High Debt Will Weaken the Economy and Hurt Americans," The Heritage Foundation (blog), Feb. 12, 2013, accessed May 27, 2020, https://www.heritage.org/budget-and-spending/report/how-the-united-states-high-debt-will-weaken-the-economy-and-hurt.

653. Government Debt as Percent of GDP, accessed May 27, 2020, https://www.google.com/publicdata/explore?ds=ds22a34krhq5p_&ctype=l&strail=false&bcs=d&nselm=h&met_y=gd_pc_gdp&scale_y=lin&ind_y=false&rdim=country_group&idim=country:el:it:de:se:es&ifdim=country_group&hl=en&dl=en&ind=false.

654. Ibid.

655. H. Plecher, Japan: National Debt from 2014 to 2024 in Relation to Gross Domestic Product (GDP)," Statista (blog), May 6, 2020, accessed May 28, 2020, https://www.statista.com/statistics/267226/japans-national-debt-in-relation-to-gross-domestic-product-gdp/.

656. Romina Boccia, "How the United States' High Debt Will Weaken the Economy and Hurt Americans," The Heritage Foundation (blog), Feb. 12, 2013, accessed May 27, 2020, https://www.heritage.org/budget-and-spending/report/how-the-united-states-high-debt-will-weaken-the-economy-and-hurt.

657. Federal Debt: Total Public Debt as Percent of Gross Domestic Product (GFDEGCQ1885), FRED, accessed May 27, 2020, https://fred.stlouisfed.org/series/GFDE-GDQ188S.

658. Ibid.

659. Ibid.

660. usdebtclock.org , accessed May 27, 2020, https://www.usdebtclock.org/index.html#.

661. Kevin Rudd, "The Coming Post-COVID Anarchy. The Pandemic Bodes Ill for Both American and Chinese Power-and for the Global Order," *Foreign Affairs* (blog), May 6, 2020, accessed May 27, 2020, https://www.foreignaffairs.com/articles/united-states/2020-05-06/coming-post-covid-anarchy.

662. Mike Patton, "The Approaching Coronavirus Debt Crisis: How Excessive Debt Reduces Economic Growth," Forbes (blog), Apr. 28, 2020, accessed May 27, 2020, https://www.forbes.com/sites/mikepatton/2020/04/28/the-approaching-covid-19-debt-crisis-how-excessive-debt-reduces-economic-growth/#c-d7296e94706.

663. *A Budget for a Better America; Promises Kept. Taxpayers First. Budget of the U.S. Government Fiscal Year 2020*, U.S Government Publishing Office (March 11, 2019: Washington, D.C.) Table S-4, accessed June 3, 2020, https://www.whitehouse.gov/wp-content/uploads/2019/03/budget-fy2020.pdf.

664. "Gross Domestic Product," Federal Reserve Bank of St. Louis, updated May 28, 2020, accessed June 3, 2020, https://fred.stlouisfed.org/series/GDP.

665. Constitution of the United States, Preamble.

666. "Florida Department of Health Updates New COVID-19 Cases, Announces Fifteen Deaths Related to COVID-19," Florida Department of Health, updated May 25, 2020, accessed May 28, 2020, http://www.floridahealth.gov/newsroom/2020/05/052520-1427-covid19.pr.html.

667. Ewen Callaway, David Cyranoski, et al, "The Coronavirus Pandemic in Five powerful Charts," *Nature* (blog) Mar. 18, 2020, accessed Mar. 26, 2020, https://www.nature.com/articles/d41586-020-00758-2.

668. Steven Sanche, Yen Ting Lin, et al., "High contagiousness and rapid spread of severe acute respiratory syndrome coronavirus 2," *Emerging Infect. Dis.* (2020) Vol. 26, No. 7, accessed May 28, 2020, https://doi.org/10.3201/eid2607.200282.

669. "Coronavirus Disease 2019: Pandemic Planning Scenarios," CDC, last reviewed May 2, 2020, accessed May 28, 2020, https://www.cdc.gov/coronavirus/2019-ncov/hcp/planning-scenarios.html.

670. Ibid.

671. Ibid.

672. Kat Stafford, Meghan Hoyer, and Aaron Morrison, "Outcry Over Racial Date Grows as Virus Slams Black Americans," AP (blog), Apr. 8, 2020, accessed May 28, 2020, https://apnews.com/71d952faad4a2a5d14441534f7230c7c?fbclid=I-wAR1plunY_qfeA2KrSU-PA1TuJobAwQh53a_QIkf5dw0dWjz-iz85GA1FOt4.

673. Bob Curley, "Why COVID-19 Is Hitting Men Harder Than Women," Healthline (blog), May 12, 2020, accessed May 28, 2020, https://www.healthline.com/health-news/men-more-susceptible-to-serious-covid-19-illnesses.

674. Ibid.

675. Kevin Rudd, "The Coming Post-COVID Anarchy. The Pandemic Bodes Ill for Both American and Chinese Power-and for the Global Order," *Foreign Affairs* (blog), May 6, 2020, accessed May 27, 2020, https://www.foreignaffairs.com/articles/united-states/2020-05-06/coming-post-covid-anarchy.

676. Michael Crowley, Edward Wong, and Ana Swanson, "Rebuking China, Trump Curtails Ties to Hong Kong and Severs Them With W.H.O.," *The New York Times* (blog), May 29, 2020, accessed May 29, 2020.

Index

Gonzalez

Gonzalez

Gonzalez

Endnotes

1 Taken from http://wjw.wuhan.gov.cn/front/web/showDetail/2020011109035, accessed Apr. 20, 2020. Translation obtained through Google.

2 "H1N1: The 2009 H1N1 Pandemic: Summary Highlights, April 2009-April 2010," CDC, Jun. 16, 2010, accessed Apr. 3, 2020, https://www.cdc.gov/h1n1flu/cdcresponse.htm.

3 Mangia A, Piazzolla V, Giannelli A, et al. SVR12 rates higher than 99% after sofosbuvir/velpatasvir combination in HCV infected patients with F0-F1 fibrosis stage: A real world experience [published correction appears in *PLoS One*. 2019 Sep 25;14(9):e0223287]. PLoS One. 2019;14(5):e0215783. Published 2019 May 15. doi:10.1371/journal.pone.0215783.

4 Apoorva Mandavilli, "H.I.V. Is Reported Cured in a Second Patient, a Milestone in the Global AIDS Epidemic," *New York Times* (blog), Mar. 4, 2019, accessed Apr. 4, 2020, https://www.nytimes.com/2019/03/04/health/aids-cure-london-patient.html.

5 "H1N1: The 2009 H1N1 Pandemic: Summary Highlights, April 2009-April 2010," CDC, Jun. 16, 2010, accessed Apr. 3, 2020, https://www.cdc.gov/h1n1flu/cdcresponse.htm.

6 Ibid.

7 Owen Jarvis, "20 of the Worst Epidemics and Pandemics in History," Live Science (blog), Mar. 20, 2020, accessed Apr. 1, 2020, https://www.livescience.com/worst-epidemics-and-pandemics-in-history.html.

8 Ibid.

9 Ibid.

10 Julio Gonzalez, *The Case for Free Market Healthcare*, (Sarasota, FL: Bardolf & Co., 2020), 32.

11 Ibid, 33

12 Ibid, 33

13 Ibid, 33

14 Owen Jarvis, "20 of the Worst Epidemics and Pandemics in History," Live Science (blog), Mar. 20, 2020, accessed Apr. 1, 2020, https://www.livescience.com/worst-epidemics-and-pandemics-in-history.html.

15 Ibid.

16 Ibid.

17 Ibid.

18 "Influenza (Flu): 1957-1958 Pandemic (H2N2 virus), CDC, accessed Apr. 4, 2020,

https://www.cdc.gov/flu/pandemic-resources/1957-1958-pandemic.html.

19 "Influenza (Flu) Burden of Influenza," CDC, accessed Apr. 13, 2020, https://www.cdc.gov/flu/about/burden/index.html.

20 Jeffrey Kahn, Kenneth McIntosh, "History and Recent Advances in Coronavirus Discovery," *The Pediatric Infections Disease Journ.*, Vol. 24, No. 11, pS223-227, Nov. 2005, digital version accessed Apr. 6, 2020, https://journals.lww.com/pidj/fulltext/2005/11001/history_and_recent_advances_in_coronavirus.12.aspx.

21 Ewen Callaway, David Cyranoski, et al, "The Coronavirus Pandemic in Five powerful Charts," Nature (blog) 579, 482-483 (2020) Mar. 18, 2020, accessed Mar. 26, 2020, https://www.nature.com/articles/d41586-020-00758-2.

22 J.S. Peiris, "Coronavirus," Ch. 57, in *Medical Microbiology A Guide to Micro-biological Infections: Pathogenesis, Immunity, Laboratory Diagnosis and Control.* (18th Ed) David Greenwood, Mike Barer, et al. ed. Elsevier, London, 2012, 590.

23 Ibid.

24 Ibid.

25 Owen Jarvis, "20 of the Worst Epidemics and Pandemics in History," Live Science (blog), Mar. 20, 2020, accessed Apr. 1, 2020, https://www.livescience.com/worst-epidemics-and-pandemics-in-history.html.

26 "H1N1: The 2009 H1N1 Pandemic: Summary Highlights, April 2009-April 2010," CDC, Jun. 16, 2010, accessed Apr. 3, 2020, https://www.cdc.gov/h1n1flu/cdcresponse.htm.

27 Ibid.

28 Ibid.

29 Ibid.

30 Ibid.

31 Ibid.

32 Ibid.

33 Ibid.

34

35

36

37

38

39

40   "Influenza (Flu) 2009 H1N1 Pandemic," CDC (blog), accessed Apr. 2, 2020, https://www.cdc.gov/flu/pandemic-re-

sources/2009-h1n1-pandemic.html.

41 Owen Jarvis, "20 of the Worst Epidemics and Pandemics in History," Live Science (blog), Mar. 20, 2020, accessed Apr. 1, 2020, https://www.livescience.com/worst-epidemics-and-pandemics-in-history.html.

42 ibid.

43 "Ebola (Ebola Virus Disease): 2014-2016 Ebola Outbreak in West Africa," CDC, accessed Apr. 4, 2020, https://www.cdc.gov/vhf/ebola/history/2014-2016-outbreak/index.html.

44 Ibid.

45 Ibid.

46 Ibid.

47 Ibid.

48 Owen Jarvis, "20 of the Worst Epidemics and Pandemics in History," Live Science (blog), Mar. 20, 2020, accessed Apr. 1, 2020, https://www.livescience.com/worst-epidemics-and-pandemics-in-history.html

49 Jeffrey Kahn, Kenneth McIntosh, "History and Recent Advances in Coronavirus Discovery," *The Pediatric Infections Disease Journ.*, Vol. 24, No. 11, pS223-227, Nov. 2005, digital version accessed Apr. 6, 2020, https://journals.lww.com/pidj/fulltext/2005/11001/history_and_recent_advances_in_coronavirus.12.aspx.

50 Ibid.

51 J.S. Peiris, "Coronavirus," Ch. 57, in *Medical Microbiology A Guide to Microbiological Infections: Pathogenesis, Immunity, Laboratory Diagnosis and Control.* (18th Ed) David Greenwood, Mike Barer, et al. ed. Elsevier, London, 2012, 590.

52 Ibid., 590.

53 Ibid., 587.

54 Ibid., 590.

55 Michelle L. Holshue, Chas DeBolt, et al., "First Case of 2019 Novel Coronavirus in the United States, NEJM, 2020;382:929-36. DOI: 10.1056/NEJMoa2001191 , Jan 31, 2020, p 929, accessed March 25, 2020, https://www.nejm.org/doi/pdf/10.1056/NEJMoa2001191.

56 Jeremy Page, Wenxin Fan, and Natasha Khan, "How it All Started: China's Early Coronavirus Missteps," *The Wall Street Journal*, March 6, 2020, accessed March 19, 2020, https://www.wsj.com/articles/how-it-all-started-chinas-early-coronavirus-missteps-11583508932.

57 Madeleine Johnson, "Diagnostic Developers Leap Into Action on Novel Coronavirus Tests," Genoweb (blog), Jan. 23, 2020, accessed Apr. 29, 2020, https://www.genomeweb.com/pcr/diagnostics-developers-leap-action-novel-coronavirus-tests.

58 "WHO Makes Field Trip to Wuhan, China," in "Rolling Updates on Coronavirus Disease (COVID-19), WHO (blog), Jan. 21, 2020, accessed Apr. 29, 2020, https://www.who.int/emergencies/diseases/novel-coronavirus-2019/events-as-they-happen.

59 Madeleine Johnson, "Diagnostic Developers Leap Into Action on Novel Coronavirus Tests," Genoweb (blog), Jan. 23, 2020, accessed Apr. 29, 2020, https://www.genomeweb.com/pcr/diagnostics-developers-leap-action-novel-coronavirus-tests.

60 Taiesha Moss, "Sona Achieves Significant Milestone in Covid-19 Test Development," Sona Nanotech, Mar. 18, 2020, accessed Apr. 28, 2020, https://sonanano.com/sona-achieves-significant-milestone-in-covid-19-test-development/.

61 Alyssa Billingsley, "The Latest in Coronavirus (COVID-19) Testing Methods and Availability," GoodRx, Apr. 21, 2020, https://www.goodrx.com/blog/coronavirus-covid-19-testing-updates-methods-cost-availability/.

62 Jamie Ducharme, "Why Ventilators May Not Be Working as Well for COVID-19 Patients as Doctors Hoped," Time (blog), Apr. 16, 2020, accessed Jun. 6, 2020, https://time.com/5820556/ventilators-covid-19/.

63 Philippe Gautret, Jean-Christopher Lagier, "Clinical and Microbiological Effect of a Combination of Hydroxychloroquine and Azithromycin in 80 COVID-19 Patients with at Least a Six-Day Follow-Up: An Observational Study," *Mediterranée Infection* (blog) accessed Apr. 5, 2020, https://www.mediterranee-infection.com/wp-content/uploads/2020/03/COVID-IHU-2-1.pdf.

64 Zhaowenu Chen, Jija Hu, et al., "Efficacy of Hydroxychloroquine in Patients with COVID-19: Results of a Randomized Clinical Trail," MedRxiv (blog), Mar 22, 2020, accessed Apr. 4, 2020, https://www.medrxiv.org/content/10.1101/2020.03.22.20040758v2.

65 Jean Michel Molina, Constance Delaugerre, et al., "No Evidence of Rapid Antiviral Clearance or Clinical Benefit with the Combination of Hydroxychloroqinie and Azithromycin in Patients with Severe COVID-19 Infection," *Médecine et Maladies Infectieuses* (blog), Mar. 30, 2020, accessed Apr. 5, 2020, https://www.sciencedirect.com/science/article/pii/S0399077X-20300858?via%3Dihub.

66 Manli Wang, Ruiyan Cao, et al., "Remdesivir and Chloroquine Effectively Inhibit the Recently Emerged Novel Coronavirus (2019-nCoV) in Vitro," Cell Research, Nature (blog), vol. 30 269-271 (2020) elct published Feb. 4, 2020, accessed Apr. 4, 2020, https://www.nature.com/articles/s41422-020-0282-0#citeas.

67 "Advisort on the Use of Hydroxy-Chloroquine as Prophylaxis for SARS-

CoV-2 Infection," National Task Force for COVID-19 in Balram Bhargava of the Indian Council for Medical Researh Open Letter, Mar. 22, 2020, accessed Apr. 22, 2020, https://www.mohfw.gov.in/pdf/AdvisoryontheuseofHydroxy-chloroquinasprophylaxisforSARSCoV2infection.pdf.

68 Kai Kupferschmidt, "Trials of Drugs to Prevent Coronavirus Infection Begin in Health Care Workers," *Science* (blog), Apr. 7, 2020, accessed Apr. 22, 2020, https://www.sciencemag.org/news/2020/04/trials-drugs-prevent-coronavirus-infection-begin-health-care-workers.

69 Joseph Magagnoli, Siddharth Narendran, et al., "Outcomes of Hydroxy-chloroquine Usage in United States Veterans Hospitalized with Covid-19," MedRxIV.org, Apr. 16, 2020, accessed Apr. 21, 2020, https://www.medrxiv.org/content/10.1101/2020.04.16.20065920v1.full.pdf.

70 Mandeep R. Mehra, Sapan S. Desai, et al., "Hydroxychloroquine or Chloroquine With or Without a Macrolide for Treatment of COVID-19: A Multinational Registry Analysis," *The Lancet*, May 22, 2020, accessed May 25, 2020, https://www.thelancet.com/journals/lancet/article/PIIS0140-6736(20)31180-6/fulltext#sec1.

71 Gerhardt SG, McDyer JF, Girgis RE, Orens JB. "Maintenance of Azith-romycin Therapy for Bronchiolitis Obliterans Syndrome," *Am. J. Respir. Crit. Care Med.*, 2003;168 :121–125, accessed Apr. 22, 2020, https://www.atsjournals.org/doi/pdf/10.1164/rccm.200212-1424BC.

72 Phillippe Gautret, Jean-Christophe Lagier, et al., "Hydroxychloroquine and Azithromycin as a Treatment of COVID-19: REsults of an Open-Label Non-Randomized Clinical Trial," *Int. J. Anitmicrob. Agents*," Mar. 20, 2020, accessed Apr. 22, 2020, https://www.ncbi.nlm.nih.gov/pmc/articles/PMC7102549/.

73 Eve Bossebouf, Maite Aubry, et al., "Azithromycin Inhibits the Replica-tion of Zika Virus," *Antivirals Antiretrovirals*. 2018;10(1):6–11, https://www.semanticscholar.org/paper/Azithromycin-Inhibits-the-Replication-of-Zika-Virus-Bosseboeuf-Aubry/52c1d80156463278c862cfea4152f5f819020bad.

74 Gerhardt SG, McDyer JF, Girgis RE, Orens JB. "Maintenance of Azithro-mycin Therapy for Bronchiolitis Obliterans Syndrome," Am. J. Respir. Crit. Care Med., 2003;168 :121–125, accessed Apr. 22, 2020, https://www.atsjournals.org/doi/pdf/10.1164/rccm.200212-1424BC.

75 Amin Gasmi, Sadaf Noor, et al., "Individual Risk Management Strategy and Potential Therapeutic Options of the COVID-19 Pandemic," *Clin. Immunol.*, Apr 7, 2020, Accessed Apr. 22, 2020, https://www.ncbi.nlm.nih.gov/pmc/articles/PMC7139252/

76 Ibid.

77 Letter from Denise M. Hinton to Ashley Rhoades, May 1, 2020, accessed May 11, 2020, https://www.fda.gov/media/137564/download.

78 Jonathan Grein, Norio Ohmagari, et al., "Compassionate Use of Remdesivir, for Patients with Severe Covid-19," *NEJM*, Apr. 10, 2020, 5, accessed Apr. 20, 2020, https://www.nejm.org/doi/pdf/10.1056/NEJMoa2007016.

79 Chenguang Shen, Zhaoqin Wang, et al., "Treatment of 5 Critically Ill Patients With COVID-19 With Convalescent Plasma," *JAMA* (blog), Mar. 27, 2020, accessed Apr. 5, 2020, https://jamanetwork.com/journals/jama/fullarticle/2763983.

80 Ibid.

81 Julio Gonzalez, *The Case for Free Market Healthcare*, (Sarasota, FL: Bardolf & Co., 2020), 86.

82 Bill Bostock, "Fauci Said It Will Take 12 to 18 Months to Get a Coronavirus Vaccine in the US. Experts Say a Quick Approval Could Be Risky," *Business Insider* (blog), Apr. 1, 2020, accessed Apr. 21 2020, https://www.businessinsider.com/coronavirus-vaccine-quest-18-months-fauci-experts-flag-dangers-testing-2020-4.

83 Ibid.

84 Ibid.

85 Alana Wise, "Trump Promises 'Warp Speed' Coronavirus Vaccine Effort With New Program," NPR (blog), May 15, 2020, accessed May 16, 2020, https://www.npr.org/sections/coronavirus-live-updates/2020/05/15/857014274/trump-touts-operation-warp-speed-coronavirus-vaccine-effort.

86 W. Huisman, B.E.E. Martina, et al.,, "Vaccine-Induced Enhancement of Viral Infections," *Vaccine*, Vol. 27, Iss 4. Jan. 22, 2009, 505-512, accessed Apr. 21, 2020, https://www.sciencedirect.com/science/article/pii/S0264410X08015053#!.

87 WHO, *Programme Budget 2020-2021*, (Switzerland, WHO 2019), accessed May 5, 2020, https://www.who.int/about/finances-accountability/budget/WHOPB-PRP-19.pdf?ua=1.

88 Yanzhong Huang, "The SARS Epicemic and Its Aftermath in China: A Political Perspective," *Learning From SARS: Preparing for the Next Disease Outbreak: Workshop Summary* (Washington, D.C., Institute of Medicine National Academies Press 2004), accessed May 5, 2020, https://www.ncbi.nlm.nih.gov/books/NBK92479/.

89 Ibid.

90 "WHO Boss Has SARS Baggage," Forbes (blog), Apr. 29, 2009, ac-

cessed May 4, 2020, https://www.forbes.com/2009/04/29/wto-marga-ret-chan-face-epidemic.html#391ebb411d34.

91 Valerie Richardson, "WHO's China Ties Scrutinized After Botched Corona-virus Response," *The Washington Times* (blog), Apr. 9, 2020, accessed May 5, 2020, https://www.washingtontimes.com/news/2020/apr/9/who-chi-na-ties-scrutinized-after-botched-coronavir/.

92 Tedros Adhanom Ghebreyesus in Andrew Joseph and Megan Thielking, "WHO Praises China's Response to Coronavirus, Will Reconvene Expert Com-mittee to Assess Global Threat," STAT (blog), Jan. 29, 2020, accessed May 5, 2020, https://www.statnews.com/2020/01/29/who-reconvene-expert-com-mittee-coronavirus/.

93 "Japan PM Abe Calls for Taiwan's Participation in WHO as Coronavirus Spreads," Kyodo News (blog), Jan. 30, 2020, accessed May 25, 2020, https://english.kyodonews.net/news/2020/01/cff2af87f289-abe-calls-for-taiwans-participation-in-who-as-coronavirus-spreads.html.

94 David Green, "WHO Bows to China Pressure, Contravenes Human Rights in Refusing Taiwan Media," The News Lens (blog), May 18, 2018, accessed May 25, 2020, https://international.thenewslens.com/article/95982.

95 Tom Grundy, "Video: Top WHO Doctor Bruce Aylward Ends Video Call After Journalist Asks About Taiwan's Status," Hong Kong Free Press, Mar. 29, 2020, accessed May 25, 2020, https://hongkongfp.com/2020/03/29/video-top-doctor-bruce-aylward-pretends-not-hear-journalists-taiwan-questions-ends-video-call/.

96 @StudioIncendo, Twitter, Mar. 28, 2020, 1034 AM, accessed May 25, 2020, https://twitter.com/studioincendo/status/1243909358133473285.

97 "Gross Domestic Product (GCP)," FRED, Apr. 29, 2020, accessed May 3, 2020, https://fred.stlouisfed.org/series/GDP.

98 Future Workers of Indiana: Projecting the Labor Force to 2040. INcontext Indiana University Kelly School of Business, vol 13, no 6 November-Decem-ber 2012, http://www.incontext.indiana.edu/2012/nov-dec/article1.asp.

99 Thomas Franck, "Job Gains for the Manufacturing industry in the Last 12 Months Are the Most Since 1995," CNBC (blog), Aug, 3, 2019, accessed May 3, 2020, https://www.cnbc.com/2018/08/03/job-gains-for-the-manufactur-ing-industry-are-the-most-since-1995.html.

100 Table 2.1 Employment by Major Industry Sector," U.S. Bureau of Labor Statistics, last modified Sept. 4, 2019, accessed May 3, 2020, https://www.bls.gov/emp/tables/employment-by-major-industry-sector.htm.

101 Shannon K. O'Neil in "The Instability of Global Supply Chains in a Pandemic, With Shannon K. O'Neil," Council on Foreign Relations (podcast),

Apr1, 2020, accessed May 4, 2020, https://www.cfr.org/podcasts/instability-global-supply-chains-pandemic-shannon-k-oneil.

102 Ana Swanson, "Coronavirus Spurs U.S. Efforts to End China's Chokehold on Drugs," *The New York Times* (blog), Mar. 11, 2020, accessed May 4, 2020, https://www.nytimes.com/2020/03/11/business/economy/coronavirus-china-trump-drugs.html.

103 Testimony of Mark Abdoo Before the US-China Economic & Security Review Commission, Jul. 31, 20219, accessed May 3, 2020, https://www.uscc.gov/sites/default/files/USCC%20Mark%20Abdoo%20FDA%20Hearing%20Statement%20073119.pdf.

104 "Chapter 3 Section 3-Growing U.S. Reliance on China's Biotech and Pharmaceutical Products," 2019 Report to Congress of the US-China Economic and Security Review Commission, November 2019, 250, accessed May 4, 2020, https://www.uscc.gov/sites/default/files/2019-11/Chapter%203%20Section%203%20-%20Growing%20U.S.%20Reliance%20on%20China%E2%80%99s%20Biotech%20and%20Pharmaceutical%20Products.pdf.

105 Testimony of Rosemary Gibson before the US-China Economic and Security Review Commission, Jul. 31, 2010, accessed May 3, 2020, https://www.uscc.gov/sites/default/files/RosemaryGibsonTestimonyUSCCJuly152019.pdf.

106 Austen Huffor and Mark Maremont, "Low Quality Masks Infiltrate U.S. Coronavirus Supply, The Wall Street Journal (blog), May 4, 2020, accessed May 4, 2020, https://www.wsj.com/articles/we-werent-protected-low-quality-masks-infiltrate-u-s-coronavirus-supply-11588528690?mod=searchresults&page=1&pos=1.

107 Julio Gonzalez, *The Case for Free Market Healthcare*, (Sarasota, FL: Bardolf & Co., 2020), 87.

108 Ibid., 88-90.

109 Olivia Waxman, "Coronavirus Is Putting the U.S. Strategic National Stockpile to the Test. Here's the Surprising Story Behind the Stash," Mar. 11, 2020, accessed May 1, 2020, https://time.com/5800393/coronavirus-national-stockpile-history/.

110 Anna Nicholson, Scott Wollek, et al., *The Nation's Medical Countermeasure Stockpile: Opportunities to Improve the Efficacy, Effecitiveness, and Sustainability of the CDC Strategic National Stockpile*, (Washington, D.C.: The National Academies Press, doi: 10.17226/23532, 2016), 1.

111 Strategic National Stockpile 12-Hour Push Pacakge Product Catalog, CDC, accessed May 1, 2020, https://ftp.cdc.gov/pub/MCMTraining/Miscellaneous%20Resources%20and%20Documents/SNS_Push%20Package%20Catalogl_2-1-12.pdf.

112 Gregg Re, "Obama Administration Sought to Cut PPE Stockpile, but Biden Team Points to GOP-Led Budget Squeeze,'" Fox News (blog), Apr. 10, 2020, accessed May 16, 2020, https://www.foxnews.com/politics/obama-administration-

sought-to-cut-ppe-stockpile-biden-gop.

113 Wolf Blitzer Staff, "troops Put Rumsfeld in the Hot Seat," CNN (blog) Dec. 8, 2004, accessed May 11, 2020, https://www.cnn.com/2004/US/12/08/rumsfeld.kuwait/index.html.

114 Jeremy Page, Wenxin Fan, and Natasha Khan, "How it All Started: China's Early Coronavirus Missteps," *The Wall Street Journal*, March 6, 2020, accessed March 19, 2020, https://www.wsj.com/articles/how-it-all-started-chinas-early-coronavirus-missteps-11583508932.

115 Ibid.

116 Ibid.

117 Ibid.

118 Ibid.

119 Ibid.

120 Ibid.

121 Ibid.

122 Ibid.

123 Kathy Gilsinan, "How China Deceived the WHO," The Atlantic (blog), Apr. 12, 2020, accessed Apr. 19, 2020, https://www.theatlantic.com/politics/archive/2020/04/world-health-organization-blame-pandemic-coronavirus/609820/.

124 Michelle L. Holshue, Chas DeBolt, et al., "First Case of 2019 Novel Coronavirus in the United States, *NEJM*, 2020;382:929-36. DOI: 10.1056/NEJMoa2001191 , Jan 31, 2020, p 929, accessed March 25, 2020, https://www.nejm.org/doi/pdf/10.1056/NEJMoa2001191.

125 Qun Li, Xuhua Guan, et al., "Early Transmission Dynamics in Wuhan, China, of Novel Coronavirus-Infected Pneumonia," *NEJM*, Jan. 29, 2020, pg. 4, accessed Mar. 25, 2020, DOI: 10.1056/NEJMoa2001316

126 Jeremy Page, Wenxin Fan, and Natasha Khan, "How it All Started: China's Early Coronavirus Missteps," *The Wall Street Journal*, March 6, 2020, accessed March 19, 2020, https://www.wsj.com/articles/how-it-all-started-chinas-early-coronavirus-missteps-11583508932.

127 Roujian Lu, Xiang Zhao, et al., "Genomic Characterization and Epidemiology of 2019 Novel Coronavirus: Implication for Virus Origins and Receptor Bonding," The Lancet, vol. 395 Iss 10224, 565-674, Feb 22, 2020, accessed Apr. 18, 2020, DOI: https://doi.org/10.1016/S0140-6736(20)30251-8.

128 Jane Qiu, "How China's 'Bat Woman' Hunted Down Viruses from SARS to the New Coronoavirus," *Scientific American* (blog), Mar. 11, 2020, accessed Apr. 18, 2020, https://www.scientificamerican.com/article/how-chinas-bat-woman-hunted-down-viruses-from-sars-to-the-new-coronavirus1/.

129 Ibid.

130 Ibid.

131 Ibif.

132 Ibid.

133 Ian Birrell, "How China Muzzled Its Bat Woman: Beiking Authorities Hushed up the Findings of a Scientist who Unlocked the Genetic Mak-Up of the Coronavirus Within Days of the Outbreak-Which Is Vital for Tests and Vaccines," Apr. 12, 2020, accessed Apr. 18, 2020, https://www.dailymail.co.uk/news/article-8210951/Beijing-authorities-hushed-findings-Chinese-scientist.html.

134 Jeremy Page, Wenxin Fan, and Natasha Khan, "How it All Started: China's Early Coronavirus Missteps," *The Wall Street Journal,* March 6, 2020, accessed March 19, 2020, https://www.wsj.com/articles/how-it-all-started-chinas-early-coronavirus-missteps-11583508932.

135 Ibid.

136 Ibid.

137 Michelle L. Holshue, Chas DeBolt, et al., "First Case of 2019 Novel Coronavirus in the United States, NEJM, 2020;382:929-36. DOI: 10.1056/NEJMoa2001191 , Jan 31, 2020, p 929, accessed March 25, 2020, https://www.nejm.org/doi/pdf/10.1056/NEJMoa2001191

138 Jeremy Page, Wenxin Fan, and Natasha Khan, "How it All Started: China's Early Coronavirus Missteps," *The Wall Street Journal,* March 6, 2020, accessed March 19, 2020, https://www.wsj.com/articles/how-it-all-started-chinas-early-coronavirus-missteps-11583508932.

139 "Wuhan Neighborhood Sees Infections after 40,000 Families Gather for Potluck," The Star (blog), Feb. 6, 2020, accessed Mar. 26, 2020, https://www.thestar.com.my/news/regional/2020/02/06/wuhan-neighbourhood-sees-infections-after-40000-families-gather-for-potluck.

140 IHME COVID-19 Health Service Utilization Forecasting Team, "Forecasting COVID-19 impact on hospital bed-days, ICU-days, ventilator-days and deaths by US state in the next 4 months," 2, accessed Apr. 8, 2020, http://www.healthdata.org/sites/default/files/files/research_articles/2020/covid_paper_MEDRXIV-2020-043752v1-Murray.pdf.

141 Bret Baier and Gregg Re, "Sources Believe Coronavirus Outbreak Originated in Wuhan Lab as Part of China's Efforts to Compete with US," Fox News (blog), Apr. 16, 2020, accessed Apr. 18, 2020, https://www.foxnews.com/politics/coronavirus-wuhan-lab-china-compete-us-sources.

142 "Early and Combined Interventions Crucial in Tackling COVID-19 Spread in China," U. of Southampton News (blog), Mar. 11, 2020, accessed Apr. 19, 2020, https://www.southampton.ac.uk/news/2020/03/covid-19-china.page.

143 Jeremy Page, Wenxin Fan, and Natasha Khan, "How it All Started: China's Early Coronavirus Missteps," *The Wall Street Journal,* March 6, 2020, accessed March 19, 2020, https://www.wsj.com/articles/how-it-all-started-chinas-early-coronavirus-missteps-11583508932.

144 Kathy Gilsinan, "How China Deceived the WHO," *The Atlantic* (blog), Apr. 12, 2020, accessed Apr. 19, 2020, https://www.theatlantic.com/politics/archive/2020/04/world-health-organization-blame-pandemic-coronavirus/609820/

145 Ibid.

146 "Statement on the Meeting of the International Health Regulations (2005) Emergency Committee Regarding the Outbreak of Novel Coronavirus (2019-nCoV)," WHO (blog), Jan. 23, 2020, accessed May 4, 2020, https://www.who.int/news-room/detail/23-01-2020-statement-on-the-meeting-of-the-international-health-regulations-(2005)-emergency-committee-regarding-the-outbreak-of-novel-coronavirus-(2019-ncov).

147 Kathy Gilsinan, "How China Deceived the WHO," *The Atlantic* (blog), Apr. 12, 2020, accessed Apr. 19, 2020, https://www.theatlantic.com/politics/archive/2020/04/world-health-organization-blame-pandemic-coronavirus/609820/

148 Tedros Adhanom Ghebreyesus in Andrew Joseph and Megan Thielking, "WHO Praises China's Response to Coronavirus, Will Reconvene Expert Committee to Assess Global Threat," STAT (blog), Jan. 29, 2020, accessed May 5, 2020, https://www.statnews.com/2020/01/29/who-reconvene-expert-committee-coronavirus/.

149 Grace Panetta, "US Officials Were Reportedly Concerned that Safety Breaches at a Wuhan Lab Studying Coronaviruses in Bats Could Cause a Pandemic," Business Insider (blog), Apr. 14, 2020, accessed Apr. 18, 2020, https://www.businessinsider.com/us-officials-raised-alarms-about-safety-issues-in-wuhan-lab-report-2020-4.

150 In Bret Baier and Gregg Re, "Sources Believe Coronavirus Outbreak Originated in Wuhan Lab as Part of China's Efforts to Compete with US," Fox News (blog), Apr. 16, 2020, accessed Apr. 18, 2020, https://www.foxnews.com/politics/coronavirus-wuhan-lab-china-compete-us-sources

151 Ibid.

152 Ibid.

153 Donald J. Trump during The Coronavirus White House Task Force briefing Apr. 19, 2020.

154 Eran Bendavid, Bianca Mulaney, et al., COVID-19 Antibody Seroprevalence in Santa Clara County, California, MedRxiv (blog), Apr. 11, 2020, accessed Apr. 18, 2020, https://www.medrxiv.org/content/10.1101/2020.04.14.20062463v1.full.pdf+html.

155 Peter Aitken, "One Third of Participants in Massachusetts Study Tested Positive for Coronavirus," Fox News (blog), Apr. 18, 2020, accessed Apr. 18,

2020, https://www.foxnews.com/science/third-blood-samples-massachu-setts-study-coronavirus.

156 Ralph Baric in Jane Qiu, "How China's 'Bat Woman' Hunted Down Viruses from SARS to the New Coronoavirus," *Scientific American* (blog), Mar. 11, 2020, accessed Apr. 18, 2020, https://www.scientificamerican.com/article/how-chinas-bat-woman-hunted-down-viruses-from-sars-to-the-new-coronavirus1/.

157 Zhao lijian, @zlj517, Twitter, Mar. 12, 2020, 10:37 AM, accessed Apr. 25, 2020, https://twitter.com/zlj517/status/1238111898828066823.

158 "Coronavirus May Have Existed in Italy Since November: Local Researcher," CGTN, Mar. 22, 2020, accessed Apr. 19, 2020, https://news.cgtn.com/news/2020-03-22/Coronavirus-may-have-existed-in-Italy-since-November-local-research-er-P4i2As2OAg/index.html.

159 Ibid.

160 WHO, Feb. 28, 2020, accessed Apr. 19, 2020, https://www.who.int/docs/default-source/coronaviruse/transcripts/who-audio-emergencies-coronavi-rus-press-conference-full-28feb2020.pdf?sfvrsn=13eeb6a4_2.

161 Kathy Gilsinan, "How China Deceived the WHO," *The Atlantic* (blog), Apr. 12, 2020, accessed Apr. 19, 2020, https://www.theatlantic.com/politics/ar-chive/2020/04/world-health-organization-blame-pandemic-coronavirus/609820/.

162 Tedros Adhanom Ghebreyesus in Jon Cohen, "'We Will Have Many Body Bags.' WHO Chief Responds to Trump's Criticisms," Science (blog), Apr. 12, 2020, accessed Apr. 19, 2020, https://www.sciencemag.org/news/2020/04/we-will-have-many-body-bags-who-chief-responds-trumps-criticisms.

163 Kathy Gilsinan, "How China Deceived the WHO," *The Atlantic* (blog), Apr. 12, 2020, accessed Apr. 19, 2020, https://www.theatlantic.com/politics/ar-chive/2020/04/world-health-organization-blame-pandemic-coronavirus/609820/.

164 Alayna Treene and Jonathan Swift, "Trump Announces U.S. Will Halt Funding for WHO Over Coronavirus Response," Axios (blog), Apr. 15, 2020, accessed May 25, 2020, https://www.axios.com/trump-world-health-organization-funding-65de2595-2d5e-4a6c-b7c6-9c18aa4cb905.html.

165 Ibid.

166 Rob Picheta and Jessie Yeung, "Trump Is Threatening to pull the US Out of the WHO. What Does That Actually Mean? CNN (blog), May 19, 2020, accessed May 25, 2020, https://www.cnn.com/2020/05/19/us/trump-who-funding-threat-ex-plainer-intl/index.html.

167 Ibid.

168 Hollie McKay, "Coronavirus: US Gives 10 Times the Amount of Money to WHO Than China," Fox News (blog), Apr. 10, 2020, accessed May 25, 2020, https://www.foxnews.com/world/coronavirus-us-china-who-world-health-organization-china.

169 Dario Cristiani, "Italy's Coronavirus Experience and the Challenge of Extreme Crises to Liberal Democracies," The German Marshall Fund of the United States, (blog) Mar. 20, 2020, accessed Apr. 25, 2020, http://www.gmfus.org/blog/2020/03/20/italys-coronavirus-experience-and-challenge-extreme-crises-liberal-democracies.

170 Helen Raleigh, "Iran and Italy Are Paying a Hefty Price for Close Ties with Communist China," The Federalist (blog), Mar. 17, 2020, accessed Apr. 26, 2020, https://thefederalist.com/2020/03/17/iran-and-italy-are-paying-a-hefty-price-for-close-ties-with-communist-china/.

171 Una Aleksander Berzina-Cerenkova, "BRI Instead of OBOR-China Edits the English Name of its Most Ambitious International Project," Latvian Institute of International Affairs (blog), Jul. 28, 2016, accessed Apr. 26, 2020, https://web.archive.org/web/20170206061842/http://liia.lv/en/analysis/bri-instead-of-obor-china-edits-the-english-name-of-its-most-ambitious-international-project-532.

172 Dario Cristani, "Italy Joins the Belt and Road Initiative: Context, Interests, and Drivers," China Brief, The Jamestown Foundation, (2020) vol. 19(8) Apr. 24, 2019, accessed Apr. 26, 2020, https://jamestown.org/program/italy-joins-the-belt-and-road-initiative-context-interests-and-drivers/

173 Independent Bureau, "Italy Becomes First G7 Nation to Join China's 'Belt & Road Initiative,'" The Indepedent (blog), Mar. 24, 2019, accessed Apr. 26, 2020, http://theindependent.in/italy-becomes-first-g7-nation-to-join-chinas-belt-road-initiative/.

174 IANS, "Corona-Hit Italy Suffers Due to Improved Ties With China?" Outlook (blog), Mar. 20, 2020, accessed May 4, 2020, https://www.outlookindia.com/newsscroll/coronahit-italy-suffering-due-to-improved-ties-with-china/1774564.

175 Naomi Xu Elegant, "China Locks Down 3 Cities and Suspends Flights: The Latest on the Deadly Wuhan Virus Outbreak," Fortune (blog), Jan. 23, 2020, accessed Apr. 26, 2020, https://fortune.com/2020/01/23/china-wuhan-lockdown-flights-suspended-virus-outbreak/.

176 Italy, Central Intelligence Agency Library, accessed Apr. 25, 2020, https://www.cia.gov/library/publications/the-world-factbook/geos/it.html.

177 Country Comparison: Median Age, Central Intelligence Agency Library, accessed Apr. 25, 2020, https://www.cia.gov/library/publications/the-world-factbook/fields/343rank.html#IT.

178 "Which Country Has the oldest Population? It Depends on How You Define 'Old,'" PRB (blog), accessed Apr. 26, 2020, https://www.prb.org/which-country-has-the-oldest-population/.

179 Dario Cristiani, "Italy's Coronavirus Experience and the Challenge of Extreme Crises to Liberal Democracies," The German Marshall Fund of the United

States, (blog) Mar. 20, 2020, accessed Apr. 25, 2020, http://www.gmfus.org/blog/2020/03/20/italys-coronavirus-experience-and-challenge-extreme-crises-liberal-democracies.

180 "Italian Residents Hug Chinese People to Encourage Them in Coronavirus Fight," Feb. 4, 2020, accessed Apr. 26, 2020, https://www.youtube.com/watch?v=mNMdg4morQs.

181 Ibid.

182 Tales Azzoni and Andrew Dampf, "Game Zero: Spread of Virus Linked to Champions League Match," Associate Press (blog), Mar. 25, 2020, accessed Apr. 25, 2020, https://apnews.com/ae59cfc0641fc63afd09182bb832ebe2.

183 Ibid.

184 Ibid.

185 Ibid.

186 COVID-19 Coronavirus Pandemic, Worldometer, updated May 6, 2020, accessed May 6, 2020, https://www.worldometers.info/coronavirus/#countries.

187 Silvia Sciorilli Borrelli, "Rome Locks Down Northern Italy Amid Surge in Coronavirus Cases, Politico (blog), Mar. 8, 2020, accessed Apr. 25, 2020, https://www.politico.eu/article/rome-locks-down-northern-italy-as-coronavirus-cases-surge/.

188 Ibid.

189 Dario Cristiani, "Italy's Coronavirus Experience and the Challenge of Extreme Crises to Liberal Democracies," The German Marshall Fund of the United States, (blog) Mar. 20, 2020, accessed Apr. 25, 2020, http://www.gmfus.org/blog/2020/03/20/italys-coronavirus-experience-and-challenge-extreme-crises-liberal-democracies.

190 Margherita Stancati, "Italy's Coronavirus Lockdown Met With Confusion, Questions About Enforcement," The Wall Street Journal, Mar. 8, 2020, accessed Apr. 25, 2020, https://www.wsj.com/articles/italy-imposes-coronavirus-lockdown-on-large-parts-of-nations-north-11583668232?mod=article_inline.

191 Eric Sylvers and Giovanni Legorano, "As Virus Spreads, Italy Locks Down Country," The Wall Street Journal, Mar. 9, 2020, accessed Apr. 25, 2020, https://www.wsj.com/articles/italy-bolsters-quarantine-checks-after-initial-lockdown-confusion-11583756737?mod=article_inline.

192 country brought thousands of ventilators, but it still faced personnel shortages. There simply weren't enough trained personnel to handle the onslaught of sick people.

193 Margherita Stancati, Italy, With Aging Population, Has World's Highest Daily Deaths From Virus," The Wall Street Journal, Mar. 9, 2020, accessed Apr. 25, 2020, https://www.wsj.com/articles/italy-with-elderly-population-has-worlds-high-

est-death-rate-from-virus-11583785086?mod=article_inline.

194 Maurizio Massari, "Italian Ambassador to the EU: Italy Needs Europe' Help," Politico (blog), Mar. 10, 2020, accessed Apr. 25, 2020, https://www.politico.eu/article/coronavirus-italy-needs-europe-help/.

195 Marcus Walker and Mark Maremont, "Lessons From Italy's Hospital Melt-down. 'Every Day You Lose, the Contagion Gets Worse,'" *The Wall Street Journal*, Mar. 17, 2020, accessed Apr. 25, 2020, https://www.wsj.com/articles/every-day-you-lose-the-contagion-gets-worse-lessons-from-italys-hospital-meltdown-11584455470?mod=article_inline.

196 Margherita Stancati, Italy, With Aging Population, Has World's Highest Daily Deaths From Virus," *The Wall Street Journal*, Mar. 9, 2020, accessed Apr. 25, 2020, https://www.wsj.com/articles/italy-with-elderly-population-has-worlds-high-est-death-rate-from-virus-11583785086?mod=article_inline.

197 Marcus Walker and Mark Maremont, "Lessons From Italy's Hospital Melt-down. 'Every Day You Lose, the Contagion Gets Worse,'" *The Wall Street Journal*, Mar. 17, 2020, accessed Apr. 25, 2020, https://www.wsj.com/articles/every-day-you-lose-the-contagion-gets-worse-lessons-from-italys-hospital-meltdown-11584455470?mod=article_inline.

198 Ibid.

199 Ibid.

200 Margherita Stancati and Eric Sylvers, "Italy's Coronavirus Death Toll Is Far High-er Than Reported," *The Wall Street Journal*, Apr. 1, 2020, accessed Apr 25, 2020, https://www.wsj.com/articles/italys-coronavirus-death-toll-is-far-higher-than-re-ported-11585767179?mod=article_inline.

201 Noemie Bisserbe and Matthew Dalton, "How Coronavirus Outmaneuvered France's Health-Care System," *The Wall Street Journal* (blog), Apr. 26, 2020, accessed Apr. 26, 2020, https://www.wsj.com/articles/how-coronavirus-outma-neuvered-frances-health-care-system-11587906000?mod=searchresults&page=1&-pos=6.

202 María Sosa Troya, "Data Shows Over 7,500 Confirmed or Probable COVID-19 Deaths at Spain's Care Homes," *El País* (blog) May 7, 2020, accessed May 28, 2020, https://english.elpais.com/society/2020-05-07/data-shows-over-17500-confirmed-or-probable-covid-19-deaths-at-spains-care-homes.html.

203 Jessie Yeung, Steve George and Ivan Kottaosvá, "First Case of Coronavirus Confirmed in Spain, CNN (blog), Jan. 31, 2020, accesses Apr. 26, 2020, https://www.cnn.com/asia/live-news/coronavirus-outbreak-02-01-20-intl-hnk/h_afc-f3a4665521aab11c721c8cc80dd03

204 Ibid.

205 Giovanni Legorano, Xavier Fontdegloria, "Spain Seized by Fast-Growing Coro-

navirus Outbreak," *The Wall Street Journal* (blog), Mar. 24, 2020, accessed Apr. 26, 2020, https://www.wsj.com/articles/spain-seized-by-fast-growing-coronavirus-out-break-11585074509?mod=searchresults&page=8&pos=1.

206 Ibid.

207 Elena Rodriguez, "Thousands March in Spain on Women's Day Despite Coronavirus Fears," Mar. 8, 2020, accessed Apr. 26, 2020, https://www.usnews.com/news/world/articles/2020-03-08/thousands-march-in-spain-on-womens-day-despite-coronavirus-fears.

208 Raphael Minder and Elian Peltier, "Spain Imposes Nationwide Lockdown to Fight Coronavirus," *The New York Times* (blog), Mar. 14, 2020, accessed Apr. 26, 2020, https://www.nytimes.com/2020/03/14/world/europe/spain-coronavirus.html.

209 Noemie Bisserbe and Matthew Dalton, "How Coronavirus Outmaneuvered France's Health-Care System," *The Wall Street Journal* (blog), Apr. 26, 2020, accessed Apr. 26, 2020, https://www.wsj.com/articles/how-coronavirus-outmaneuvered-frances-health-care-system-11587906000?mod=searchresults&page=1&-pos=6.

210 Ibid.

211 Matthew Dalton and Nick Kostov, "ICUs on Rails: How France Coped With a Surge of Coronavirus Patients," The Wall Street Journal (blog), Apr. 25, 2020, accessed Apr, 26, 2020, https://www.wsj.com/articles/icus-on-rails-how-france-coped-with-a-surge-of-coronavirus-patients-11587807002?mod=article_inline

212 Noemie Bisserbe and Matthew Dalton, "How Coronavirus Outmaneuvered France's Health-Care System," *The Wall Street Journal* (blog), Apr. 26, 2020, accessed Apr. 26, 2020, https://www.wsj.com/articles/how-coronavirus-outmaneuvered-frances-health-care-system-11587906000?mod=searchresults&page=1&-pos=6.

213 Ibid.

214 Max Colchester, "Boris Johnson Set to Return to Work After Recovery From Covid-19," *The Wall Street Journal* (blog), Apr. 26, 2020, accessed Apr. 27, 2020, https://www.wsj.com/articles/boris-johnson-set-to-return-to-work-after-recovery-from-covid-19-11587907303?mod=searchresults&page=1&pos=5.

215 H.J. Mai, "Stockholm Expected to Reach Herd Immunity in May, Swedish Ambassador Says," NPR (blog), Apr. 26, 2020, accessed Apr. 27, 2020, https://www.npr.org/2020/04/26/845211085/stockholm-expected-to-reach-herd-immunity-in-may-swedish-ambassador-says.

216 Ibid.

217 COVID-19 Coronavirus Pandemic, Worldometer, updated May 6, 2020, accessed May 6, 2020, https://www.worldometers.info/coronavirus/#countries.

218 Ibid.

219 Ibid.

220 iH.J. Mai, "Stockholm Expected to Reach Herd Immunity in May, Swedish Ambassador Says," NPR (blog), Apr. 26, 2020, accessed Apr. 27, 2020, https://www.npr.org/2020/04/26/845211085/stockholm-expected-to-reach-herd-immunity-in-may-swedish-ambassador-says.

221 Kate Baggaley, "Covid-19 Herd Immunity Isn't Happening Any Time Soon," Popular Science (blog), Apr. 22, 2020, accessed May 6, 2020, https://www.popsci.com/story/health/herd-immunity-covid-19-coronavirus/.

222 Benoir Faucon, Sune Engel Rasmussen, and Jeremy Page, "Strategic Partnership With China Lies at Root of Iran's Coronavirus Outbreak," *The Wall Street Journal* (blog), Mar. 11, 2020, accessed May 2, 2020, https://www.wsj.com/articles/irans-strategic-partnership-with-china-lies-at-root-of-its-coronavirus-outbreak-11583940683/.

223 Covid-19 Coronavirus Pandemi, Worldometer, updted May 2, 2020, accessed May 2, 2020, https://worldometers.info/coronavirus/#countries

224 Coronavirus Singapore, Worldometer, last updated May 2, 2020, accessed May 2, 2020, https://www.worldometers.info/coronavirus/country/singapore/.

225 Holly Secon, "Singapore's Coronavirus Response, Marked by Digital Surveillance and Quarantines in Hospitals Was Initially Successful. But It's Reaching a Tipping Point," *Business Insider* (blog), Apr. 8, 2020, accessed May 2, 2020, https://www.businessinsider.com/singapore-coronavirus-containment-new-challenges-2020-4.

226 H

227 Ibid.

228 Ibid.

229 Coronavirus Singapore, Worldometer, last updated May 2, 2020, accessed May 2, 2020, https://www.worldometers.info/coronavirus/country/singapore/.

230 Ibid.

231 Ibid.

232 Dewey Sim and Kok Xighui, "Coronavirus: Why So Few Deaths Among Singapore's 14,000 Covid-19 Infections?" South China Morning Post (blog), Apr. 27, 2020, https://www.scmp.com/week-asia/health-environment/article/3081772/coronavirus-why-so-few-deaths-among-singapores-14000.

233 Singapore, The World Factboook, CIA, May 3, 2020, accessed May 3, 2020, https://www.cia.gov/library/publications/the-world-factbook/geos/sn.html.

234 Dewey Sim and Kok Xighui, "Coronavirus: Why So Few Deaths Among Singapore's 14,000 Covid-19 Infections?" South China Morning Post (blog), Apr. 27, 2020, https://www.scmp.com/week-asia/health-environment/article/3081772/coronavi-

rus-why-so-few-deaths-among-singapores-14000.

235 Coronavirus COVID-19 Coronavirus Pandemic, Worldometer, last updated May 6, 2020, accessed May 6, 2020, https://www.worldometers.info/coronavirus/#countries.

236 Coronavirus Hong Kong, Worldometer, last updated May 6, 2020, accessed May 6, 2020, https://www.worldometers.info/coronavirus/country/china-hong-kong-sar/.

237 Suzanne Staline, "Covid-19's Resurgence in Hong Kong Holds a Lesson: Defeating It Demands Presistnece," STAT (blog) Mar. 26, 2020, accessed May 6, 2020, https://www.statnews.com/2020/03/26/coronavirus-hong-kong-resur-genece-holds-lesson-defeating-it-demands-persistence/.

238 Ibid.

239 Ibid.

240 Jessie Yeung, "Two Weeks of Zero Local Infections: How Hong Kong Contained Its Second Wave of COVID-19," CNN (blog), May 5, 2020, accessed May 6, 2020, https://www.cnn.com/2020/05/05/asia/hong-kong-coronavirus-recovery-in-tl-hnk/index.html.

241 Coronavirus Hong Kong, Worldometer, last updated May 6, 2020, accessed May 6, 2020, https://www.worldometers.info/coronavirus/country/china-hong-kong-sar/.

242 Jessie Yeung, "Two Weeks of Zero Local Infections: How Hong Kong Contained Its Second Wave of COVID-19," CNN (blog), May 5, 2020, accessed May 6, 2020, https://www.cnn.com/2020/05/05/asia/hong-kong-coronavirus-recovery-intl-hnk/index.html.

243 Ibid.

244 Coronavirus COVID-19 Coronavirus Pandemic, Worldometer, last updated May 17, 2020, accessed May 17, 2020, https://www.worldometers.info/coronavirus/#countries.

245 Ibid.

246 Anup Malani, Arpit Gupta and Reuben Abraham, "Why Does India Have so Few Covid-19 Cases and Deaths?" Quartz India (blog), Apr. 16, 2020, accessed May 3, 2020, https://qz.com/india/1839018/why-does-india-have-so-few-coronavirus-covid-19-cases-and-deaths/.

247 ibid.

248 Ibid.

249 Neetu Chandra Sharma, "Why India's COVID Count Remains High Despite Lockdown, LiveMint (blog), updated May 12, accessed May 17, https://www.livemint.com/news/india/why-india-s-covid-count-remains-high-despite-lock-

down-11589300259404.html.

250 "Advisort on the Use of Hydroxy-Chloroquine as Prophylaxis for SARS-CoV-2 Infection," National Task Force for COVID-19 in Balram Bhargava of the Indian Council for Medical Researh Open Letter, Mar. 22, 2020, accessed Apr. 22, 2020, https://www.mohfw.gov.in/pdf/AdvisoryontheuseofHydroxychloroquinasprophy-laxisforSARSCoV2infection.pdf.

251 Shaj Rahti, Pranav Ish, et al., "Hydroxychloroquine Prophylaxis for COVID-19 Contact in India," *The Lancet*, Apr. 17, 2020, accessed May 3, 2020, https://www.thelancet.com/journals/laninf/article/PIIS1473-3099(20)30313-3/fulltext.

252 IANS, "India Bans Exports of Wonder Drug Used to Treat Covid-19 Patients," *Business Insider* (blog), Mar 25, 2020, accessed May 3, 2020, https://www.businessinsider.in/india/news/india-bans-exports-of-wonder-drug-used-to-treat-covid-19-patients/articleshow/74802892.cms.

253 Lauren Frayer, "India Reverses Export Ban on Hydrozychloroquine, Other Drugs Following Trump Pressure," NPR (blog), Apr. 8, 2020, accessed May 3, 2020, https://www.npr.org/2020/04/08/830205883/india-reverses-export-ban-on-hy-droxycloroquine-other-drugs-following-trump-press.

254 Aniruddha Ghosal, "India Scraps Plan to Test Hydorxyxhloroquine in Mumbai Slums," *The Washington Times* (blog), Apr. 29, 2020, accessed May 3, 2020, https://www.washingtontimes.com/news/2020/apr/29/india-scraps-plan-test-hy-droxychloroquine-mumbai-s/.

255 Anup Malani, Arpit Gupta and Reuben Abraham, "Why Does India Have so Few Covid-19 Cases and Deaths?" Quartz India (blog), Apr. 16, 2020, accessed May 3, 2020, https://qz.com/india/1839018/why-does-india-have-so-few-coronavirus-covid-19-cases-and-deaths/.

256 Tuberculosis, BCG Vaccine, CDC, last reviewed May 4, 2020, accessed May 3, 2020, https://www.cdc.gov/tb/publications/factsheets/prevention/bcg.htm.

257 Nigel Curtis, Annie Sparrow, et al., "Considering BCG Vaccination to Reduce the Impact of COVID-19," The Lancet, Apr. 30, 2020, accessed May 3, 2020, https://www.thelancet.com/journals/lancet/article/PIIS0140-6736(20)31025-4/fulltext.

258 Nicole L. Messina, Kaya Gardiner, et al., "Study Protocol for the Melbourne Infant Study: BCG for Allergy and Infection Reduction (MIS BAIR), A Randomized Controlled Trial to Determine the Non-Specific Effects of Neonatal BCG Vaccination in a Lw-Mortality Setting," BMJ Open, (2019) Vol. 9, Iss. 12, https://bmjopen.bmj.com/content/bmjopen/9/12/e032844.full.pdf.

259 Coronavirus COVID-19 Coronavirus Pandemic, Worldometer, last updated May 3, 2020, accessed May 3, 2020, https://www.worldometers.info/coronavi-rus/#countries.

260 South Korea, The World Factboook, CIA, May 3, 2020, accessed May 3, 2020, https://www.cia.gov/library/publications/the-world-factbook/geos/ks.html

261 Coronavirus South Korea, Worldometer, last updated May 3, 2020, accessed May 3, 2020, https://www.worldometers.info/coronavirus/country/south-korea/.

262 Charlie Campbell, "South Korea's Health Minister on How His Country Is Beating Coronavirus Without a Lockdown," *Time* (blog), Apr 30, 2020, accessed May 3, 2020, https://time.com/5830594/south-korea-covid19-coronavirus/.

263 Park Neung-hoo in Charlie Campbell, "South Korea's Health Minister on How His Country Is Beating Coronavirus Without a Lockdown," *Time* (blog), Apr 30, 2020, accessed May 3, 2020, https://time.com/5830594/south-korea-covid19-coronavirus/

264 Park Neung-hoo in Charlie Campbell, "South Korea's Health Minister on How His Country Is Beating Coronavirus Without a Lockdown," Time (blog), Apr 30, 2020, accessed May 3, 2020, https://time.com/5830594/south-korea-covid19-coronavirus/

265 Alice Zwerling, Marcel A. Behr, et al., "The BCG World Atlas of Global BCG Vaccination Policies and Practicies," *PLoS Med*, (2011) 8(3): e 1001012, Mar. 22, 2011, accessed May 3, 2020, https://www.ncbi.nlm.nih.gov/pmc/articles/PMC3062527/.

266 Ibid.

267 COVID-19 Coronavirus Pandemic, Worldometer, last updated May 3, 2020, accessed May 3, 2020, https://www.worldometers.info/coronavirus/#countries.

268 Alice Klein, "Australia Seems to Be Keeping a Lid on COVID-19-How is It Doing It?" New Scientist (blog) Apr. 8, 2020, accessed May 3, 2020, https://www.newscientist.com/article/2240226-australia-seems-to-be-keeping-a-lid-on-covid-19-how-is-it-doing-it/.

269 Ibid.

270 Rosie Perper, "Australia and New Zealand Have Been Able to keep Their Number of Coronavirus Cases Low Thanks to Early Lockdown Efforts. Experts Say It's 'Probably Too Late' for Other Countries to Learn From Them," *Business insider* (blog), Apr. 17, 2020, accessed May 3, 2020, https://www.businessinsider.com/experts-australia-new-zealand-examples-how-to-slow-coronavirus-2020-4.

271 Ibid.

272 Alice Zwerling, Marcel A. Behr, et al., "The BCG World Atlas of Global BCG Vaccination Policies and Practicies," *PLoS Med*, (2011) 8(3): e 1001012, Mar. 22, 2011, accessed May 3, 2020, https://www.ncbi.nlm.nih.gov/pmc/articles/PMC3062527/.

273 Rosie Perper, "Australia and New Zealand Have Been Able to keep Their Number of Coronavirus Cases Low Thanks to Early Lockdown Efforts. Experts Say

It's 'Probably Too Late' for Other Countries to Learn From Them," *Business insider* (blog), Apr. 17, 2020, accessed May 3, 2020, https://www.businessinsider.com/experts-australia-new-zealand-examples-how-to-slow-coronavirus-2020-4.

274 Coronavirus Brazil, Worldometer, last updated May 6, 2020, accessed May 6, 2020, https://www.worldometers.info/coronavirus/country/brazil/.

275 Ibid.

276 Ibid.

277 Coronavirus COVID-19 Coronavirus Pandemic, Worldometer, last updated May 6, 2020, accessed May 6, 2020, https://www.worldometers.info/coronavirus/#countries.

278 Lucian Magalhaes and Christiana Sciaudone, "Coronavirus Sweeps Across Brazil, a Land Ill-Equipped to Fight It," *The Wall Street Journal* (blog), May 4, 2020, accessed May 6, 2020, https://www.wsj.com/articles/coronavirus-sweeps-across-brazil-a-land-ill-equipped-to-fight-it-11588603847.

279 Ibid.

280 Jair Bolsonaro in Lucian Magalhaes and Christiana Sciaudone, "Coronavirus Sweeps Across Brazil, a Land Ill-Equipped to Fight It," *The Wall Street Journal* (blog), May 4, 2020, accessed May 6, 2020, https://www.wsj.com/articles/coronavirus-sweeps-across-brazil-a-land-ill-equipped-to-fight-it-11588603847

281 Lucian Magalhaes and Christiana Sciaudone, "Coronavirus Sweeps Across Brazil, a Land Ill-Equipped to Fight It," *The Wall Street Journal* (blog), May 4, 2020, accessed May 6, 2020, https://www.wsj.com/articles/coronavirus-sweeps-across-brazil-a-land-ill-equipped-to-fight-it-11588603847.

282 Ibid.

283 Coronavirus COVID-19 Coronavirus Pandemic, Worldometer, last updated May 6, 2020, accessed May 6, 2020, https://www.worldometers.info/coronavirus/#countries.

284 Coronavirus Peru, Worldometer, last updated May 6, 2020, accessed May 6, 2020, https://www.worldometers.info/coronavirus/country/peru/.

285 Coronavirus Argentina, Worldometer, last updated May 6, 2020, accessed May 6, 2020, https://www.worldometers.info/coronavirus/country/argentina/.

286 Coronavirus COVID-19 Coronavirus Pandemic, Worldometer, last updated May 6, 2020, accessed May 6, 2020, https://www.worldometers.info/coronavirus/#countries.

287 Ibid.

288 Coronavirus Ecuador, Worldometer, last updated May 6, 2020, accessed May 6, 2020, https://www.worldometers.info/coronavirus/country/ecuador/.

289 Eisuke Nakasawa, Hiroyasu, Ino, and Akira Akabayashi, "Chronology of COVID-19 Cases on the Diamond Princess Cruise Ship and Ethical Considerations: A Report From Japan," *Disaster Med. Pub. Health Prep.*, Mar 24, 2020, accessed Apr. 22, 2020, https://www.ncbi.nlm.nih.gov/pmc/articles/PMC7156812/.

290 Smriti, Mallapaty, "What the Cruis-Ship Outbreaks Reveal About COVID-19, *Nature* (blog), Mar. 26, 2020, accessed Apr. 22, 2020, https://www.nature.com/articles/d41586-020-00885-w.

291 Eisuke Nakasawa, Hiroyasu, Ino, and Akira Akabayashi, "Chronology of COVID-19 Cases on the Diamond Princess Cruise Ship and Ethical Considerations: A Report From Japan," *Disaster Med. Pub. Health Prep.*, Mar 24, 2020, accessed Apr. 22, 2020, https://www.ncbi.nlm.nih.gov/pmc/articles/PMC7156812/.

292 Smriti, Mallapaty, "What the Cruis-Ship Outbreaks Reveal About COVID-19, *Nature* (blog), Mar. 26, 2020, accessed Apr. 22, 2020, https://www.nature.com/articles/d41586-020-00885-w.

293 Ibid.

294 Eisuke Nakasawa, Hiroyasu, Ino, and Akira Akabayashi, "Chronology of COVID-19 Cases on the Diamond Princess Cruise Ship and Ethical Considerations: A Report From Japan," Disaster Med. Pub. Health Prep., Mar 24, 2020, accessed Apr. 22, 2020, https://www.ncbi.nlm.nih.gov/pmc/articles/PMC7156812/.

295 Ibid.

296 Timothy Russell, Joel Hellewell, et al., "Estimating the Infection and Case Fatality Ration for Coronavirus Disease (COVID-19) Using Age-Adjusted Date from the Outbreak on the Diamond Princess Cruise Shipe, February 2020," Eurosurvelllance, 2020;25(12), Mar. 26, 2020, accessed Apr. 22, 2020, https://www.eurosurveillance.org/content/10.2807/1560-7917.ES.2020.25.12.2000256#t2.

297 Smriti, Mallapaty, "What the Cruis-Ship Outbreaks Reveal About COVID-19, *Nature* (blog), Mar. 26, 2020, accessed Apr. 22, 2020, https://www.nature.com/articles/d41586-020-00885-w.

298 Timothy Russell, Joel Hellewell, et al., "Estimating the Infection and Case Fatality Ration for Coronavirus Disease (COVID-19) Using Age-Adjusted Date from the Outbreak on the Diamond Princess Cruise Shipe, February 2020," Eurosurvelllance, 2020;25(12), Mar. 26, 2020, accessed Apr. 22, 2020, https://www.eurosurveillance.org/content/10.2807/1560-7917.ES.2020.25.12.2000256#t2.

299 Kenji Mizumoto, Katsushi Kagaya, et al., "Estimating the Asymptomatic Proportion of Coronavirus Disease 2019 (COVID-19) Cases on Board the Diamond Princess Cruise Ship, Yokohama, Japan, 2020," *Eurosurveillance*, 2020;25 (10), Mar. 12, 2020, accessed Apr. 22, 2020, https://www.eurosurveillance.org/con-

tent/10.2807/1560-7917.ES.2020.25.10.2000180.

300 Smriti, Mallapaty, "What the Cruis-Ship Outbreaks Reveal About COVID-19, *Nature* (blog), Mar. 26, 2020, accessed Apr. 22, 2020, https://www.nature.com/articles/d41586-020-00885-w.

301 Richard Paddock, Sui-Lee Wee, and Roni Caryn Rabin, "Coronavirus Infection Found After Cruise Ship Passengers Disperse," *The New York Times* (blog), Feb. 16, 2020, updated Feb. 20, 2020, accessed Apr. 22, 2020, https://www.nytimes.com/2020/02/16/world/asia/coronavirus-cruise-americans.html.

302 Ibid.

303 Ibid.

304 Tomoya Onishi, "Cambodia's Hun Sen Welcomes Passengers from Shunned *Westerdam*," Nikkei Asian Review (blog), Feb. 15, 32020, accessed May 8, 2020, https://asia.nikkei.com/Spotlight/Coronavirus/Cambodia-s-Hun-Sen-welcomes-passengers-from-shunned-Westerdam.

305 Coronavirus: How Did Cambodia's Cruise Ship Welcome Go Wrong?" BBC News (blog), Feb. 20, 2020, accessed Apr. 22, 2020, https://www.bbc.com/news/world-asia-51542241.

306 Richard Paddock, Sui-Lee Wee, and Roni Caryn Rabin, "Coronavirus Infection Found After Cruise Ship Passengers Disperse," *The New York Times* (blog), Feb. 16, 2020, updated Feb. 20, 2020, accessed Apr. 22, 2020, https://www.nytimes.com/2020/02/16/world/asia/coronavirus-cruise-americans.html.

307 Ibid.

308 Julie, "Updated Statement Regarding Westerdam," Holland America Cruise Line (blog) Mar. 4, 2020, accessed Apr. 22, 2020, https://www.hollandamerica.com/blog/ships/ms-westerdam/statement-regarding-westerdam-in-japan/.

309 Public Health Responses to COVID-19 Outbreaks on Cruise Ships-Worldwide, February-March 2020, *MMWR* (blog), CDC, Mar. 27, 2020, accessed Apr. 23, 2020, https://www.cdc.gov/mmwr/volumes/69/wr/mm6912e3.htm.

310 Katie Canales, "Two-Thirds of Passengers from the Coronavirus-Stricken Grand Princess Cruise Ship Declined to be Tested While Quarantined at a California Miltary Base so They Could Go Home Sooner," *Business Insider* (blog), Mar. 19, 2020, accessed Apr. 23, 2020, https://www.businessinsider.com/coronavirus-grand-princess-cruise-ship-passengers-decline-testing-2020-3.

311 "Public Health Responses to COVID-19 Outbreaks on Cruise Ships-Worldwide, February-March 2020, *MMWR* (blog), CDC, Mar. 27, 2020, accessed Apr. 23, 2020, https://www.cdc.gov/mmwr/volumes/69/wr/mm6912e3.htm.

312 Katie Canales, "Two-Thirds of Passengers from the Coronavirus-Stricken Grand Princess Cruise Ship Declined to be Tested While Quarantined at a California Miltary Base so They Could Go Home Sooner," *Business Insider* (blog), Mar.

19, 2020, accessed Apr. 23, 2020, https://www.businessinsider.com/coronavirus-grand-princess-cruise-ship-passengers-decline-testing-2020-3.

313 "Public Health Responses to COVID-19 Outbreaks on Cruise Ships-Worldwide, February-March 2020, *MMWR* (blog), CDC, Mar. 27, 2020, accessed Apr. 23, 2020, https://www.cdc.gov/mmwr/volumes/69/wr/mm6912e3.htm.

314 Morgan Hines and Andrea Mandell, "Two Grand Princess Cruise Passengers with Coronavirus Die; 103 Have Tested Positive for COVID-19, USA Today (blog), Mar. 25, 2020, accessed Apr. 23, 2020, https://www.usatoday.com/story/travel/cruises/2020/03/25/coronavirus-cruise-grand-princess-two-passenger-deaths/5081851002/.

315 Alex Harris, Taylor, Dolven, and Michelle Kaufman, "Zaandam Was Cruising tot he 'End of the world.' Then COVID-19 Spread Across the Ship," *Miami Herald* (blog), Apr. 12, 2020, updated Apr. 15, 2020, accessed Apr. 23, 2020, https://www.miamiherald.com/news/business/tourism-cruises/article241740696.html.316

317 Ibid.

318 Ibid.

319 Ibid.

320 Ibid.

321 Ibid.

322 Ibid.

323 U.S. HHS and CDC, "Order Under Sections 361 & 365 of the Public Health Service Act (USC §§ 264,268) and 42 Code Federal Regulations Part 70 (Interstate) and Part 71 (Foreign): No Sail Order and Other Measures Related to Operations," 1, Mar. 14, 2020, accessed Apr. 22, 2020, https://www.cdc.gov/quarantine/pdf/signed-manifest-order_031520.pdf.

324 Brad Lendon, "Coronavirus May Be Giving Beijing an Opening in the South China Sea," CNN (blog), Apr. 7, 2020, accessed Apr. 25, 2020, https://www.cnn.com/2020/04/07/asia/coronavirus-china-us-military-south-china-sea-intl-hnk/index.html.

325 Matthias Gafni and Joe Garofoli, "Exclusive: Captain of Aircraft Carrier with Growing Coronavirus Outbreak Pleads for Help from Navy," *San Francisco Chronicle*, Mar. 30, 2020, accessed Apr. 24, 2020, https://www.sfchronicle.com/bayarea/article/Exclusive-Captain-of-aircraft-carrier-with-15167883.php.

326 Brad Lendon, "Coronavirus May Be Giving Beijing an Opening in the South China Sea," CNN (blog), Apr. 7, 2020, accessed Apr. 25, 2020, https://www.cnn.com/2020/04/07/asia/coronavirus-china-us-military-south-china-sea-intl-hnk/index.html.

327 Matthias Gafni and Joe Garofoli, "Exclusive: Captain of Aircraft Carrier with

Growing Coronavirus Outbreak Pleads for Help from Navy," *San Francisco Chronicle*, Mar. 30, 2020, accessed Apr. 24, 2020, https://www.sfchronicle.com/bayarea/article/Exclusive-Captain-of-aircraft-carrier-with-15167883.php.

328 Gina Harkins, "Modly Resigns as Acting SecNav Amid Backlash Over Carrier Captain's Firing," Military.com (blog), Apr. 7, 2020, accessed May 8, 2020, https://www.military.com/daily-news/2020/04/07/acting-navy-secretary-offers-resign-amid-growing-backlash-reports.html.

329 U.S. Pacific Fleet Public Affairs, "Navy Identifies USS Theodore Roosevelt Sailor Who Died of COVID-19," U.S. Navy, Apr. 16, 2020, accessed Apr. 24, 2020, https://www.navy.mil/submit/display.asp?story_id=112672.

330 Barbara Starr and Ryan Crowne, "Sailor from USS Teddy Roosevelt Found Unconscious, Transferred to Intensive Care," CNN Politics, Apr. 10, 2020, accessed Apr. 24, 2020, https://www.cnn.com/2020/04/09/politics/sailor-teddy-roosevelt-unconcious-covid-modly/index.html.

331 Ibid.

332 U.S. Pacific Fleet Public Affairs, "Navy Sailor Assigned to USS Theodore Roosevelt Dies of COVID-Related Complications," U.S. Navy, Apr. 13, 2020, accessed Apr. 24, 2020, https://www.navy.mil/submit/display.asp?story_id=112614.

333 "Daily Update: Apr. 23, 2020. Key Developments," Navy Line (blog), Apr. 23, 2020, accessed Apr. 24, 2020, https://navylive.dodlive.mil/2020/03/15/u-s-navy-covid-19-updates/.

334 Lolita C. Baldor, "Five USS Theodore Roosevelt Sailors Test Positive for Coronavirus a Second Time," *Time* (blog), May 15, 2020, accessed May 20, 2020, https://time.com/5837531/sailors-coronavirus-second-time/.

335 Brad Lendon, "Coronavirus May Be Giving Beijing an Opening in the South China Sea," CNN (blog), Apr. 7, 2020, accessed Apr. 25, 2020, https://www.cnn.com/2020/04/07/asia/coronavirus-china-us-military-south-china-sea-intl-hnk/index.html.

336 Cheng Chi-Wen, editor-in-chief Asia-Pacific Defense in John Xie, "China Claims Zero Infections in Its Military," VOA Cambodia (blog), Apr. 7, 2020, accessed Apr. 24, 2020. https://www.voacambodia.com/a/5362985.html.

337 "China Confirms No Cases of Coronavirus Infection in Military," China Military (blog), Mar. 3, 2020, accessed Apr. 25, 2020, http://eng.chinamil.com.cn/view/2020-03/03/content_9758336.htm.

338 Brad Lendon, "Chinese State Media Claims Country's Navy Is Not Affected by Coronavirus," CNN (blog), Apr. 15, 2020, accessed Apr. 17, 2020, https://www.cnn.com/2020/04/13/asia/china-coronavirus-aircraft-carrier-deployment-dp-hnk-intl/index.html.

339 Paul Shinkman, "Military Warns of Coronavirus 'Breakouts' Aboard the

USS Nimitz," *U.S. News & World Report* (blog), Apr. 9, 2020, accessed Apr. 24, 2020, https://www.usnews.com/news/national-news/articles/2020-04-09/military-warns-of-coronavirus-breakouts-aboard-uss-nimitz-aircraft-carrier.

340 Reuters, "EXCLUSIVE-US Navy Destroyer in Caribbean Sees Significant Coronavirus Outbreak-Officials," Thomson Reuters Foundation News (blog), Apr. 24, 2020, accessed Apr. 25, 2020, https://news.trust.org/item/20200424140331-zrivo.

341 Lolita C. Baldor, "Five USS Theodore Roosevelt Sailors Test Positive for Coronavirus a Second Time," *Time* (blog), May 15, 2020, accessed May 20, 2020, https://time.com/5837531/sailors-coronavirus-second-time/.

342 "COCVID-19 in China," CDC Travelers' Health (blog), CDC, Jan. 6, 2020, accessed Mar. 25, 2020, https://wwwnc.cdc.gov/travel/notices/warning/novel-coronavirus-china.

343 Michelle L. Holshue, Chas DeBolt, et al., "First Case of 2019 Novel Coronavirus in the United States, NEJM, 2020;382:929-36. DOI: 10.1056/NEJMoa2001191 , Jan 31, 2020, p 929, accessed March 25, 2020, https://www.nejm.org/doi/pdf/10.1056/NEJMoa2001191.

344 Ibid.

345 Ibid.

346 Ibid.

347 First Travel-Related Case of 2019 Novel Coronavirus detected in United States, *CDC Newsroom* (blog), CDC, Jan. 21, 2020, accessed Mar. 25, 2020, https://www.cdc.gov/media/releases/2020/p0121-novel-coronavirus-travel-case.html.

348 Michelle L. Holshue, Chas DeBolt, et al., "First Case of 2019 Novel Coronavirus in the United States, NEJM, 2020;382:929-36. DOI: 10.1056/NEJMoa2001191 , Jan 31, 2020, p 929, accessed March 25, 2020, https://www.nejm.org/doi/pdf/10.1056/NEJMoa2001191.

349 "Public Health Screening to Begin at 3 U.S. Airports for 2019 Novel Coronavirus ("2019-nCoV")," *CDC Newsroom* (blog), CDC, Jan. 17, 2020, accessed Mar. 25, 2020, https://www.cdc.gov/media/releases/2020/p0117-coronavirus-screening.html.

350 Michelle L. Holshue, Chas DeBolt, et al., "First Case of 2019 Novel Coronavirus in the United States, NEJM, 2020;382:929-36. DOI: 10.1056/NEJMoa2001191 , Jan 31, 2020, p 929, accessed March 25, 2020, https://www.nejm.org/doi/pdf/10.1056/NEJMoa2001191.

351 Ibid.

352 "First Travel-Related Case of 2019 Novel Coronavirus detected in United States, *CDC Newsroom* (blog), CDC, Jan. 21, 2020, accessed Mar. 25, 2020, https://www.cdc.gov/media/releases/2020/p0121-novel-coronavirus-travel-case.html.

353 Steve Eder, Henry Fountain, et al., "430,000 People Have Traveled From China to S.S. Since Coronavirus Surfaced," *New York Times* (blog), Apr. 4, 2020, accessed Apr. 4, 2020, https://www.nytimes.com/2020/04/04/us/coronavirus-china-travel-restrictions.html?referringSource=articleShare.

354 Ibid.

355 Elvia Malagón, Lauren Zumbach, and Dawn Rhodes, "Chicago Woman Who Traveled to China Diagnosed with Coronavirus, Health Officials Say," Chicago Tribune (blog), Jan. 25, 2020, accessed Mar. 26, 2020, https://www.chicagotribune.com/news/breaking/ct-coronavirus-china-epidemic-illinois-case-20200124-yx2x-d3yeovar3o25ei6bfvvbze-story.html.

356 Ibid.

357 David Jackson, "Trump Administration Declare Coronavirus Emergency, Orders First Quarantine in 50 Years," *USA Today* (blog) Jan. 31, 2020, accessed Apr. 14, 2020, https://www.usatoday.com/story/news/politics/2020/01/31/coronavirus-donald-trump-declares-public-health-emergency/4625299002/.

358 Ibid.

359 "Could the Electoral College Elect Hillary Clinton Instead of Donald Trump?" *USA Today* (blog), updated Dec. 20, 2016, accessed Apr. 16, 2020, https://www.usatoday.com/story/news/politics/elections/2016/2016/11/16/fact-check-could-electoral-college-elect-hillary-clinton-instead-donald-trump/93951818/.

360 Kirstein Schmidt and Wilson Andrews, "A Historic Number of Electors Defected, and Most Were Supposed to Vote for Clinton," *The New York Times* (blog), Dec. 19, 2016, accessed Apr. 16, 2020, https://www.nytimes.com/interactive/2016/12/19/us/elections/electoral-college-results.html.

361 Matea Gold, "The Campaign to Impeach Trump Has Begun," *The Washington Post* (blog), Jan. 20, 2017, accessed Apr. 16, 2020, https://www.washingtonpost.com/news/post-politics/wp/2017/01/20/the-campaign-to-impeach-president-trump-has-begun/.

362 Melissa Chan, "There's Already a Campaign to Impeach President Donald Trump," *Time*, Jan. 20, 2017, accessed Apr. 16, 2020, https://time.com/4641233/donald-trump-inauguration-impeach/.

363 Kevin Breuninger, "Robert Mueller's Russia Probe Cost Nearly $32 Million in Total, Justice Department Says," CNBC (blog), Aug. 2, 2019, accessed Apr. 16, 2020, https://www.cnbc.com/2019/08/02/robert-muellers-russia-probe-cost-nearly-32-million-in-total-doj.html.

364 Susan Jones, "Mueller Probe: 22 Months, 19 Lawyers, 40 FBI, 2,800 Subpoenas, 500 Search Warrants, and 500 Witnesses, CNBC (blog), Mar. 29, 205, accessed Apr. 16, 2020, https://www.cnsnews.com/news/article/susan-jones/you-paid-22-months-19-lawyers-40-fbi-2800-subpoenas-500-search-warrants-500.

365 Rick Bright in interview with Norah O'Donnell, *60 Minutes*, May 17, 2020, accessed May 18, 2020, https://www.cbsnews.com/video/rick-bright-whistleblower-virologist-coroanvirus-pandemic-drug-research-60-minutes/.

366 Alex Azar in Stephanie Soucheray, "Officials Say Most Americans Not at Risk of Coronavirus," Center for Infectious Disease Research and Policy, Jan. 28, 2020, accessed Apr. 14, 2020, https://www.cidrap.umn.edu/news-perspective/2020/01/officials-say-most-americans-not-risk-coronavirus.

367 Nancy Messonier in Stephanie Soucheray, "Officials Say Most Americans Not at Risk of Coronavirus," Center for Infectious Disease Research and Policy, Jan. 28, 2020, accessed Apr. 14, 2020, https://www.cidrap.umn.edu/news-perspective/2020/01/officials-say-most-americans-not-risk-coronavirus.

368 Logan Ratick, "Jan. Flashback: Dr. Fauci Said coronavirus 'Is Not a Threat to the People of the United States," SARA (blog), Apr. 3, 2020, accessed Apr. 14, 2020, https://saraacarter.com/jan-flashback-dr-fauci-said-coronavirus-is-not-a-major-threat-to-the-people-of-the-united-states.

369 Alex Azar in David Jackson, "Trump Administration Declare Coronavirus Emergency, Orders First Quarantine in 50 Years," *USA Today* (blog) Jan. 31, 2020, accessed Apr. 14, 2020, https://www.usatoday.com/story/news/politics/2020/01/31/coronavirus-donald-trump-declares-public-health-emergency/4625299002/.

370 Pelosi Tours San Francisco's Chinatown To Quell Coronavirus Fears," KPX CBS SF BayArea (blog), Feb. 24, 2020, accessed Apr. 13, 2020, https://sanfrancisco.cbslocal.com/2020/02/24/coronavirus-speaker-house-nancy-pelosi-tours-san-franciscos-chinatown/.

371 Vox tweet in Gregg Re, "After Attacking Trump's Coronavirus-Related China Ban as Xenophobic, Dem and Media Have Changed Tune," Fox News (blog), Apr. 1, 2020, https://www.foxnews.com/politics/dems-media-change-tune-trump-attacks-coronavirus-china-travel-ban.

372 Nancy Pelosi in "Pelosi Statement on President Trump's Expanded Travel Ban," Nancy Pelosi Speaker of the House Newsroom (blog), Jan. 31, 2020, accessed Apr. 30, 2020, https://www.speaker.gov/newsroom/13120-2.

373 Joe Biden, @JoeBiden, Feb. 1, 2020, accessed Apr. 30, 2020, https://twitter.com/JoeBiden/status/1223727977361338370.

374 "About Us," STAT, accessed Apr. 30, 2020, https://www.statnews.com/about/.

375 Megan Thielking, "Health Experts Warn China Travel Ban Will Hinder Coronavirus Response," STAT (blog), Jan. 31, 2020, accessed Apr. 30, 2020, https://www.statnews.com/2020/01/31/as-far-right-calls-for-china-travel-ban-health-experts-warn-coronavirus-response-would-suffer/.

376 Michael Corkery and Annie Karni, "Trump Administration Restricts Entry Into U.S. From China," Jan. 31, 2020, *The New York Times* (blog) Jan. 31, 2020, accessed Apr. 30, 2020, https://www.nytimes.com/2020/01/31/business/china-travel-coronavirus.html.

377 Jessie Yeung, "As the Coronavirus Spreads, Fear is Fueling Racism and Xenophobia," CNN (blog), Jan. 31, 2020, accessed Apr. 30, 2020, https://www.cnn.com/2020/01/31/asia/wuhan-coronavirus-racism-fear-intl-hnk/index.html.

378 Eric Carter in Catherine E. Schoichet, The U Coronavirus Travel Ban Could Backfire. Here's How," CNN (blog), Feb. 7, 2020, accessed Apr. 30, 2020, https://www.cnn.com/2020/02/07/health/coronavirus-travel-ban/index.html.

379 Tom Howell, Jr., "Dems Ding Trump's $2.5 billion coronavirus request as 'too little, too late,'" *The Washington Times* (blog), Feb. 24, 2020, accessed May 1, 2020, https://www.washingtontimes.com/news/2020/feb/24/donald-trump-requests-25-billion-coronavirus-fight/.

380 Lauren Hirsch and Kevin Breuninger, "Trump Signs $8.3 billion Emergency Coronavirus Spending Package," CNCBC (blog), Mar. 6, 2020, accessed Apr. 30, 2020, https://www.cnbc.com/2020/03/06/trump-signs-8point3-billion-emergency-coronavirus-spending-package.html.

381 Donald J. Trump, "Oval Office Address to the Union," Mar. 11, 2020.

382 Ibid.

383 Ibid.

384 Olivia Niland, "Trump Is Extending the Europe Travel Ban to the UK and Ireland as the Coronavirus Pandemic Escalates," *BuzzFeed News* (blog), Mar. 14, 2020, accessed Apr. 15, 2020, https://www.buzzfeednews.com/article/olivianiland/trump-uk-ireland-travel-ban-europe-coronavirus.

385 Ibid.

386 Ibid.

387 Coronavirus Disease 2019: Social Distancing, CDC, Apr. 4, 2020, accessed Apr. 26, 2020, https://www.cdc.gov/coronavirus/2019-ncov/prevent-getting-sick/social-distancing.html.

388 Ibid.

389 Ibid.

390 Sheri Fink, "Worst-Case Estimates for U.S. Coronavirus Deaths," *The New York Times* (blog), Mar. 13, 2020, accessed Apr. 9, 2020, https://www.nytimes.com/2020/03/13/us/coronavirus-deaths-estimate.html.

391 Ibid.

392 Meredith McGraw," *"Trump's New Coronavirus Argument: 2 Million People Are Being Saved,"* Politico, Apr. 1, 2020, accessed Apr. 13, 2020, https://www.

politico.com/news/2020/04/01/trump-coronavirus-millions-saved-160814.

393 Doug Palmer, "U.S. Medical Stockpile Wasn't Built to Handle Current Crisis, Former Director Says," *Politico* (blog), Apr. 8, 2020, accessed May 1, 2020, https://www.politico.com/news/2020/04/08/national-stockpile-coronavirus-crisis-175619.

394 Ibid.

395 Sarah Kliff, Adam Stariano, et al., "There Aren't Enough Ventilators to Cope With the Coronavirus, *The New York Times* (blog), Mar. 18, 2020, accessed May 1, 2020, https://www.nytimes.com/2020/03/18/business/coronavirus-ventilator-shortage.html.

396 Anthony Fauci interview in *State of the Union With Jake Tapper*, CNN, Mar. 15, 2020, memorialized in @CNNSotu, Twitter, Mar. 15, 2020, 6:33 PM, accessed May 2, 2020, https://twitter.com/CNNSotu/status/1239318789856034817.

397 Peter Loftus, "Ventilator Makers Ramp Up Production Amid Coronavirus Crunch," *The Wall Street Journal* (blog), Mar. 19, 2020, accessed May 1, 2020, https://www.wsj.com/articles/ventilator-makers-ramp-up-production-amid-coronavirus-crunch-11584626858?mod=searchresults&page=4&pos=8.

398 Sarah Kliff, Adam Stariano, et al., "There Aren't Enough Ventilators to Cope With the Coronavirus, *The New York Times* (blog), Mar. 18, 2020, accessed May 1, 2020, https://www.nytimes.com/2020/03/18/business/coronavirus-ventilator-shortage.html.

399 Brett Samuels, "Trump Uses Defense Production Act to Require GM to Make Ventilators," The Hill (blog), Mar. 27, 2020, accessed May 2, 2020, https://thehill.com/homenews/administration/489909-trump-uses-defense-production-act-to-require-gm-to-make-ventilators.

400 Memorandum on Order Under the Defense Production Act Regarding 3M Company, Apr. 2, 2020, §2.

401 Rachel Sandler, "Trump Ends Feud With Mask Maker 3M, Announces Deal for 55 Million U.S. Masks per Month." *Forbes* (blog), Apr. 6, 2020, accessed May 2, 2020, https://www.forbes.com/sites/rachelsandler/2020/04/06/trump-ends-feud-with-mask-maker-3m-announces-deal-for-55-million-us-masks-per-month/#637691ce1209.

402 "President Donald J. Trump Has Led a Historic Mobilization to Combat the Coronavirus," The White House (blog), Apr. 14, 2020, accessed May 2, 2020, https://www.whitehouse.gov/briefings-statements/president-donald-j-trump-led-historic-mobilization-combat-coronavirus/

403 "Coronavirus Disease 2019 Diagnostic Testing," CDC, last reviewed Apr. 14, 2020, accessed May 7, 2020, https://www.cdc.gov/coronavirus/2019-ncov/php/testing.html.

404 Ibid.

405 Adam Bernheim, Xueyan Mei, et al., "Chest CT Findings in Coronavirus Disease- 19 (COVID-19): Relationship to Duration of Infection," *Radiology*, Feb. 20, 2020, accessed May 7, 2020, https://pubs.rsna.org/doi/10.1148/radi-ol.2020200463.

406 Maria Rachal, "Abbott Touts Speed, Scale of POC Coronavirus Test," Medtech Dive (bog), Mar. 30, 2020, accessed May 8, 2020, https://www.medtechdive.com/news/abbott-touts-speed-scale-of-poc-coronavirus-test/575092/

407 "Abbott Launches Molecular Point-of Care Test to Detect novel Coronavirus," Abbott Newsroom (blog), Mar. 27, 2020, accessed May 8, 2020, https://abbott.mediaroom.com/2020-03-27-Abbott-Launches-Molecular-Point-of-Care-Test-to-Detect-Novel-Coronavirus-in-as-Little-as-Five-Minutes.

408 Scott Gottlieb, @ScottGottliebMD, Twitter, Mar. 27, 2020, 8:26 PM, accessed May 8, 2020, https://twitter.com/ScottGottliebMD/status/1243696001958981632.

409 "Abbott Launches Molecular Point-of Care Test to Detect novel Coronavirus," Abbott Newsroom (blog), Mar. 27, 2020, accessed May 8, 2020, https://abbott.mediaroom.com/2020-03-27-Abbott-Launches-Molecular-Point-of-Care-Test-to-Detect-Novel-Coronavirus-in-as-Little-as-Five-Minutes.

410 Ibid.

411 Letter from Uwe Scherf to Christian Bixby, Re: EUA200090, Apr. 10 2020, accessed May 7, 2020, https://www.fda.gov/media/136876/download.

412 "Cleveland Company Approved to Make Swabs for Coronavirus Testing," Cleveland.com (blog), Apr. 24, 2020, accessed May 8, 2020, https://www.cleve-land.com/open/2020/04/cleveland-company-approved-to-make-swabs-for-coro-navirus-testing.html.

413 John Huotari, "ORNL Making Molds to Help Produce COVID-19 Test Tubes," Oak Ridge Today (blog), Apr. 21, 2020, accessed May 8, 2020, https://oakridgeto-day.com/2020/04/21/ornl-making-molds-to-help-produce-covid-19-test-tubes/.

414 Brad Smith in "Remarks by President Trump, Vice President Pence, and Mem-bers of the Coronavirus Task Force in Press Briefing, Apr. 20, 2020, accessed May 8, 2020, https://www.whitehouse.gov/briefings-statements/remarks-president-trump-vice-president-pence-members-coronavirus-task-force-press-briefing-29/.

415 Coronavirus Disease 2019: Testing in US, CDC, updated May 7, 2020, ac-cessed May 8, 2020, https://www.cdc.gov/coronavirus/2019-ncov/cases-updates/testing-in-us.html.

416 COVID-19 Coronavirus Pandemic, Worldometer, updated May 8, 2020, ac-cessed May 8, 2020, https://www.worldometers.info/coronavirus/#countries.

417 COVID-19 Coronavirus Pandemic, Worldometer, updated May 17, 2020, ac-

cessed May 18, 2020, https://www.worldometers.info/coronavirus/#countries.

418 U.S. Constitution, Art. I, Sxn. 9, Cl 2.

419 U.S. Constitution, Art. V, Sxn. 4, Cl 1.

420 Taryn Luna, John Myers, "Large Gatherings Should Be Canceled Due to Coronavirus Outbreak, California Gov. Gavin Newsom Says," *Los Angeles Times* (blog), Mar. 11, 2020, accessed Apr. 15, 2020, https://www.latimes.com/california/story/2020-03-11/coronavirus-outbreak-large-gatherings-canceled-governor-gavin-newsom-california.

421 Order of the State Public Health Officer, Mar. 19, 2020.

422 Executive Department State of California, Executive Order N-33-20.

423 Sarah Mervosh, Denise Lu, and Venessa Seales, "See Which States and Cities Have Told Resident to Stay at Home," *The New York Times* (blog), Apr. 7, 2020, accessed Apr. 15, 2020, https://www.nytimes.com/interactive/2020/us/coronavirus-stay-at-home-order.html.

424 Justine Coleman, "All 50 States Under Disaster Declaration for First Time in US History," *The Hill* (blog), Apr. 12, 2020, accessed Apr. 15, 2020, https://thehill.com/policy/healthcare/public-global-health/492433-all-50-states-under-disaster-declaration-for-first.

425 Michigan Executive Order 2020-42 (COVID-19)

426 Andrew O'Reilly, "Drivers Swarm Michigan Capital to Protest Coronavirus Lockdown Measures, Fox News (blog), Apr. 15, 2020, accessed Apr. 15, 2020, https://www.foxnews.com/politics/drivers-swarm-michigan-capital-to-protest-coronavirus-lockdown-measures.

427 Ibid.

428 State of Wisconsin Executive Order #74 Relating to Suspending In-Person Voting on April 7, 2020, due to the COVID-19 Pandemic," Apr. 6, 2020.

429 Natasha Korecki and Zack Montellaro, "Wisconsin Supreme Court Overturns Governor. Orders Tuesday Elections to Proceed," *Politico* (blog), Apr. 6, 2020, accessed Apr. 19, 2020, https://www.politico.com/news/2020/04/06/wisconsin-governor-orders-stop-to-in-person-voting-on-eve-of-election-168527.

430 State of New York Executive Order 202.10, Mar. 7, 2020.

431 Scott Neuman, "Man Dies, Woman Hospitalized After Taking Form of Chloroquine to Prevent COVID-19," NPR (blog), Mar. 24, 2020, accessed Apr. 15, 2020, https://www.npr.org/sections/coronavirus-live-updates/2020/03/24/820512107/man-dies-woman-hospitalized-after-taking-form-of-chloroquine-to-prevent-covid-19.

432 2020-03-23 - COVID-19 Emergency Regulation Board of Pharmacy.

433 Letter from Deb Gagliardi and Forrest to Licensed Prescribers & Dispensers,

Mar. 24, 2020.

434 Chuck Goudie, Bob Markoff, et al., "Coronavirus: New Questions About how Many Illinois State Prison Inmates Are Being Released Due to COVID-19," ABC7 (blog), Apr. 28, 2020, accessed May 18, 2020, https://abc7chicago.com/coronavirus-update-cases-illinois/6135977/; John Eligon, "'It's a Slap in the Face': Victims Are Angered as Jails Free Inmates," *The New York Times* (blog), Apr. 24, 2020, accessed May 18, 2020, https://www.nytimes.com/2020/04/24/us/coronavirus-jail-inmates-released.html.

435 State of Florida Executive Order No. 20-91, Apr. 1, 2020.

436 State of Florida Executive Order No. 20-70, Mar. 20, 2020.

437 State of Florida Executive Order No. 20-71, Mar. 20, 2020.

438 State of Florida Executive Order No. 20-68, Mar. 17, 2020.

439 State of Florida Executive Order No. 20-89, Mar. 30, 2020.

440 State of Florida Executive Order No. 20-72, Mar. 20, 2020.

441 State of Florida Executive Order No. 20-91, Apr. 1, 2020.

442 State of Florida Executive Order No. 20-91, Apr. 1, 2020.

443 Ellen Barry, "Days After a Funeral in a Georgia Town, Coronavirus 'Hit Like a Bomb," *The New York Times*, Mar. 30, 2020, accessed Mar. 30, 2020, https://www.nytimes.com/2020/03/30/us/coronavirus-funeral-albany-georgia.html?action=click&module=Top%20Stories&pgtype=Homepage.

444 Ibid.

445 Lee Brown, "New York City's First Coronavirus Patient Is a Healthcare Worker; Cuomo Says," *New York Post* (blog), Mar. 2, 2020, accessed May 8, 2020, https://nypost.com/2020/03/02/new-york-citys-first-coronavirus-patient-is-a-healthcare-worker-cuomo-says/.

446 Tamer Lapin, "Coronavirus in NY: A Timeline of How the Disease Spread Through the Metro Area," *New York Post* (blog), Mar. 12, 2020, accessed May 8, 2020, https://nypost.com/2020/03/12/coronavirus-in-ny-a-timeline-of-how-the-disease-spread-through-the-metro-area/.

447 "Coronavirus in NY: Cases, Maps, Charts, and Resources," Syracuse.com (blog), last updated May 7, 2020, accessed May 8, 2020, https://www.syracuse.com/coronavirus-ny/.

448 Lee Brown, "New York City's First Coronavirus Patient Is a Healthcare Worker; Cuomo Says," *New York Post* (blog), Mar. 2, 2020, accessed May 8, 2020, https://nypost.com/2020/03/02/new-york-citys-first-coronavirus-patient-is-a-healthcare-worker-cuomo-says/.

449 ibid.

450 "Coronavirus in NY: Cases, Maps, Charts, and Resources," Syracuse.com (blog),

last updated May 7, 2020, accessed May 8, 2020, https://www.syracuse.com/coronavirus-ny/.

451 Jimmy Vielkind, Leslie Brody, and Costas Paris, "Containment Area Planned for New York Suburb to Stem Coronavirus Spread," *The Wall Street Journal* (blog), Mar. 10, 2020, accessed May 8, 2020, https://www.wsj.com/articles/containment-area-planned-for-new-york-suburb-to-stem-coronavirus-spread-11583858117?mod=article_inline.

452 "Coronavirus in NY: Cases, Maps, Charts, and Resources," Syracuse.com (blog), last updated May 7, 2020, accessed May 8, 2020, https://www.syracuse.com/coronavirus-ny/.

453 Kyle Smith, "The Ventilator Shortage That Wasn't," *National Review* (blog), Apr. 17, 2020, accessed May 8, 2020, https://www.nationalreview.com/2020/04/coronavirus-crisis-ventilator-shortages-have-not-come-to-pass/.

454 Ibid.

455 Donald J. Trump in "Remarks by President Trump, Vice President Pence, and Members of the Coronavirus Task Force in Press Briefing, Apr. 20, 2020, accessed May 8, 2020, https://www.whitehouse.gov/briefings-statements/remarks-president-trump-vice-president-pence-members-coronavirus-task-force-press-briefing-29/.

456 Michael R. Sisak, "Many Field Hospitals Went Largely Unused, Will Be Shut Down," *Military Times* (blog), Apr. 29, 2020, accessed May 8, 2020, https://www.militarytimes.com/news/coronavirus/2020/04/29/many-field-hospitals-went-largely-unused-will-be-shut-down/.

457 Ibid.

458 Elizabeth Koh, Jon Kamp, and Dan Froshc, "One Nursing Home, 35 Coronavirus Deaths: Inside the Kirkland Disaster," *The Wall Street Journal* (blog), Mar. 23, 2020, accessed Apr. 27, 2020, https://www.wsj.com/articles/one-nursing-home-35-coronavirus-deaths-inside-the-kirkland-disaster-11584982494.

459 Kate Feldman, "Life Care Center in Kirkland Epicenter of Washington's Coronavirus Outbreak, Sued for Wrongful Death," *New York Daily News* (blog), Apr. 12, 2020, accessed May 8, 2020, https://www.nydailynews.com/coronavirus/ny-coronavirus-kirkland-nursing-home-lawsuit-washington-20200412-ngbkjj7rffg2ld4f2s345lltii-story.html.

460 "State Data and Policy Actions to Address Coronavirus," The Henry J. Kaiser Foundation (blog) Apr. 23, 2020, Table: State Report of Long-Term Care Facility Cases and Deaths Related to COVID-19 (as of May 7, 2020), accessed May 8, 2020, https://www.kff.org/health-costs/issue-brief/state-data-and-policy-actions-to-address-coronavirus/.

461 Ibid.

462 Ibid.

463 Ibid.

464 Ibid.

465 Jim Mustian, Jennifer Peltz, and Bernard Condon, "NY's Cuomo Criticized Over Highest Nursing Home Death Toll," Spectrum News, Bay News 9 (blog), May 9, 2020, accessed May 9, 2020, https://abcnews.go.com/Health/wireStory/nys-cuomo-criticized-highest-nursing-home-death-toll-70596950.

466 "New Count Reveals 1,600 More Nursing Home Deaths in N.Y.," *The New York Times* (blog), May 5, 2020, accessed May 9, 2020, https://www.nytimes.com/2020/05/05/nyregion/covid-ny-update.html.

467 Ibid.

468 Jim Mustian, Jennifer Peltz, and Bernard Condon, "NY's Cuomo Criticized Over Highest Nursing Home Death Toll," Spectrum News, Bay News 9 (blog), May 9, 2020, accessed May 9, 2020, https://abcnews.go.com/Health/wireStory/nys-cuomo-criticized-highest-nursing-home-death-toll-70596950.

469 Ibid.

470 Carolyn J. Berdzik, Jonathan Berkowitz, Lisa M. Robinson., "New York State Department Releases Advisory Prohibiting Nursing Homes From Denying Admissions Due to Coronavrius," Goldberg Segalla Knowledge (blog), Mar. 27, 2020, accessed May 8, 2020, https://www.goldbergsegalla.com/news-and-knowledge/knowledge/nys-health-dept-releases-coronavirus-advisory.

471 ibid.

472 Jim Mustian, Jennifer Peltz, and Bernard Condon, "NY's Cuomo Criticized Over Highest Nursing Home Death Toll," Spectrum News, Bay News 9 (blog), May 9, 2020, accessed May 9, 2020, https://abcnews.go.com/Health/wireStory/nys-cuomo-criticized-highest-nursing-home-death-toll-70596950.

473 ibid.

474 Jared Moskowitz, State of Florida Division of Emergency Management DEM ORDER NO. 20-006, Mar. 15, 2020, accessed May 8, 2020, https://s33330.pcdn.co/wp-content/uploads/2020/03/DEM-ORDER-NO.-20-006-In-re-COVID-19-Public-Health-Emergency-Issued-March-15-2020.pdf.

475 ibid.

476 "Nursing Homes," Florida COVID-19 Response, accessed May 8, 2020, https://floridahealthcovid19.gov/nursing-homes/.

477 "State Data and Policy Actions to Address Coronavirus," The Henry J. Kaiser Foundation (blog) Apr. 23, 2020, Table: State Report of Long-Term Care Facility Cases and Deaths Related to COVID-19 (as of May 7, 2020), accessed May 8, 2020, https://www.kff.org/health-costs/issue-brief/state-data-and-policy-ac-

tions-to-address-coronavirus/.

478 Ibid.

479 Anjeanette Damon, "COVID-19 cases and Death in Nevada Nursing Homes Continue to Climb," *Reno Gazette Journal* (blog), Apr. 30, 2020, accessed May 8, 2020, https://www.rgj.com/story/news/2020/05/01/nevada-coronavirus-covid-19-cases-nursing-homes-deaths/3061863001/.

480 Memo from Nevada Department of Health and Human Services to Health Care Providers-Read Receipt Requested, "Coronavirus Disease 2019 (COVID-19)-REVISED, Mar. 25, 2020, accessed May 8, 2020, https://nvhealthresponse.nv.gov/wp-content/uploads/2020/03/COVID-19-TB-3.23.20-1.pdf.

481 Christopher Helman, "Bloodbath for America's Oil Frackers as Saudis Declare Price War on Russia," *Forbes* (blog), Mar. 9, 2020, accessed May 10, 2020, https://www.forbes.com/sites/christopherhelman/2020/03/09/bloodbath-for-oil-frackers-as-saudis-declare-price-war-on-russia/#22ceb5892198.

482 Rosie Perper, Sarah Al-Arshani, and Holly Secon, "More Than Half of the US Population Is Now Under Orders to Stay Home-Here's a List of Xoronavirus Lockdowns in US States and Cities," *Business Insider* (blog), Mar. 15, 2020, last updated Apr. 1, 2020, accessed May 8, 2020, https://www.businessinsider.com/states-cities-shutting-down-bars-restaurants-concerts-curfew-2020-3.

483 Jack Kelly, "A Record-Setting 3.3 Million People Filed for Unemployment," *Forbes* (blog), Mar. 26, 2020, accessed May 8, 2020, https://www.forbes.com/sites/jackkelly/2020/03/26/a-record-setting-33-million-people-filed-for-unemployment/#54e2f3597ccf.

484 Ibid.

485 Matt Krantz, "These 13 Stock Completely Erase Their Massive Coronavirus Losses," *Investors Business Daily* (blog), Apr. 9, 2020, accessed May 11, https://www.investors.com/etfs-and-funds/sectors/sp500-stocks-completely-erase-massive-coronavirus-losses-bounce/.

486 Jack Brewster, "Trump Signs $2 Trillion Coronavirus Relief Bill Into Law, Largest Aid Package in U.S. History," *Forbes* (blog), Mar. 27, 2020, accessed May 9, 2020, https://www.forbes.com/sites/jackbrewster/2020/03/27/trump-signs-2-trillion-stimulus-bill-into-law-largest-aid-package-in-us-history/#6e3d83ab4ea5.

487 Ibid.

488 Joseph Zeballos-Roig, "Trump Signs the $2 Trillion Coronavirus Economic Relief Bill Into Law, Which Includes Checks for Americans and Business Loans," *Business Insider* (blog), Mar. 27 2020, accessed May 8, 2020, https://www.businessinsider.com/trump-signs-coronavirus-economic-relief-aid-bill-checks-for-americans-2020-3.

489 Ebony Bowden and Steven Nelson, "President Trump Sign Into Law $2 Trillion

Coronavirus Bailout," *New York Post* (blog), Mar. 27, 2020, accessed May 8, 2020, https://nypost.com/2020/03/27/president-trump-signs-into-law-2-trillion-corona-virus-bailout/.

490 "The CARES Act Provides Assistance to Small Businesses," U.S. Department of the Treasury, accessed May 8, 2020, https://home.treasury.gov/policy-issues/cares/assistance-for-small-businesses.

491 Andrew Duehren, "Funding Exhausted for $350 Billion Small-Business Pay-check Protection Program, *The Wall Street Journal* (blog), Apr. 16, 2020, accessed May 10, 2020, https://www.wsj.com/articles/funding-exhausted-for-350-bil-lion-small-business-paycheck-protection-program-11587048384.

492 Jeffrey Bartash, "U.S. Unemployment Rate Has Likely Reached 15% Econ-omists Say," MarketWatch (blog), Apr. 16, 2020, accessed May 8, 2020, https://www.marketwatch.com/story/jobless-claims-soar-again-by-525-million-as-coro-navirus-pushes-unemployment-to-15-2020-04-16.

493 Natalie Andrews, "Trump Signs Coronavirus Stimulus Bill as Focus Shifts to State Funding," *The Wall Street Journal* (blog), Apr. 24, 2020, May 10, 2020, https://www.wsj.com/articles/trump-signs-coronavirus-stimulus-bill-as-focus-shifts-to-state-funding-11587749963.

494 Jeff Cox, "Here Is Everything the Fed Has Done to Save the Economy," CNCBC (blog), Apr. 13, 2020, accessed May 13, 2020, https://www.cnbc.com/2020/04/13/coronavirus-update-here-is-everything-the-fed-has-done-to-save-the-economy.html.

495 Kimberly Amadeo, "Reserve Requirement and How It Affects Interest Rates," The Balance (blog), Mar. 16, 2020, accessed May 13, 2020, https://www.thebal-ance.com/reserve-requirement-3305883.

496 Jeff Cox, "Here Is Everything the Fed Has Done to Save the Economy," CNCBC (blog), Apr. 13, 2020, accessed May 13, 2020, https://www.cnbc.com/2020/04/13/coronavirus-update-here-is-everything-the-fed-has-done-to-save-the-economy.html.

497 Sarah Chaney and Eric Morath, "April Unemployment Rate Rose to a Record 14%, *The Wall Street Journal* (blog), May 8, 2020, accessed May 11, 2020, https://www.wsj.com/articles/april-jobs-report-coronavirus-2020-11588888089.

498 Patricia Cohen and Tiffany Hsu, "For Workers, No Sign of 'What Normal Is Going to Look Like,'" *The New York Times* (blog), May 7, 2020, accessed May 11, 2020, https://www.nytimes.com/2020/05/07/business/economy/coronavirus-un-employment-claims.html.

499 Patricia Mazzei, "Florida Pastor Arrested AFter Defying Virus Orders," *The New York Times* (blog), Mar. 30, 2020, accessed Apr. 14, 2020, https://www.ny-times.com/2020/03/30/us/coronavirus-pastor-arrested-tampa-florida.html.

500 Ibid.

501 Ibid.

502 Executive Order of the Hillsborough County Emergency Policy Group Safer-At-Home Order in Response to a County Wide Threat from the COVID-19 Virus, § 3.ii, Mar. 27, 2020, accessed May 12, 2020, https://www.hillsboroughcounty.org/library/hillsborough/media-center/documents/administrator/epg/saferathomeorder.pdf.

503 Michael Ruiz, "Mississippi City's Coronavirus Shutdown Bans Drive-In Church Services Ahead of Easter," Fox News (blog), Apr. 11, 2020, accessed May 11, 2020, https://www.foxnews.com/us/mississippi-coronavirus-shutdown-city-bans-drive-in-church-services-easter.

504 Sophie O'Hara, "Report: Judge Overrules Democrat Mayor Who Banned Easter Drive-In Church Services," Wayne Dupree (blog), Apr. 11, 2020, accessed May 8, 2020, https://www.waynedupree.com/louisville-mayor-church/.

505 William Barr, "Attorney General William P. Barr Issues Statement on Religious Practice and Social Distancing; Department of Justice Files Statement of Interest in Mississippi Church Case," Department of Justice Office of Public Affairs, Fn. 1., Apr. 14, 2020, accessed May 21, 2020, https://www.justice.gov/opa/pr/attorney-general-william-p-barr-issues-statement-religious-practice-and-social-distancing-0.

506 Ibid.

507 "Governor Northam Announces New Measures to Combat COVID-19 and Support Impacted Virginians," Virginia Governor Ralph S. Northam, Mar. 17, 2020, accessed Apr. 14, 2020, https://www.governor.virginia.gov/newsroom/all-releases/2020/march/headline-854487-en.html.

508 Executive Order 2020-11 (COVID-19).

509 "Coronavirus, Executive Order 2020-11 FAQs," Michigan.gov, accessed Apr. 15, 2020, https://www.michigan.gov/coronavirus/0,9753,7-406-98178_98455-522357--,00.html.

510 Letter Eric S. Dreiband to Gavin Newsom, May 19, 2020, in @KerriKupecDOJ, Twitter, May 19, 2020, 7:57 PM, accessed May 21, 2020, https://twitter.com/KerriKupecDOJ/status/1262895160318480384.

511 Ibid.

512 State of Florida Office of the Governor Executive Order 20-91, (Essential Services and Activities During Covid-19, §3.A.i.

513 Lee Brown, "Virginia Pastor Who Defiantly Held Church Service Dies of Coronavirus," New York Post (blog), Apr. 13, 2020, accessed Apr, 14, 2020, https://nypost.com/2020/04/13/virginia-pastor-who-held-packed-church-service-dies-of-coronavirus/.

514 Deliverance Evangelistic Church, Facebook Post of April 12, 0744, accessed Apr. 14, 2020, https://www.facebook.com/OfficialNDEC/videos/233789087982971/?__tn__=-R.

515 Neil Ferguson, Daniel Laydon, et al., "COVID-19 Impact of Non-Pharmaceutical Intervention (NPIs) to Reduce COVID-19 Mortality and Healthcare Demand," Imperial College COVID-19 Response Team, Mar. 16, 2020, accessed May 13, 2020, https://www.imperial.ac.uk/media/imperial-college/medicine/sph/ide/gida-fellowships/Imperial-College-COVID19-NPI-modelling-16-03-2020.pdf.

516 Lydia Ramsey, "A Leaked Presentation Reveals the document US Hospitals Are Using to Prepare for a Major Coronavirus Outbreak. It Estimates 96 Million US Coronavirus Cases and 480,000 Deaths, *Business Insider* (blog), Mar. 6, 2020, accessed Apr. 13, 2020, https://www.businessinsider.com/presentation-how-hospitals-are-preparing-for-us-coronavirus-outbreak-2020-3.

517 "IHME COVID-19 model FAQs," healthdata.org (blog), accessed Apr. 8, 2020, http://www.healthdata.org/covid/faqs#differences%20in%20modeling.

518 Ibid.

519 IHME COVID-19 Health Service Utilization Forecasting Team, "Forecasting COVID-19 impact on hospital bed-days, ICU-days, ventilator-days and deaths by US state in the next 4 months," accessed Apr. 8, 2020, http://www.healthdata.org/sites/default/files/files/research_articles/2020/covid_paper_MEDRXIV-2020-043752v1-Murray.pdf.

520 Ibid.

521 Ibid.

522 Video in Ian Schwartz, CNN's Acosta: Trump 'Propaganda' Video 'Looked Straight Out of Beijing or Pyongyang," Real Clear Politics (blog), Apr. 13, accessed May 13, 2020, https://www.realclearpolitics.com/video/2020/04/13/cnns_acosta_trump_propaganda_video_looked_straight_out_of_beijing_or_pyongyang.html.

523 Jim Acosta in transcript of *Anderson Cooper 360 Degrees*, Apr. 13, 2020, accessed May 13, 2020, http://transcripts.cnn.com/TRANSCRIPTS/2004/13/acd.01.html.

524 Sean Collins, "Fauci Acknowledged a Delay in the US Coronavirus Response. Trump Then Retweeted a Call to Fire Him," Vox (blog), Apr. 13, 2020, accessed Apr. 16, 2020, https://www.vox.com/covid-19-coronavirus-us-response-trump/2020/4/13/21218922/coronavirus-fauci-trump-fire-tweet.

525 Eric Lipton, David E. Sanger, et al., "He Could Have Seen What Was Coming: Behind Trump's Failure on the Virus," *The New York Times* (blog) Apr. 11, 2020, updated, Apr. 14, 2020, accessed Apr. 16, 2020, https://www.nytimes.com/2020/04/11/us/politics/coronavirus-trump-response.html.

526 Grace Panetta, "Trump Reportedly Squandered 3 Crucial Weeks to Miti-

Not at Risk of Coronavirus," Center for Infectious Disease Research and Policy, Jan. 28, 2020, accessed Apr. 14, 2020, https://www.cidrap.umn.edu/news-perspective/2020/01/officials-say-most-americans-not-risk-coronavirus.

537 Logan Ratick, "Jan. Flashback: Dr. Fauci Said coronavirus 'Is Not a Threat to the People of the United States," SARA (blog), Apr. 3, 2020, accessed Apr. 14, 2020, https://saraacarter.com/jan-flashback-dr-fauci-said-coronavirus-is-not-a-major-threat-to-the-people-of-the-united-states.

538 Philippe Gautret, Jean-Christopher Lagier, " Hydroxychloroquine and Azithromycin as a Treatment of COVID-19: Results of an Open-Label Non-Randomized Clinical Trial," medrxiv.org (blog) Mar. 16, 2020, accessed Apr. 21, 2020, https://www.medrxiv.org/content/10.1101/2020.03.16.20037135v1.full.pdf.

539 Author, personal observation of Gregory Rigano in *Tucker Carlson Tonight*, Fox News, Mar. 18, 2020; Tim Pierce, "Malaria Drug See Promising Signs as Future Coronavirus Treatment," *Washington Examiner* (blog), March 18, 2020, accessed Apr. 20, 2020, https://www.washingtonexaminer.com/news/malaria-drug-sees-promising-signs-as-future-coronavirus-treatment.

540 Aude Lecruvier, "COVID-19: Could Hydroxychloroquine Really Be an Answer? *Medscape* (blog), Mar. 18, 2020, accessed Apr. 21, 2020, https://www.medscape.com/viewarticle/927033.

541 Author, personal observation of Gregory Rigano in *Tucker Carlson Tonight*, Fox News, Mar. 18, 2020; Tim Pierce, "Malaria Drug See Promising Signs as Future Coronavirus Treatment," *Washington Examiner* (blog), March 18, 2020, accessed Apr. 20, 2020, https://www.washingtonexaminer.com/news/malaria-drug-sees-promising-signs-as-future-coronavirus-treatment.

542 Mary Beth Pfeiffer, "Researchers Look to Old Drug for a Possible Coronavirus Treatment-It Might Just Work," *Forbes* (blog), Mar. 18, 2020, accessed Apr. 21, 2020, https://www.forbes.com/sites/marybethpfeiffer/2020/03/18/science-works-to-use-old-cheap-drugs-to-attack-coronavirus--it-might-just-work/#41b380655c49.

543 Tal Axelrod, "Trump Steps up Effort to Tout Malaria Drug as Coronavirus 'game changer' Despite Doubts from FDA," *The Hill* Mar. 21 2020, accessed Apr. 21, 2020, https://thehill.com/homenews/administration/488796-trump-steps-up-effort-to-tout-malaria-drug-as-coronavirus-game.

544 Donald J. Trump, @realDonaldTrump, Twitter, Mar. 21, 2020, in Joe Palca, "NIH Panel Recommends Against Drug Combination Promoted By Trump For COVID-19," NPR (blog), Apr. 21, 2020, accessed Apr. 21, 2020, https://www.npr.org/sections/coronavirus-live-updates/2020/04/21/840341224/nih-panel-recommends-against-drug-combination-trump-has-promoted-for-covid-19.

545 Anna Edney, "Trump Touts Drug That FDA Says Isn't Yet Approved for Virus," *Bloomberg* (blog) Mar. 19, 2020, accessed Apr. 17, 2020, https://www.bloomberg.com/news/articles/2020-03-19/trump-touts-malaria-drug-as-potential-coronavi-

rus-treatment.

546 *Business Insider* (blog) Apr. 9, 2020, accessed Apr. 17, 2020, https://www.businessinsider.com/trump-unproven-coronavirus-treatment-chloroquine-dangerous-expert-2020-4.

547 Sarah Owermohle, "What You Need to Know About the Malaria Drugs Trump Keeps Touting," *Politico*, Apr. 6, 2020, accessed Apr. 17, 2020, https://www.politico.com/news/2020/04/06/malaria-drug-coronavirus-trump-hydroxychloroquine-169103.

548 David Barrett, "Anti-Malarial rug Touted by Trump Was Subject of CIA Warning to Employees," *The Washington Post* (blog), Apr. 13, 2020, accessed Apr. 17, 2020, https://www.washingtonpost.com/; Marina Pitofsky, "CIA Warned Employees Against Using Hydroxychloroquine for Coronavirus: Report," *The Hill* (blog), Apr. 14, 2020, accessed Apr. 17, 2020, https://thehill.com/homenews/administration/492649-internal-cia-document-warns-against-using-hydroxychloroquine-for.

549 "Management of Persons with COVID-19," NIH, accessed Apr. 21, 2020, https://covid19treatmentguidelines.nih.gov/overview/management-of-covid-19/.

550 "Therapeutic Options for COVID-19 Currently Under Investigation," NIH, accessed Apr. 21, 2020, https://covid19treatmentguidelines.nih.gov/therapeutic-options-under-investigation/.

551 Ibid.

552 Ibid.

553 Ibid.

554 Joe Palca, "NIH Panel Recommends Against Drug Combination Promoted By Trump For COVID-19," NPR (blog), Apr. 21, 2020, accessed Apr. 21, 2020, https://www.npr.org/sections/coronavirus-live-updates/2020/04/21/840341224/nih-panel-recommends-against-drug-combination-trump-has-promoted-for-covid-19.

555 Rachel Sandler, "NIH Panel Recommends Against Using Hydroxychloroquine and Azithromycin, Drug Combination Touted By Trump." *Forbes* (blog), Apr. 21, 2020, accessed Apr. 21, 2020, https://www.forbes.com/sites/rachelsandler/2020/04/21/nih-panel-recommends-against-using-drug-combination-touted-by-trump-outside-clinical-trials/#506477d4b405.

556 Joseph Guzman, "NIH Panel Recommends Against Use of Hydroxychloroquine and Azithromycin to Treat COVID-19." *The Hill* (blog), Apr. 21, 2020, accessed Apr. 21, 2020, https://thehill.com/changing-america/well-being/prevention-cures/493995-nih-panel-recommends-against-use-of.

557 Susan Swindells in Joe Palca, "NIH Panel Recommends Against Drug Combination Promoted By Trump For COVID-19," NPR (blog), Apr. 21, 2020, accessed Apr. 21, 2020, https://www.npr.org/sections/coronavirus-live-updates/2020/04/21/840341224/nih-panel-recommends-against-drug-combination-

trump-has-promoted-for-covid-19.

558 "NIH Begins Clinical Trial of Hydroxychloroquine and Azithromycin to Treat COVID-19," NIH (blog), May 14, 2020, accessed May 19, 2020, https://www.nih. gov/news-events/news-releases/nih-begins-clinical-trial-hydroxychloroquine-azithromycin-treat-covid-19.

559 Brad Lendon, "Chinese State Media Claims Country's Navy Is Not Affected by Coronavirus," CNN (blog), Apr. 15, 2020, accessed Apr. 17, 2020, https://www.cnn. com/2020/04/13/asia/china-coronavirus-aircraft-carrier-deployment-dp-hnk-intl/ index.html.

560 Tom Cotton Letter to Mike Pompeo, Alex Azar, and Chad Wolf, Jan 28, 2020.

561 ibid.

562 Nick Robins-Early, "Don't Listen to Sen. Tom Cotton About Coronavirus," Huffpost (blog) Jan. 31, 2020, accessed Apr. 16, 2020, https://www.huffpost.com/ entry/tom-cotton-coronavirus-china_n_5e34a3b7c5b6f26233294378.

563 ibid.

564 ibid.

565 Ashley Kirzinger, Audrey Kearney, et al., "KFF Tracking Poll-Early April 2020: The Impact of Coronavirus on Life in America," KFF (blog), Apr. 2, 2020, accessed May 14, 2020, https://www.kff.org/coronavirus-covid-19/report/kff-health-tracking-poll-early-april-2020/.

566 Peter Grinspoon, "A Tale of Two Epidemics: When COVID-19 and Opioid Addiction Collide," Harvard Health Publishing (blog), Apr. 20, 2020, accessed May 14, 2020, https://www.health.harvard.edu/blog/a-tale-of-two-epidemics-when-covid-19-and-opioid-addiction-collide-2020042019569.

567 Olivia Goldhill, "Cancer Screenings Are Way Down During the Coronavirus," Quartz (blog), May 8, 2020, accessed May 14, 2020, https://qz.com/1853670/cancer-screenings-are-way-down-during-coronavirus/.

568 Emma Reynolds, "Lockdowns Shouldn't Be Fully Lifted Until Coronavirus Vaccine Found, New Study Warns," CNN (blog), Apr. 9, 2020, accessed May 8, 2020, https://www.cnn.com/2020/04/09/world/lockdown-lift-vaccine-coronavirus-lancet-intl/index.html.

569 Terri Whitcraft, Bill Hutchinson, and Nadine Shubailat, "'Road Map' to Recovery Report: 20 Million Coronavirus Tests per Day Needed to Fully Open Economy," ABC News (blog), Apr. 20, 2020, accessed May 14, 2020, https://abcnews.go.com/ US/road-map-recovery-report-20-million-coronavirus-tests/story?id=70230097.

570 Ed O'Keefe and Kathryn Watson, "'You're Gonna Call Your Own Shots,'" Trump Tell Governors About Guidelines to Reopen States," CBS News (blog), Apr. 16, 2020, accessed May 14, 2020, https://www.cbsnews.com/news/trump-guidelines-on-opening-up-america-leave-much-up-to-governors/.

gate the Coronavirus Outbreak after a CDC Official's Blunt Warnings Spooked the Stock Market," *Business Insider* (blog) Apr. 12, 2020, accessed Apr. 16, 2020, https://www.businessinsider.com/trump-wasted-3-weeks-coronavirus-mitigation-time-february-march-nyt-2020-4.

527 Ed Pilkington, Victoria Bekiempis, and Oliver Laughland, "Pelosi Accuses Trump of Costing US Lives with Coronavirus Denials and Delays," *The Guardian* (blog), Mar. 29, 2020, accessed Apr. 14, 2020, https://www.theguardian.com/us-news/2020/mar/29/pelosi-trump-coronavirus-response-inaction-delays

528 Mark von Rennenkampff, "Trump's Hubris and Ideological Rigidity Will Cost American Lives," *The Hill* (blog), Mar. 30, 2020, accessed Apr. 14, 2020, https://thehill.com/opinion/white-house/490045-trumps-hubris-and-ideological-rigidity-will-cost-american-lives.

529 David Remnick in "Remnick: Cost of Trump's Delays Will Be 'Paid in Human Lives,'" *CNN Business* (blog), accessed Apr. 13, 2020, https://www.cnn.com/videos/business/2020/03/29/remnick-cost-of-trumps-delays-will-be-paid-in-human-lives.cnn

530 David Frum, "This Is Trump's Fault; The President Is Failing, and Americans Are Paying for His Failures," *The Atlantic* (blog), Apr. 7, 2020; accessed Apr. 14, 2020, https://www.theatlantic.com/ideas/archive/2020/04/americans-are-paying-the-price-for-trumps-failures/609532/.

531 Mary Petrone and Nathan Grubaugh, "Coronavirus Mutations: Much Ado About Nothing," CNN Health (blog), Mar. 7, 2020, accessed, Apr. 16, 2020, https://www.cnn.com/2020/03/07/health/coronavirus-mutations-analysis/index.html.

532 Michael Crowley, "Some Experts Worry as a Germ-Phobic Trump Confronts Growing Epidemic," *The New York Times* (blog), Feb. 10, 2020, accessed Apr. 16, 2020, https://www.nytimes.com/2020/02/10/us/politics/trump-coronavirus-epidemic.html.

533 Vox in Timothy P. Carney, "Coronavirus Revisionism: When the Media Pretends Their Narrative is 'Reality'," *Washington Examiner* (blog), March 31, 2020, accessed Apr. 16, 2020, https://www.washingtonexaminer.com/opinion/coronavirus-revisionism-when-the-media-pretends-their-narrative-is-reality.

534 Nick Robins-Early, "Don't Listen to Sen. Tom Cotton About Coronavirus," Huffpost (blog) Jan. 31, 2020, accessed Apr. 16, 2020, https://www.huffpost.com/entry/tom-cotton-coronavirus-china_n_5e34a3b7c5b6f26233294378.

535 Alex Azar in Stephanie Soucheray, "Officials Say Most Americans Not at Risk of Coronavirus," Center for Infectious Disease Research and Policy, Jan. 28, 2020, accessed Apr. 14, 2020, https://www.cidrap.umn.edu/news-perspective/2020/01/officials-say-most-americans-not-risk-coronavirus.

536 Nancy Messonier in Stephanie Soucheray, "Officials Say Most Americans

571 White House and CDC, "Guidelines Opening Up America Again," whitehouse.gov, accessed May 14. 2020, https://www.whitehouse.gov/openingamerica/.

572 Ibid.

573 Ibid.

574 Ibid.

575 Ibid.

576 Ibid.

577 Ibid.

578 Ibid.

579 Ibid.

580 Ibid.

581 David Smith, "Trump's 'Science Based' Reopening Strategy Is Still Full of Unanswered Questions," The (blog), Apr. 16, 2002, accessed May 14, 2020, https://www.theguardian.com/world/2020/apr/16/trumps-science-based-reopening-strategy-is-still-full-of-unanswered-questions.

582 Teri Whitcraft, Bill Hutchinson, and Nadine Shubailat, "'Road Map' to Recovery Report: 20 Million Coronavirus Tests per Day Needed to Fully Open Economy," ABC News (blog) Apr. 20, 2020, accessed May 7, 2020, https://abcnews.go.com/US/road-map-recovery-report-20-million-coronavirus-tests/story?id=70230097.

583 James C. Capretta, "Opinion: This Conservative Economist Says President Trump's Plan to Reopen the Economy Fails in Crucial Ways," MarketWatch (blog), Apr. 26, 2020, accessed May 14, 2020, https://www.marketwatch.com/story/this-conservative-economist-says-president-trumps-plan-to-reopen-the-economy-fails-in-crucial-ways-2020-04-24.

584 ABC News/Ipsos Poll, May 6-7, 2020, accessed May 14, 2020, https://www.ipsos.com/sites/default/files/ct/news/documents/2020-05/topline-abc-coronavirus-wave-8.pdf.

585 Kendall Karson, "Reopening the Country Seen as Greater Risk Among Most Americans: POLL," ABC News (blog), May 8, 2020, accessed May 14, 2020, https://abcnews.go.com/Politics/reopening-country-greater-risk-americans-poll/story?id=70555060.

586 Brian Kempf, The State of Georgia Executive Order Providing Flexibility for Healthcare Practices, Moving Certain Businesses to Minimum Operation and Providing for Emergency Response, Apr. 20, 2020, accessed May 14, 2020, https://gov.georgia.gov/executive-action/executive-orders/2020-executive-orders.

587 Russ Bynum, "Georgia Lets Clos-Contact Businesses Reopening Despite Rise in Coronavirus Cases," Time (blog), Apr. 24, 2020, accessed May 14, 2020,

588 Brian Kempf, The State of Georgia Executive Order Providing Flexibility for

Healthcare Practices, Moving Certain Businesses to Minimum Operation and Providing for Emergency Response, Apr. 20, 2020, accessed May 14, 2020, https://time.com/5826943/georgia-reopen-coronavirus/.https://gov.georgia.gov/executive-action/executive-orders/2020-executive-orders.

589 Fig. COVID-19 Cases Over Time, Georgia Department of Public Health Daily Status Report, Georgia Department of Public Health, accessed May 14, 2020, https://dph.georgia.gov/covid-19-daily-status-report.

590 Ibid.

591 Jiachuan Wu, Robin Muccari, et al., "Reopening America Some States Are Staring to Reopen and Lift Lockdowns, Even as the Battle Against the Coronavirus Rages on," NBC News (blog), updated May 11, 2020, accessed May 14, 2020, https://www.nbcnews.com/news/us-news/reopening-america-see-what-states-across-u-s-are-starting-n1195676.

592 Ibid.

593 Ibid.

594 Ibid.

595 Sarah Mervosh, Kasmine C. Lee, et al., "See Which States Are Reopening and Which Are Still Shut Down," *The New York Times* (blog), updated May 13, 2020, accessed May 14, 2020, https://www.nytimes.com/interactive/2020/us/states-reopen-map-coronavirus.html.

596 Jill Filipovic, "Governors Reopening Their States Are Endangering American Lives," CNN (blog), Apr. 21, 2020, accessed May 14, 2020.

597 Ibid.

598 Yaneer Bar-Yam, "Don't Let Governors Fool You About Reopening," CNN (blog), May 12, 2020, accessed May 14, 2020, https://www.cnn.com/2020/05/12/opinions/governors-reopen-states-opinion-bar-yam/index.html.

599 Sonia Y Angell, Order of the State Public Health Officer, May 7, 2020, accessed May 15, 2020, https://www.cdph.ca.gov/Programs/CID/DCDC/CDPH%20Document%20Library/COVID-19/SHO%20Order%205-7-2020.pdf.

600 Ibid.

601 Kellie Hwang, "Los Angeles to Extend Stay-At-Home Order, While Some California Counties Are Cleared to Reopen," *San Francisco Chronicle* (blog), May 14, 2020, accessed May 15, 2020, https://www.sfchronicle.com/bayarea/article/LA-to-extend-stay-home-through-July-while-two-15265751.php.

602 Gretchen Whitmer, Executive Order 2020-68 (COVID-19), "Declaration of States of Emergency and Disaster Under the Emergency Management Act, 176 PA 390, Apr. 30, 2020, accessed May 15, 2020, https://www.michigan.gov/whitmer/0,9309,7-387-90499_90705-527716--,00.html.

603 David Eggert, "Hundred Protest Stay-At-Home Order Outside Michigan Capitol, *The News Tribune* (blog), May 14, 2020, accessed May 15, 2020, https://www.thenewstribune.com/news/nation-world/national/article242737811.html.

604 Ivan Pereira, "Protester With Ax Involved in Clash at Michigan Rally Against Stay-At-Home Orders, May 14, 2020, accessed May 15, 2020, https://abc7.com/protester-with-ax-involved-in-clash-at-michigan-rally-against-stay-at-home-orders/6183213/.

605 David Eggert, "Hundred Protest Stay-At-Home Order Outside Michigan Capitol, The News Tribune (blog), May 14, 2020, accessed May 15, 2020, https://www.thenewstribune.com/news/nation-world/national/article242737811.html.

606 Gus Burns, "Judge to Determine if Michigan's Extended Coronavirus State of Emergency Is Legal," MLive (blog), updated May 15, 2020, accessed May 15, 2020, https://www.mlive.com/public-interest/2020/05/judge-to-determine-if-michigans-extended-coronavirus-state-of-emergency-is-legal.html.

607 Ibid.

608 State of Wisconsin Department of Health Emergency Order #28 Safer at Home Order, Apr. 16, 2020, accessed Apr. 19, 2020, https://content.govdelivery.com/attachments/WIGOV/2020/04/16/file_attachments/1428995/EMO28-SaferAtHome.pdf.

609 Tony Evers in Scott Bauer, "Wisconsin Gov. Tony Evers Extends Stay-at Home Orders for Another Month, Closes Schools for Remainder of Academic Year," *Hartford Courant*, Apr. 16, 2020, accessed Apr. 19, 2020, https://www.courant.com/coronavirus/ct-nw-wisconsin-stay-at-home-order-extended-20200416-eajw46fjqvegpf4x43yenweqfm-story.html.

610 *Wisconsin Legislature v. Secretary-Designee Andre Palm, et al.*, Wisc. No. 2020AP765-OA, May 13, 2020, accessed May 15, 2020, https://www.wicourts.gov/sc/opinion/DisplayDocument.pdf?content=pdf&seqNo=260868&mod=article_inline.

611 State of Wisconsin Executive Order #74 Relating to Suspending In-Person Voting on April 7, 2020, due to the COVID-19 Pandemic," Apr. 6, 2020.

612 Jason Calvi and AP Wire Service, "Wisconsin Republicans to Challenge Extension of 'Safer at Home' Order; Interest in Rally Explodes, Fox6Now.com (blog), Apr. 17, 2020, accessed Apr. 19, 2020, https://fox6now.com/2020/04/17/interest-in-rally-explodes-after-gov-evers-extension-of-safer-at-home-order/.

613 Christopher Schmaling Media Release, Apr. 17, 2020, accessed Apr. 19, 2020, https://www.racinecounty.com/government/sheriff-s-office.

614 Ibid

615 *Wisconsin Legislature v. Secretary-Designee Andre Palm, et al.*, Wisc. No. 2020AP765-OA, May 13, 2020, accessed May 15, 2020, https://www.wicourts.gov/

sc/opinion/DisplayDocument.pdf?content=pdf&seqNo=260868&mod=article_in-line.

616 Ed White, "Michigan Barber Who Pledged to Stay Open 'Until Jesus Comes' Has License Suspended for Defying Coronavirus Orders," *Time* (blog), May 13, 2020, accessed May 16, 2020, https://time.com/5836393/michigan-barber-license-suspended/.

617 Karl Manke in Ed White, "Michigan Barber Who Pledged to Stay Open 'Until Jesus Comes' Has License Suspended for Defying Coronavirus Orders," *Time* (blog), May 13, 2020, accessed May 16, 2020, https://time.com/5836393/michigan-barber-license-suspended/.

618 Madeline Holcombe, "New York Tourist Is Arrested in Hawaii After Posting Beach Pictures on Instagram," CNN (blog), May 16, 2020, accessed May 16, 2020, https://www.cnn.com/2020/05/16/us/hawaii-arrest-coronavirus-trnd/index.html.

619 Ibid.

620 @theCJPearson, Twitter, May 14, 1227 PM, accessed May 17, 2020, https://twitter.com/thecjpearson/status/1260969917345603586?s=12.

621 Robert Levin in Ventura County presentation, KTLA 5, YouTube, May 4, 2020, at 3:20-5:20, accessed May 22, 2020, https://www.youtube.com/watch?v=0Kf_gWrBio4.

622 Ibid.

623 Neil Vigdor, "Dallas Salon Owner Is Jailed for Defying Order of Stay Closed," *The New York Times* (blog), Apr. 24, accessed May 15, 2020, https://www.nytimes.com/2020/05/05/us/dallas-salon-opens-coronavirus.html.

624 Shelley Luther in Neil Vigdor, "Dallas Salon Owner Is Jailed for Defying Order of Stay Closed," *The New York Times* (blog), Apr. 24, accessed May 15, 2020, https://www.nytimes.com/2020/05/05/us/dallas-salon-opens-coronavirus.html.

625 Manny Fernandez and David Montgomery, "Dallas Salon Owner Who Was Jailed for Reopening Is Released," *The New York Times* (blog), May 7, 2020, accessed May 15, 2020, https://www.nytimes.com/2020/05/07/us/dallas-salon-owner-shelley-luther.html.

626 Neil Vigdor, "Dallas Salon Owner Is Jailed for Defying Order of Stay Closed," *The New York Times* (blog), Apr. 24, accessed May 15, 2020, https://www.nytimes.com/2020/05/05/us/dallas-salon-opens-coronavirus.html.

627 Emily Czachor, "GoFundMe Raises More Than $500,000 for Dallas Hair Salon Owner Arrested fro Opening Business Despite Coronavirus Restrictions," *Newsweek* (blog), May 12, 2020, accessed May 15, 2020, https://www.newsweek.com/gofundme-raises-more-500000-dallas-hair-salon-owner-arrested-opening-business-despite-1503496.

628 Manny Fernandez and David Montgomery, "Dallas Salon Owner Who Was

Jailed for Reopening Is Released," *The New York Times* (blog), May 7, 2020, accessed May 15, 2020, https://www.nytimes.com/2020/05/07/us/dallas-salon-owner-shelley-luther.html.

629 Ibid.

630 Letter from various Dallas Circuit Court Judges to Ken Paxton, undated, in @ HowertonNews, Twitter, May 6, 2020, 710 PM, accessed May 15, 2020, https://twitter.com/HowertonNews/status/1258172318414770181.

631 Greg Abbott, Executive Order GA 21 Relating to the Expanded Reopening of Services as Part of the Sage, Strategic Plan to Open Texas in Response to the COVID-19 Disaster, May 5, 2020, accessed May 16, 2020, https://www.cityofazle.org/DocumentCenter/View/6692/EO-GA-21-expanding-Open-Texas-COVID-19-salons-barber-shops-05-05-2020?bidId=.

632 GDP per Capita, The World Bank, May 2020, https://data.worldbank.org/indicator/NY.GDP.PCAP.CD.

633 Physicians per 1,000 People, The World Bank, May 2020, https://data.worldbank.org/indicator/SH.MED.PHYS.ZS.

634 Population density (people per sq. km of land area), The World Bank, May 2020, https://data.worldbank.org/indicator/EN.POP.DNST?end=2018&start=1961.

635 Life expectancy at birth, total (years), The World Bank, May 2020, https://data.worldbank.org/indicator/SP.DYN.LE00.IN.

636 COVID-19 Coronavirus Pandemic, Worldometer, updated May 2, 2020, accessed May 3, 2020, https://www.worldometers.info/coronavirus/#countries.

637 Tableau.com, accessed Amy 23, 2020, https://www.tableau.com/trial/tableau-software?utm_campaign_id=2017049&utm_campaign=Prospecting-CORE-ALL-ALL-ALL-ALL&utm_medium=Paid+Search&utm_source=-Google+Search&utm_language=EN&utm_country=USCA&kw=tableau&adgroup=CTX-Brand-Priority-Core-E&adused=RESP&matchtype=e&placement=&gclid=CjwKCAjwk6P2BRAIEiwAfVJ0rEgswhgXWmCm2qDVwTwn3JjDE-Sl-65deGiqtc2IDX18-RTwd-GGacRoCf7wQAvD_BwE&gclsrc=aw.ds.

638
639
640
641
642
643
644
645

646
647
648
649
650
651
652
653
654
655
656
657
658
659
660
661
662
663
664
665
666
667
668
669
670
671
672
673
674
675
676
677
T. J. Rodgers. "Do Lockdowns Save Many Lives? In Most Places, the Data Say No," The Wall Street Journal, Apr. 26, 2020, accessed May 24, 2020, https://www.wsj.com/articles/

Gonzalez

Gonzalez

www.ingramcontent.com/pod-product-compliance
Lightning Source LLC
Chambersburg PA
CBHW031458270326
41930CB00006B/146